Interpretive
Phenomenology

This book is dedicated to Richard Benner, who has participated in, inspired, and supported every stage of this book.

Interpretive Phenomenology

Embodiment, Caring, and Ethics in Health and Illness

Patricia Benner
editor

SAGE Publications
International Educational and Professional Publisher
Thousand Oaks   London   New Delhi

For information address:

SAGE Publications, Inc.
2455 Teller Road
Thousand Oaks, California 91320
SAGE Publications Ltd.
6 Bonhill Street
London EC2A 4PU
United Kingdom
SAGE Publications India Pvt. Ltd.
M-32 Market
Greater Kailash I
New Delhi 110048 India

Printed in the United States of America

Library of Congress Cataloging-in-Publication Data

Main entry under title:

Interpretive phenomenology: embodiment, caring, and ethics in health and illness/edited by Patricia Benner.
    p. cm.
  Includes bibliographical references and index.
  ISBN 0-8039-5722-X (cl).—ISBN 0-8039-5723-8 (pb)
  1. Nursing—Philosophy. 2. Phenomenology. 3. Nursing ethics.
I. Nurse—Patient Relations. II. Benner, Patricia E.
  [DNLM: 1. Philosophy, Nursing. 2. Ethics, Nursing. 3. Nursing Care—psychology. WY 86 1994]
RT84.5.I58   1994
610.73'01—dc20
DNLM/DLC   94-4229

94 95 96 97 10 9 8 7 6 5 4 3 2 1

Sage Production Editor: Diane S. Foster

Contents

Preface

HUBERT L. DREYFUS

The authors in this collection of essays and studies collectively demonstrate the power of Heideggerian or Interpretive phenomenology for areas of study related to lifeworld, meanings, skilled know-how, clinical knowledge and everyday skillful ethical comportment. The background of this work and its philosophical underpinnings are described in Part I. Part II demonstrates how the powers of understanding and the skills, of allowing the text and the transitions in thinking that naturally occur when questioning and interpreting texts, shape the studies. The authors use *Interpretive Phenomenology* to study these everyday aspects of the world and give new access and vision to interpretive human studies. While each of the interpretive studies has a family resemblance, they are uniquely shaped by the questions asked and responses given by the participants. The family resemblance is not based on uniformly trying to get structures, processes, or functions of human capacities explained or described in the same ways. The similarities come from a shared *understanding* of what it means to be an embodied human-being that is self-interpreting and that takes a stand on being a particular finite human being in particular communities at a particular time in history.

These authors reverse the usual hierarchical relationship between theory and practice. The relation between theory and practice and between reason and intuition has concerned our culture since our Western way of being human was first defined in ancient Greece. To understand the complicated relation between theory and practice and between reason and intuition illustrated in these studies, we have to go back to the time when Hippocrates was trying to move medicine from folk wisdom to a scientific art of healing, while, at the same time, Socrates, born 9 years after Hippocrates in 469 B.C., was trying to understand this new intellectual achievement, of which medicine was only one example. Around 400 B.C., physics, astronomy, and geometry had taken off from everyday, practical, measuring and counting and thinkers were asking: What is special about these new disciplines? The answer proposed by Socrates and refined by the philosophical tradition was that these new disciplines were based on theory.

Descartes and Kant completed the Socratic account of theory by insisting that theory must be stated in terms of context-free elements, which we now call features, factors, attributes, data points, cues, and so on—isolable elements which make no reference to human interests, traditions, institutions, and so on. A theory must be a new whole in which decontextualized elements are related to each other by rules or laws. Plato clairvoyantly expressed all five characteristics in the myth of the cave: The theorist must remove his object of knowledge from the everyday, perceptual, social world in order to see the universal relations between the explicit and abstract elements, in this case the ideas. Freed from all context, the elements form a system of their own—all ideas are organized by the idea of the Good. Plato saw that while everyday understanding is implicit, concrete, local, holistic, and partial, theories, by contrast, are explicit, abstract, universal, and range over elements organized into a new total whole.

What the authors in this book have done is revisit this monolithic assumption about the primacy of theory as being the source of knowledge and a meaningful human world and examine actual meanings and patterns of everyday, skilled, ethical comportment. For example, Socrates assumes in his dialogue, **Euthyphro,** that Euthyphro, a religious prophet, is an expert at recognizing piety, and so asks Euthyphro for his piety recognizing rule:

"I want to know what is characteristic of piety . . . to use as a standard whereby to judge your actions and those of other men"(6e3-6). He wanted a principle that would ground piety in theory and so make it knowledge.

A generation after Plato, Aristotle already suspected that something crucial had been left out of Plato's theory-based model of knowledge. Rather than being able to give reasons for their actions as the test of expertise, Aristotle sees, precisely, the immediate, unreasoned, intuitive response as characteristic of an expert craftsman. "Art (techne) does not deliberate" he says in **Physics,** Bk. II, Moreover, Aristotle was clear that even if there were universal principles based on a theory, intuitive skill was needed to see how the principles applied in each particular case. He (Thomson, 1953) derives an illustration from ethics, which Plato thought must be based on universal rules:

[I]t is not easy to find a formula by which we may determine how far and up to what point a man may go wrong before he incurs blame. [Aristotle notes, and then adds:] But this difficulty of definition is inherent in every object of perception: such questions of degree are bound up with the circumstances of the individual case, where our only criterion *is* the perceptions.(p. 75)

The same would, of course, apply to thinking about disease, health, and illness. Disease is a dysfunction of the body, a physical object governed by physical laws, so it should come as no surprise that Hippocrates' vision of the physician as scientist is finally being achieved. But it would be a mistake characteristic of our rationalistic culture to think that the success of medicine in any way suggests that there can be a theory of nursing as a caring practice. Caring, in the context of illness, consists in keeping open the possibilities that can be saved in the world of the sick person, while aiding the person in letting go of possibilities that are no longer realistic. If human beings were simply rational animals, as the Greeks thought, then it might be possible to reduce the world to theories about having a world and how to keep it. But as the existential thought of Soren Kierkegaard, points out human beings cannot be understood as some combination of body and mind. Human beings, Martin Heidegger, the most famous philosopher in existential phenomenology points out, are defined by their self-understandings and the stand they take upon themselves, which in turn sets up the range of possibilities open to them. On this view, human being is a unique way of being in that human experience and actions follow from their self-interpretation. The meaning of a whole life is basic and determines what possibilities show up and how they make sense to a person. Moreover, we are not objective, theoretical spectators of our lives and of the world, but involved participants. Things show up as mattering to us. Heidegger's project is to demonstrate that human being does not have fixed properties, like an object or animal, but that the basic human way of being is care. These papers show that care is a way of being that must be understood, preserved and enhanced in health care in general and by nursing as a caring practice.

There can be no abstract, analytical theory of the human way of being in all its cultural and historical diversity and because it is holistic skilled practice, there can be no abstract, analytical theory of it. Caring is what one might call an existential skill. It is, indeed, what Socrates would have called a knack, but because, unlike cooking, it is a matter of life and death and involves the whole person, that term hardly seems appropriate. It shows the power of a tradition based on the theory of disease that the existential skills of caring have no traditional name that does honor to their importance and uniqueness, and we seem to have no appropriate word for them in our vocabulary. The best I can come up with is that caring, as a way of helping people by entering their world, is a higher kind of knowledge, which we can call understanding and the potential for what Aristotle called practical wisdom. Individually and collectively, the studies in this volume demonstrate the power of understanding for revealing human concerns.

These studies show that much can be said about the tact involved in world preserving. They describe the general structure of human being, the way care consists of mattering, possibilities and inhabiting a shared world. This is what Heidegger calls an existential account of human being. They also describe in detail how specific cultures, families, and individuals structure their worlds. Because meanings are shared, one can also select and describe paradigm cases, laying out what matters and what possibilities are opened and closed in typical situations. One can then make qualitative distinctions between more and less successful interventions. They also examine the knowledge and skills residing in caring practices, growth and healing. Experts in caring know that they cannot be guided by principles or any pseudo-sciences of the psyche but must enter into the situation of the patient and be guided by participation and intuition.

In this domain there can be no clinical *knowledge* as Plato would define it, but there can and must be clinical *understanding*. Thus in caring, as in the case of the *application* of medical theory, one finds a practice requiring involvement for which there can be no theory. But there is an important difference between the treatment of disease and the care of illness. Those engaged in caring must be able to take on the perspective of the patient and make his or her peace with the situation and its suffering in order to be touched by the situation of a fellow human being. They must have the tact to enable that person to face, surmount or weather his or her illness. Only by combining both technological and existential skills can we approach healing the embodied person.

For the past 18 years, nurses have come to my courses in Kierkegaard, Heidegger, and interpretive methodology for the human sciences and they seem to have found there a language for the concerns, meanings, and practices of nursing. Few have had the usual philosophical background for taking existential phenomenology, but because of the concerns that are central to their practice they have contributed to class discussion and shown that they have found new ways of thinking about and articulating what they know in their practice. Typically they discover a new way of describing and understanding what it means to be human being, who is finite and always situated in a world with a history and concerns. In exchange, I have come to see that nursing draws on a mixture of natural and medical sciences and that in addition to the human sciences nurses need a way to criticize the Cartesian view of the person as a private subject standing up against an objective world. They need to be able to describe and legitimize the person in relation with others for coherence in their own self understanding as nurses engaged in caring practices. Finally, studying Heideggerian phenomenology seems to enable them to understand human beings in their physical and cultural diversity and not only as private, autonomous Cartesian selves.

References

Euthyphro, 6e3-6.

Thomas. J. A. K. (trans.). (1953). Aristotle, *Nicomachean Ethics* as *The Ethics of Aristotle* (p. 75). New York: Penguin.

Introduction

PATRICIA BENNER

M ost agree in this postpositivistic era that significant distinctions between the natural and human sciences exist, but debate continues about over where and what the distinctions are (Hiley, Bohman, & Shusterman, 1991). Some argue that the physical sciences are far closer to the human sciences in their holism, whereas others argue for distinctions between the holism of the physical sciences and the human sciences. Dreyfus (1991) argues for scientific realism, attributing the particular kind of holism that exists in the natural sciences to an inability to account for the background habits, practices, and skills that create the science. For Dreyfus, holism in the human sciences is different in that it stems from not being able to account adequately for the malleability of human "nature" and embodiment shaped by cultural understandings, habits, skills, practices, and environment. The atom and the quark do not change their physical properties or responses because the physical scientist introduces a new description and interpretation of them. The authors in this book hold that the particular methodological assumptions of logical positivism and the preference for disengaged criteria-based reasoning (Taylor, 1993) in the human sciences cause a systematic bias for the study of breakdown and a systematic blindness to embodied, lived experience in learning, health, illness, and any human transformation that includes transitions and experiential learning.

The chapters in this book reflect the work of a scholarly community who have worked out what interpretive phenomenology has to offer nursing science, nursing practice, the lived experience of health and illness, and health care ethics and policy. It was not possible to include all those who have participated in this dialogue, and where possible references to these works are made to extend the dialogue (see Appendix for a list of dissertations using interpretive phenomenology). Throughout the work, the teachings of Hubert L. Dreyfus (1979, 1991; Dreyfus & Rubin, 1991), Jane Rubin (1984), and Charles Taylor (1985, 1989, 1991, 1993) are evident. Each has sustained a conversation with nurses doing interpretive phenomenology over the past 11 years, teaching courses, giving lectures, and commenting on manuscripts. Because the chapters come from a community of scholars engaged in an ongoing project of developing interpretive phenomenology, the careful reader will sense the family resemblances and even the conversations between the contributors. The goal of this collection is to illustrate how this research tradition is worked out by different researchers with different lines of inquiry.

The book has three aims: (a) to offer a philosophical introduction to interpretive phenomenology, (b) to guide the reader in understanding the strategies and processes of this approach to human science, and (c) to provide a wide range of high-quality interpretive studies so that the reader can see the family resemblance in the method while examining the variance created by the phenomenon being studied. The terms *interpretive* and *hermeneutical* are used interchangeably, though admittedly the term *interpretive* is more accessible. Part 1 presents theoretical and philosophical foundations as well as practical guidance for conducting interpretive phenomenological studies. Part 2 presents excellent examples of interpretive phenomenological studies that address a diverse range of questions.

This work stands in the hermeneutical tradition found in the study of biblical texts, jurisprudence, historical studies, literary criticism, and anthropology (Geertz, 1973, 1983), but it is also shaped by the existential phenomenology of Kierkegaard (1843/1985), Heidegger (1975), Merleau-Ponty (1962), Wittgenstein (1980), Dreyfus (1979, 1991), and Taylor (1964, 1985, 1989, 1991) and thus goes beyond the strictly rationalist tradition in early hermeneutical methods. The commentary and articulation of interpretive phenomenology are similar to the kind of reasoning in transitions that occurs in particular practices such as nursing, medicine, practical moral reasoning, and law (see Thomasma, chapter 5 of this book; Taylor, 1993). By engaging in the interpretive process, the researcher seeks to understand the world of concerns, habits, and skills presented by participants' narratives and situated actions. These understandings are then used to contrast similarities to and differences from other participants' narratives and situated actions. Understanding human concerns, meanings, experiential learning, and practical everyday skillful comportment, when they are functioning smoothly *or* are in breakdown, is the goal as opposed to explanation or prediction through causal laws and formal theoretical propositions. It is posited that understanding is more powerful than explanation for prediction in the human sciences because it stands more fully in the human world of self-understandings, meanings, skills, and tradition. Prediction is possible only in limited ways for human beings who are self-interpreting and subject to change by the very interpretations offered by research. Prediction in the human sciences resists single-factor theories and explanations because human action and world always contain incomplete and multiple levels of meanings. The understanding sought in interpretive phenomenology considers historical change, transformations, gains, losses, temporality, and context. As in any human science, predictions are offered with qualifiers such as "all things being equal" or "barring no major changes in self-understandings and context, this is what may be expected" (see Plager, chapter 4 of this book; Dreyfus, 1991).

The reader is challenged to consider the power of understanding for becoming more effectively, skillfully, or humanely engaged in practice. The ethos embedded in existential phenomenology is respect for the social and cultural nature of being human. Human practices, skills, habits, meanings, and, in particular, recognition practices allow for the other to be encountered and made visible (MacIntyre, 1981; Taylor, 1992). When unarticulated, taken-for-granted practices and meanings fade from our social ecology and the social fabric of our lives, and we lose what they enable us to see, create, and represent. This constitutive role of background meanings, practices, and skills is, according to Dreyfus (1991), the distinction between the physical and human sciences:

> Not just any cultural interpretation will disclose entities. If, instead of encountering heroes or saints, a culture begins to develop practices for encountering aliens that are round and give off beams of light, it may well be that nothing will show up at all. But there are no clear limits as to what kinds of cultural entities can be encountered [in the human sciences]. In physical science, however, there seems to be one right answer as far as physical causality is concerned. Radically different theories than those proposed by modern science presumably would not reveal physical causal powers. (1991, p. 38)

The ethical issues of our understanding of a good life and what we consider to be an equal opportunity for the freedom to pursue health and happiness are central to whether our human science practices allow us to reveal, critique, and preserve a range of diversity in a pluralistic society. If our human science is monolithically patterned on the physical sciences, it will allow only decontextualized, elemental, rational, atomistic agents or overdetermined, radically unfree objects to be revealed. Aspects of being human related to being constituted by membership, participation, relationship, and human concerns will be covered over by the methods of the physical sciences. In the study of health and illness, we run the risk of medicalizing more and more spheres of human existence if our science allows us to study only disease, cellular processes, biochemistry, and treatments. We also exclude the possibility of studying health and smooth functioning.

The works in this book struggle to uncover and restore to visibility and credibility of marginalized practices and other voices encountered in everyday skillful comportment. All chapters share a deep respect for the primacy of practice and the primacy of caring (Benner & Wrubel, 1989). Charles Taylor (1991) points out that what the works of Martin Heidegger (1927/1962), Maurice Merleau-Ponty (1962), and Ludwig Wittgenstein (1980) have in common is that

> they see the agent, not primarily as the locus of representations, but as engaged in practices, as a being who acts in and on a world. . . .
>
> To situate our understanding in practices is to see it as implicit in our activity, and hence as going well beyond what we manage to frame representations of. We do frame representations: We explicitly formulate what our world is like, what we aim at, what we are doing. But much of our intelligent action in the world, sensitive as it usually is to our situation and goals, is carried on unformulated. It flows from an understanding that is largely inarticulate.
>
> This understanding is more fundamental in two ways: (1) it is always there, whereas we sometimes frame representations and sometimes do not, and (2) the representations we do make are comprehensible only against the background provided by this inarticulate understanding. It provides the context within which alone they make the sense they do. Rather than representations being the primary locus of understanding, they are just islands in the sea of our unformulated grasp of the world. . . .
>
> This puts the role of the body in a new light. Our body is not just the executant of the goals we frame, nor just the locus of causal factors shaping our representations. Our understanding is itself embodied. That is, our bodily know how, and the way we act and move, can encode components of our understanding of self and world. I know my way around a familiar environment in being able to get from any place to any place with ease and assurance. I may be at a loss when asked to draw a map, or even give explicit directions to a stranger. I know how to manipulate and use the familiar instruments in my world, usually in the same inarticulate fashion.
>
> But it is not only my grasp on the inanimate environment which is thus embodied. My sense of myself, of the footing I am on with others, are in large part also. The deference I owe you is carried in the distance I stand from you, in the way I fall silent when you start to speak, in the way I hold myself in

your presence. Or alternatively, the sense I have of my own importance is carried in the way I swagger. Indeed, some of the most pervasive features of my attitude to the world and to others is encoded in the way I carry myself and project in public space, whether I am "macho," or timid, or eager to please, or calm and unflappable. (pp. 308-309)

I have cited this long passage to allow the reader to trace the influence of Taylor's project of articulation in the tradition of philosophers who have studied the primacy of practices, world, and the relationship between body and world (see also Dreyfus, 1991). Social meanings and their embodied social postures, stances, habits, skills, and practices are relevant for recovery and rehabilitation, for nursing practice, and for skillful ethical comportment in caring for the ill (see especially SmithBattle, Chapter 8, and Doolittle, Chapter 11). Nurses deal with not only normality and pathophysiology but also with the lived social and skilled body in promoting health, growth, and development and in caring for the sick and dying. However, we have focused more on the mind than on the body and have not developed adequate language for the experience of skilled, responsive psychosocial bodies because of our "representational" Cartesian bias. Our medical metaphors have more to do with repairing and treating failed bodies than with promoting health or nurturing and facilitating the recovery of socially engaged, skilled bodies.

Interpretive phenomenology cannot be reduced to a set of procedures and techniques, but it nevertheless has a stringent set of disciplines in a scholarly tradition associated with giving the best possible account of the text presented. The interpretation must be auditable and plausible, must offer increased understanding, and must articulate the practices, meanings, concerns, and practical knowledge of the world it interprets. Good interpretation is guided by an ethic of understanding and responsiveness. One must not read into the text what is not there. Self-knowledge is required to limit the interpreter's projection of his or her own world onto the text. The extremes of idealizing and villainizing are to be avoided. As with interpretive studies in literary criticism, readers can judge the fidelity, clarity, insightfulness, and comprehensiveness of the interpretation of the text (MacIntyre, 1993). The reader plays an active role in critically reading the interpretive work, judging the textual evidence presented by the author, and judging the interpretation against the reader's own knowledge of the subject and text, including aesthetic appreciation. The lines of inquiry of any particular study, plus the discoveries and dialogue within data collection, interpretive analysis, and writing, comprise the ongoing evolution and design of the study. The dialogue with the participants and situation must make claims on the researcher's understanding and shape the dialogue. A controlled, completely predesigned study is not a dialogue in which the study design is altered as new lines of inquiry develop from the text. The interpretive researcher is constrained by the demands of the text—carefully listening, hearing the voices and concerns inherent in the text, giving the fullest possible account. The interpretive account should illuminate the world of the participants, articulating taken-for-granted meanings, practices, habits, skills, and concerns. Thus, as Dreyfus (1991) points out in his lectures on human science methods, the validity of an interpretation is demonstrated when participants say, "You have put into words what I have always known, but did not have the words to express."

Although the interpretation may be critical, the interpretive tradition presented here is not a hermeneutics of suspicion that offers a particular theoretical framework to reveal a reality behind or beyond the text such as a psychoanalytic or Marxist reading of the text—though once an interpretation of a text is developed, one may engage in a comparison of that interpretation with any other level of theoretical or cultural discourse offering critical reflection and comparison with the interpretive commentary. Each interpreter enters the interpretive circle by examining preunderstandings and confronting otherness, silence, similarities, and commonalities from his or her own particular historical, cultural, and personal stance. Though the interpreter begins to set up the inquiry with as much reflection and clarity as is available to him or her, the actual study is required to make visible and to challenge aspects of the researcher's preunderstanding that are not noticed prior to engaging in a dialogue with the text. The researcher must enter study with the intent and practices of staying open to the text and expecting that the text will reveal blind spots, mysteries, and otherness. Participants (where possible), research colleagues, a community of scholars, and eventually readers of the research must serve as enriching and corrective voices to augment the interpreter's finite and perspectival grasp. In working with dissertation students, I always read some raw data, both cases that are highly informative and accessible to the doctoral researcher and cases that are puzzling or troubling or that create resistance, rejection, or even moral outrage. This gives me access to the students' strategies of inclusion and exclusion, powers of understanding, and even resistances and blind spots. Multiple dialogues with dissertation advisers and research colleagues help reveal the stance of the researcher and the text over time. The discipline and intent is to avoid projecting one's own world onto the world of another. Though the horizon and similarities from one's own world provide the necessary positive bias that projects questions and provides access to the text, the text must also confront and expose these projections, questions, and access (Gadamer, 1960/1975). The interpretive researcher's questions (like those of all researchers) inadvertently shape and foretell the possible answers to the question (Dreyfus, 1991). The questions raised before and during the study become a source of reflection for the interpretive project. Why these questions and not others? The other's world is encountered through dialogue based upon shared and distinct horizons of meaning (Gadamer, 1960/1975): that is, taken-for-granted common and divergent meanings, habits, skills, and practices. Common and distinct taken-for-granted meanings are accessible through embodiment, strong situations, shared cultural and linguistic heritage, dialogue, and translation that allow differences and controversies to show up (Kesselring, 1990). But this gets ahead of the story and depends upon a philosophical critique of the Cartesian understanding of the person as a private subject, radically separate from an objective world, a topic taken up in Chapters 1 and 3 and illustrated in all the interpretive research presented.

Methodological rigor is based upon the rationality of articulation (Taylor, 1985, 1989, 1991) and a strong perspective on what it is to be a human being skillfully embodied and dwelling in a world that is constituted by taken-for-granted background meanings, concerns, practices, habits, relationships, and understandings of self and other (see Leonard, Chapter 3 of this book; Benner, 1984; Dreyfus, 1991; Heidegger, 1962). The issue of rigor is taken up in chapter 6 and in various ways by each of the chapters.

A growing concern with social engineering and human sciences designed to shape social policy is that they overlook life world, meanings, practical knowledge (skilled know-how), transition, and experiential learning. The strategies of objectification are strategies designed to decontextualize social and psychological data so that generalizations can be made across a range of situations without regard for context, temporality, transitions, and multiple meanings. As Bellah (1982) has pointed out, social engineering fails to consider communities and the constitutive meanings that shape social reality, particular communities, and social action. For example, in health care, the goal is to design a health care system based upon systems analysis and economic incentives and patterns. Consequently the system is designed and controlled based upon treatments and procedures that can be easily counted and priced. Caring practices, healing relationships, and attentiveness that prevent illness and complications are not easily counted and tend to get marginalized as the focus intensifies on treatment techniques and procedures. What shows up in the system is what can be paid for fairly equally. But this economism is parasitical on the skillful ethical comportment of health care practitioners with notions of good about what is required to adequately care for particular patients. The bureaucratic controls, economic planning, and costing are dependent on a background of practices by health care providers and participants that lend concern and attentiveness to the health care situation. Without these the system would become so adversarial and mistrusting that even basic interactions would become bogged down. (Taylor, 1992). Interpretive phenomenology offers an alternative to quantitative social science studies geared toward social engineering because it is concerned with life world, human concerns, habits, skills, practices, experiential learning, and notions of the good that fuel health care practices, help seeking, and receiving.

The interpretive studies in Part 2 offer understandings of life worlds that open new ways of community development, public policy design, and clinical practice based upon dialogue, recognition of differences, articulation, understanding, and extending of situated possibility, as opposed to the control and identification of pathologies evident in breakdown (see particularly SmithBattle, Chapter 8; Doolittle, Chapter 11; and Stuhlmiller, Chapter 15). In a democracy that wants to honor pluralism and limit domination and coercion, methods that seek understanding and recognition of others' desires, aspirations, and concerns are basic requirements (Taylor, 1992). And social policy strategies must be linked up to these studies in ways that further these projects and do not unduly limit the freedoms of others. Though we cannot do without procedural justice and negotiations based upon the rights of generalized others, we need public strategies that allow for coordinating notions of the good life, community, and particularity ("positive freedoms to") while protecting from coercion and oppression ("negative freedoms from").

In Chapter 1, Ragnar Fjelland and Eva Gjengedal discuss the constitutive relationships between theory and practice—theory being derived and constituted by practice, and practice being altered and guided by theory. They provide a condensed intellectual history of the development of hermeneutics and phenomenology without tracing the interpretive turn in phenomenology by Heidegger and Merleau-Ponty. As they point out, the limitation of traditional hermeneutics was that it assumed that actions and language were rational until proven otherwise. However, theories of rationality, particularly scientific rationality, and rational calculation (a cost-benefit analysis of two or more choices) exclude many aspects of the human world that are based upon meanings, commitments, and concerns that cannot be reduced to simple rational calculations about advantages that maximize pleasure or utility. Phenomenology, as developed by Husserl (1964, 1936/1970), offered a vision of the life world, the world of practical reasoning, human concerns, and meanings. Heidegger, a student of Husserl, offered a critique of the Cartesian understanding of the subjective and objective distinctions that traditionally separated the traditions of the physical and human sciences, or explanation and understanding. Fjelland, a philosopher from Norway, and Gjengedal, a nurse ethicist who is also from Norway, provide a provocative introduction to the current philosophy of science, mind-body philosophy, and the relationships between practice and theory. They make an argument for a science of the particular (prudence or phronesis) as a basis for nursing theory and practice.

In Chapter 2, Margaret J. Dunlop takes up a feminist perspective on science, asking whether it is possible to have a science of caring. She proposes a broadening of our notions of science to include caring practices, life world, and interpretation. She too argues for including serious study of the care of the body and the embodiment of health and illness. Rather than blunting or distorting the knowledge and voice of caring—practices traditionally relegated to women's work and therefore privatized—she argues for developing a language and science capable of making this knowledge and skill visible without sentimentalizing or trivializing these practices.

In the third chapter, Victoria W. Leonard examines views of the person embedded in rational empiricism and endemic in the Cartesian view of the person. She extends the critique of traditional theory/method distinctions raised in the first two chapters and the discussion of the links between ontological concerns—that is, what it means to be a person or a thing and how these assumptions are inextricably linked to methods and ways of knowing (epistemology). Linkages between hermeneutics and phenomenology in the work of Heidegger are drawn. Leonard points to a way to get beyond a fruitless oppositional debate between "subjective" and "objective" framing of research methods in terms of choosing between quantitative and qualitative research methods. She expands the discussion of world, care, embodiment, and temporality.

In Chapter 4, Karen A. Plager introduces the use of interpretive phenomenology in studying the family (or any natural grouping and community). Drawing on Heidegger's notion of "the clearing"—the possibilities and concerns that are made accessible by shared history, practices, and meanings—she describes focal and local clearings created by rituals, celebrations, and human events. She outlines the modes of engagement for interpretive phenomenology, explicating an approach to studying smoothly functioning social practices and human excellence, not just breakdown. She raises the problem with theory that "present-at-hand" accounts tend to be accounts of breakdown and emphasizes the danger of constructing smooth functioning or health from studying situations of breakdown. Her concern is to understand health promotion, illness prevention, and primary health care as they are practiced in families. She extends the previous discussions of rigor in evaluating interpretive phenomenological studies.

In Chapter 5, David C. Thomasma points to the similarity between clinical reasoning and practical moral reasoning as a ground for developing a nursing ethic that is true to the caring and healing practices of nurses. Thomasma gives a brief historical overview of the development of biomedical ethics and suggests ways that nursing ethics might diverge from bioethics.

Chapter 6 by Patricia Benner shifts the discussion to practical considerations and guidelines for designing and carrying out interpretive phenomenological studies. Benner explores the ethics of conducting interpretive studies and the role of narrative and participant observation for uncovering and articulating taken-for-granted concerns, meanings, and notions of the good. She also explores sources of text and strategies for data collection and interpretation.

Benner's practical discussion is extended in Chapter 7 by Diekelmann, Schuster, and Lam, who present a computer program designed to aid in the formation and writing of interpretive studies. This computer program was piloted by many of the authors in this text, and their commentary shaped some of the design. Though it is still in the developing stages, it has the marked advantages of allowing others to follow the interpreter's reasoning, patterns, and associations so that joint work on a large text and consensual validation are facilitated. The program is discovery oriented, and the retrieval is based upon the text itself. A search of interpretive terms is possible and the interpreter never has to retype a portion of text, a decided advantage of this program.

Part 2 of the book comprises actual interpretive studies. These studies were selected to demonstrate a range of interpretive investigations. In chapter 8, Lee SmithBattle brilliantly illustrates the power of the use of narrative to allow marginalized others to be heard and seen in their own terms. Lee SmithBattle is an expert community health nurse, and her own expert practice in community development and community health promotion allows her to be in diverse situations in nonintrusive, attentive ways. Her interviews and observations of teenage mothers and their significant others take place in the community where suspicion of outsiders is reasonable. She argues for a new form of health and social services and offers a critique of normalizing science that identifies deficits without examining the strengths, possibilities, and learning inherent in most experiential transitions. Interpretive talent and an ethic of responsiveness are evident in her ability to allow us to hear the voice of a teenage mother and her family.

In Chapter 9, Catherine A. Chesla examines and describes four major patterns of care constituted by parental caregiving concerns of parents with schizophrenic offspring. She uses these patterns of care to critically reflect on the existing theories of family caregiving in families with schizophrenic members. Chesla then raises her level of commentary to consider the ways in which these caregiving patterns reflect dominant societal concerns about parenting. This study demonstrates the critical powers that can be gained from in depth studies of actual practices. The Enlightenment tradition contains a bias that only theory liberates and creates innovation and that theoretical reflection is the primary source of critique and cultural design. Chesla's work powerfully demonstrates that the influence goes in both directions and that practice is richer and more varied than decontextualized theories can describe. Her work raises new challenges for thinking about caregiving practices for all parents.

In chapter 10, Philip Darbyshire reflects with candor upon his developing understanding of the distinctions between grounded theory (Glaser & Strauss, 1967) and interpretive phenomenology as he proceeded in his research project of studying parents' participation and involvement in the care of their hospitalized child. He gains a critical and reflective perspective by comparing dissonance between parental practices and understandings, public policy understandings, and nurses' practices and understandings of parental involvement. In each case, he uses narratives and observations of practice.

In Chapter 11, Nancy Doolittle presents an excellent example of clinical ethnography, an anthropological form of interpretive phenomenology that allows for a "thick description" (Geertz, 1973) of the lived experience of an illness, a phenomenological account of the social and embodied experience of the illness and manifestations of the disease, and a descriptive account of the transitions encountered during recovery. Doolittle presents paradigm cases to illustrate the meanings of recovery and the evolution of embodied skilled know-how throughout recovery. One gains an appreciation of the experiential learning and practical knowledge of the person recovering from a stroke. Reading such a work, the clinician is forced to confront the patient's perspective and possibilities in other than medical and nursing terms. Such work provides new understandings and access to compassionate responses on the part of the clinician as well as providing direction for the development of new rehabilitation therapies. Doolittle's interpretation of nursing's project recalls Thomasma's comment (Chapter 5) that "the theory underlying nursing practice suggests that the proper ethics be a relational ethic, one that targets the problems patients have with their disease, with family, with disruptions in their social and work structure, and in relation to their values, including their ultimate values." This chapter and Chapter 12 illustrate an approach to exploring these multiple levels of interpretation within one study.

In Chapter 12, Benner, Janson-Bjerklie, Ferketich, and Becker explore the moral dimensions of illness through narrative self-understandings and identity in relation to having asthma as a chronic illness. A thematic analysis of interviews yielded four different self-described relationships to the illness: an extremely adversarial relationship to the disease, rejection of the illness, a transition in self-understanding, and acceptance of the illness as a part of one's identity. The taken-for-granted projects of autonomy and mind over matter go hand in hand to create systems of responsibility, shame, blame, and guilt for causing and recovering from an illness. Acceptance and nonacceptance ways of relating to an illness are explored with their attendant tacit assumptions about responsibility, guilt, and shame. The self-described relationship to the illness is mirrored in social relationships. This is a large study that combined qualitative and quantitative strategies (Janson-Bjerklie, Ferketich, & Benner, 1993; Janson-Bjerklie, Ferketich, Benner, & Becker, 1992). The interpretive portion of the study for such a large number of participants ($N = 95$) was made possible by federal funding for a team of qualitative researchers who developed the thematic analysis of interviews obtained from the study participants.

In Chapter 13, Peggy L. Wros examines the ethics embedded in the care of particular patients. Her study includes the observation of the nursing care of dying patients and families in critical care units and the interviewing of nurses and families. She presents a paradigm case that encompasses many of the ethical concerns discovered in the study and describes "(a) characteristics of an ethic of care, (b) the role of judicial ethics in decision making, and (c) specific moral concerns expressed by nurses." Wros's chapter illustrates the philosophical directions recommended by Thomasma in Chapter 5 and exemplifies clinical and practical moral reasoning from an engaged stance and within a transition. It provides an excellent example of articulating moral concerns and notions of the good embedded in expert nursing practice.

In Chapter 14, Deborah R. Gordon describes the cultural practices and experiences that shape the health care practices of telling and not telling the diagnosis of cancer. Gordon constructs the local background of this tradition in Florence, Italy. Currently local, national, and international background forces are pushing for change. But as Gordon shows, changes toward clear communication of a cancer diagnosis and prognosis, based on the "right" of informed consent, confront many background practices concerning relationships to authority; relationships between couples and family members; gender relationships; taboos on sex, death, and emotion; and many self-understandings that remain at odds with "informed consent." These background practices and meanings create difficulty and uncertainty for people, even people seeking to change their practices and self-understandings.

Gordon constructs a story by tacking back and forth between general and local practices and particular medical practices. As an American anthropologist living in Florence, Italy, she engages in dialogue between her distinctly American practices and Italian practices. Very strong in the Italian "not telling, not knowing" practice is a way of being fundamentally social that makes not telling and not knowing show up as the kindest thing to do and the kindest way to behave. Gordon finds a conflict between universal language about what is right to do and the Italian sense of a good way to be. The Italian way of experiencing the present highlights North American and Italian differences in temporality and the dramatic individualistic self-understanding prevalent in the North American practices of telling and knowing. This chapter sheds light on the North American experience of illness and death described in chapters 12 and 13.

In Chapter 15, Cynthia Stuhlmiller presents and interprets the narratives of two groups of emergency workers—paratroopers and firefighters—who rescued survivors trapped in the collapsed Cypress Freeway following the 1989 Loma Prieta earthquake, articulates the common meanings and sustaining narratives used by these two distinct groups of rescue workers who were exposed to life-threatening conditions. In the narratives of both groups she uncovers shared cultural meanings related to "personal commitment, dedication to saving human lives, avoiding suffering, facing death, and comforting families and friends." The data sources for her study of the lived experience of the rescue workers included participant observation, document analysis, and interpretive analysis of semistructured interviews. Her study provides a contrast and point of critique for post-traumatic stress disorder theory, the predominant perspective guiding disaster studies.

Taken together, these studies present a lively account of a relatively new research tradition within nursing, nursing ethics, health, and illness. Parts 1 and 2 illustrate an interpretive turn in research related to human concerns, practical knowledge, reasoning in transitions, embodiment, and ethics. Interpretive phenomenology seeks to preserve the participant's engaged action in the world and to understand human actions in everyday skillful comportment and in breakdown. These studies offer new directions in health care ethics and policy and offer a critique of human sciences modeled on the natural sciences. They show promise for recovering a discourse on healing arts and practices that can create new therapies and enrich the increasingly highly technical, cure-oriented, commodified discourse on health and illness.

References

Bellah, R. (1982). Social science as practical reason. *Hastings Center Report, 12*(5), 32-39.

Benner, P. (1984). *Stress and satisfaction on the job: Work meanings and coping of mid-career men*. New York: Praeger.

Benner, P., & Wrubel, J. (1989). *The primacy of caring: Stress and coping in health and illness*. Reading, MA: Addison-Wesley.

Dreyfus, H. L. (1979). *What computers can't do: The limits of artificial intelligence* (rev. ed.). New York: Harper & Row.

Dreyfus, H. L. (1991). *Being-in-the-world: A commentary on "Being and time," Division I*. Cambridge: MIT Press.

Dreyfus, H. L., & Rubin, J. (1991). Kierkegaard, Division II, and later Heidegger. In H. L. Dreyfus, (Ed.), *Being-in-the-world: A commentary on "Being and time," Division I* (pp. 283-340). Cambridge: MIT Press.

Gadamer, H. J. (1975). *Truth and method* (G. Barden & J. Cumming, Trans.). New York: Seabury. (Original work published 1960)

Geertz, C. (1973). *The interpretation of cultures*. New York: Basic Books.

Geertz, C. (1983). *Local knowledge*. New York: Basic Books.

Glaser, B. G., & Strauss, A. (1967). *The discovery of grounded theory: Strategies for qualitative research*. Chicago: Aldine.

Heidegger, M. (1962). *Being and time* (J. Macquarried & E. Robinson, Trans.). New York: Harper & Row. (Original work published 1927)

Heidegger, M. (1975). *The basic problems of phenomenology* (A. Hofstadter, Trans.). Bloomington: University of Indiana Press.

Hiley, D. R., Bohman, J. F., & Shusterman, R. (1991). *The interpretive turn: Philosophy, science, culture*. Ithaca, NY: Cornell University Press.

Husserl, E. (1964). *The idea of phenomenology* (W. Alston & G. Nakhnikian, Trans.). The Hague: Nijhoff.

Husserl, E. (1970). *The crisis of European sciences* (D. Carr, Trans.). Evanston, IL: Northwestern University Press. (Original work published 1936)

Janson-Bjerklie, S., Ferketich, S., & Benner, P. (1993). Predicting the outcomes of living with asthma. *Research in Nursing and Health, 16*, 241-250.

Janson-Bjerklie, S., Ferketich, S., Benner, P., & Becker, G. (1992). Clinical markers of asthma severity and risk: Importance of subjective as well as objective factors. *Heart and Lung, 21*(3), 265-272.

Kesselring, A. (1990). *The experienced body: When taken-for-grantedness fails*. Unpublished dissertation, University of California, San Francisco.

Kierkegaard, S. (1985). *Fear and trembling* (A. Hannay, Trans.). New York: Penguin. (Original work published 1843)

MacIntyre, A. (1981). *After virtue*. Notre Dame, IN: University of Notre Dame Press.

MacIntyre, R. (1993). *Sex, power, death and symbolic meanings of T-cell counts in HIV+ gay men*. Unpublished doctoral dissertation, University of California, San Francisco.

Merleau-Ponty, M. (1962). *Phenomenology of perception* (C. Smith, Trans.). London: Routledge & Kegan Paul.

Rubin, J. (1984). *Too much of nothing: Modern culture, the self, and salvation in Kierkegaard's thought*. Unpublished doctoral dissertation, University of California, Berkeley.

Taylor, C. (1964). *The explanation of behaviour*. London: Routledge & Kegan Paul.

Taylor, C. (1985). *Philosophical papers* (2 vols). Cambridge, UK: Cambridge University Press.

Taylor, C. (1989). *Sources of the self: The making of modern identity.* Cambridge, MA: Harvard University Press.

Taylor, C. (1991). *The ethics of authenticity.* Boston: Harvard University Press.

Taylor, C. (1992). The politics of recognition. In A. Gutmann (Ed.), *Multiculturalism and the "politics of recognition"* (pp. 25-73). Princeton, NJ: Princeton University Press.

Taylor, C. (1993). Explanation and practical reason. In M. C. Nussbaum & A. Sen (Eds.), *The quality of life* (pp. 208-241). Oxford, UK: Clarendon.

Wittgenstein, L. (1980). *Remarks on the philosophy of psychology* (2 vols.). Chicago: University of Chicago Press.

Part I

**Interpretive Phenomenology:
Theory and Practice**

1

❖

A Theoretical Foundation
for Nursing as a Science

RAGNAR FJELLAND

EVA GJENGEDAL

The Aim of a Science of Nursing

During the last three decades theoretical disciplines have grown out of several professional activities that were once regarded as mainly practical. The aim of the theoretical efforts has been to lay a theoretical foundation for the practical activity. One of these activities is nursing. In the United States nursing has for years been taught at the university level, and several theories of nursing have been developed. But does nursing, which is basically a practical activity, really need these theories? One justification for the development of theories and research is that they are necessary components in a professional education. On the other hand, it is sometimes argued that theories may create a gap between those engaged in practical nursing and those working with theories.

Hence one might be tempted to ask, Is science good? However, this question, asked in a rather general and imprecise way, has no simple and unambiguous answer. We cannot assume that science is simple and unambiguous, and in particular we should not assume that science has just one function. It is therefore a better starting point to assume that *some* science is good for *some purposes*. What works well, what does not work so well, and what may even turn out to be harmful must be investigated in each particular case. In evaluating the result, the scientist cannot claim to be specially competent. The general public, which both pays for research and is often affected by it, should also have something to say.

As far as the usefulness of a science of nursing is concerned, there seems to be a simple procedure for deciding the issue. A starting point that all involved parties might accept is that a science of nursing is good if it produces better practical nursing. Hence we will formulate the following aim for a science of nursing: *The aim of a science of nursing is to contribute to better practical nursing.*

The question of whether theory can improve practice is not new. It has been raised on several occasions in the history of science. For example, around 1386 the city council of Milano decided to build a cathedral that was bigger than all existing cathedrals to symbolize the prosperity and power of the city. In the Gothic tradition rules for the construction of churches had been developed. One such rule said that the height of the church should equal its width (quadratic cross section). However, the city council decided not to use a Gothic construction because it did not fit into the Roman style. They decided to build a cathedral for which the relation between the height and width would correspond to the height and width of an equilateral triangle.

But the decision to deviate from the Gothic construction, which was the best developed at that time, caused several problems. The first problem was that the architects of Milano were not able to calculate the height of an equilateral triangle. The city council had to engage a mathematician from outside the city to solve the problem. But then they faced two problems of statics. Once they had decided to deviate from the Gothic construction, the Gothic principles of support by beams had to be abandoned. The architects of Milano had experience only with smaller Gothic churches, and so no one knew whether the cathedral was constructed well enough not to collapse. A collapsed cathedral would not have been a good symbol of the prosperity and power of Milano.

Experts from abroad were called to Milano. One of these was the Frenchman Jean Mignon, who asserted that the construction was not sufficiently solid. He argued that the architects of Milano were not competent to carry out the project because they lacked the required theoretical knowledge, and concluded, "Ars sine scientia nihil est" ("Art without science is worthless"). But the architects and engineers of Milano used the opposite argument in their defense: "Scientia sine arte nihil est" ("Science without art is worthless"). They prevailed, and the cathedral of Milano was constructed according to their instructions.

As we know, the cathedral still stands and might be used to support the view that practical experience should be preferred to theory. But it is not that simple. The cathedral stands out of sheer luck. Statics in the Middle Ages generally gave too large dimensions to constructions, leaving a rather generous margin of error. Hence the construction was reliable, but the justification was not (Böhme, Daele, & Krohn, 1978, pp. 341-344).

Building cathedrals and nursing are similar in the sense that both, with or without theory, are basically practical disciplines. In this sense they are arts. In the arts we have criteria for what is good and bad independently of theories. Hence we can distinguish between good and bad practice. For instance, when a cathedral collapses, we may conclude that either the construction was defective or the work was not properly done. Of course, it may not always be easy to judge if professional performance is good or bad, but in principle the distinction is clear enough.

The same applies to nursing. Normally it is fairly easy to see the difference between good and bad nursing. Even patients who are hospitalized for the first time will often be able to recognize a novice nurse. They may notice that the performance is hesitant and unsteady, that the bandage is too loose, or that the information given does not inspire confidence.

But normally it is not easy to determine if the lack of competence is due to lack of theory or the lack of practical experience. The relation between theoretical knowledge, knowledge obtained by experience, and the achieved end product is complicated. In the case of the cathedral of Milano practical skills seemed to triumph, but that turned out to be a coincidence. To determine the contributions of theoretical knowledge versus practical experience in achieving a special goal, one has to demonstrate in detail how the goal is achieved. Investigating these matters in more detail raises several theoretical problems. In itself this is an argument in favor of theory.

However, nursing faces a more fundamental problem. The builders of cathedrals work in stone and wood, but nurses "work on" people. The question of good nursing is not exclusively a technical problem, like the building of cathedrals. What is good nursing also depends on what is *morally right.* Nursing may be technically perfect, but it is not good nursing if it is morally unacceptable. Hence what is good nursing is itself a problem. It is a theoretical problem, if "theory" is taken in a broad sense, including ethics.

It is not sufficient to say that the aim of a science of nursing is to contribute to better nursing practice. The question of what constitutes good nursing is in itself a theoretical and ethical question. The aim of a science of nursing should consequently be expanded to comprise (a) contributing to better practical nursing and (b) exploring what good nursing is.

Good Nursing Practice as a
Basis for the Science of Nursing

If the aim of nursing theory is improved practical nursing, the idea that practical nursing must be its starting point as well immediately suggests itself. This point is stressed by Patricia Benner and Judith Wrubel in their book *The Primacy of Caring*: "A theory is needed that describes, interprets, and explains not an imagined ideal of nursing, but actual expert nursing as it is practiced day to day" (Benner & Wrubel, 1989, p. 5).

Benner and Wrubel do not try to construct a theory of nursing on the model of natural science. They build their theory on another ideal, one inspired by Søren Kierkegaard, Martin Heidegger, and Maurice Merleau-Ponty.

Even if this is a good starting point, we face at least one problem. The aim of a theory of nursing is to tell what good nursing is. But if the starting point is good practical nursing, must we not already know what good nursing is? How can we, in the first place, distinguish between good and not good nursing? One solution to the problem is that we take as our starting point what is agreed upon by nurses as good nursing and try to describe the knowledge involved in the actual performance. But if the only aim of a theory of nursing is to articulate as exactly as possible what is already taken for granted in good practical nursing, then we do not need a theory of nursing because it does not produce any new knowledge. However, we shall restrict ourselves to pointing out that good practical nursing is only the starting point for the theory. Hence our first aim is to demonstrate how a theory can take the essential attributes of good practical nursing into consideration. The second aim is to demonstrate how such a theory can improve the practice of nursing. We shall start with the first task.

The Unity of Science and Scientism

It is sometimes argued that the distinguishing mark of science is the application of a special *method,* which is therefore *the* scientific method. This implies that there is one method common to all sciences, from physics to literary science. The assertion that there is such a method is often called the thesis of the unity of science, and it was maintained by the logical empiricists, who held this to be an inductive method. Others, especially Karl Popper, argued that it was the hypothetico-deductive method. Still others spoke of "the problem-solving method." But because Popper argued that the hypothetico-deductive method was nothing but the method of trial and error (or, to be more specific, the method of trial and elimination of error) applied to theoretical problems, the hypothetico-deductive method and the problem-solving method may be regarded as identical.

The thesis of the unity of science has been criticized, especially during what has been known as "the positivist struggle." The critics argued that there is no one scientific method, but that on the contrary each field must develop its own method. In particular they argued against the application of "the method of natural science" to the social sciences and the humanities. Some of the critics argued that the hypothetico-deductive method may be adequate to the natural sciences, but that it cannot—and in particular *should not*—be applied as the only method in the social sciences and the humanities.

Advocates of the thesis of the unity of science have argued that the hypothetico-deductive method does not make any presuppositions, in particular any presuppositions that restrict its validity to the natural sciences. If the method is nothing but the systematic use of trial and error applied to theoretical problems, this view is obviously correct. The method of trial and error is used in all activities. But then it can be argued that if the scientific method is nothing more than this, there is really no general scientific method.

However, the proponents of the thesis of the unity of science often have more in mind. During the last two decades there has been a tendency among nursing theorists to attempt to construct a science of nursing on the model of natural science. The development of different instruments for measuring the quality of nursing care is one illustration of this tendency. By *the scientific method* theorists mean the method developed in the natural sciences, characterized by the use of measurements, mathematics, and experiments. Hence a discipline becomes a science by applying the same method. We shall call this view *scientism*. It is normally related to a mechanistic world view and can be traced back to two of the founders of modern science, Galileo and Descartes.

It is a popular view that modern science is characterized by being observational and experimental. This is in general correct, but it should be understood correctly. If by *observation* one means the observation of simple sense perception, most natural science is not based on observation. The investigation of nature presupposes the language in which the questions are to be posed and the answers interpreted. This is the language of mathematics, or rather the language of geometry. But this language, or the decision to use it, cannot be the outcome of observation or experiments. It is rather a result of "a change of metaphysical attitude" (Koyré, 1978, p. 2).

It is a historical fact that the emergence of modern science is intimately connected with a mechanistic world view. When Galileo founded a mathematical science, he argued that only that which can be described mathematically has an objective existence. According to Galileo, the world of science is a world of mathematical bodies.

Descartes, who was fundamentally influenced by Galileo, maintained that the only property that remains as objectively existing is the extension of things. All material things are *res extensa,* and extension is their essential property. When he had already presupposed a world solely consisting of mathematical bodies, Descartes also had to regard the human body as a material body, which like other material bodies is governed by the laws of mechanics. However, he was aware that human beings have a consciousness. Indeed, this fact was the very starting point of his philosophy. The only thing he kept outside the material realm was consciousness, that is, the human soul. But he had to pay a rather high price, for he had to divide our existence into two parts, material body and soul, which are essentially different. Material bodies are *res extensa,* pure matter, and consciousness is *res cogitans,* pure consciousness.

The advocates of scientism normally argue in favor of quantification, the use of mathematics and experiments where possible. They accept a discipline as a science only if it satisfies the requirements of the natural sciences. Hence the humanities should not be accepted as science unless they satisfy these requirements. In this paper we are not going to criticize scientism. Rather, we want to present an alternative way of thinking that we think may provide a useful foundation for nursing theory.

The Humanistic Tradition

Another tradition claims the same cognitive status for the humanities as for the natural sciences. It states that the distinguishing features of the humanities must be considered and that the humanities are essentially different from the natural sciences. This view goes back to Aristotle, who argued that a method of investigation must take into consideration the nature of the objects to be investigated. Later this view was maintained by Giambattista Vico. Vico was 16 years younger than Newton. Accordingly, he lived at a time when modern natural science rode the crest of the wave. In his main work, *Scienza nuova,* he outlined the principles of a new science of the humanities. Basically he made a distinction between human-made things and nature, which is not human-made. Human beings can understand only what is human-made, such as language, institutions, and works of art—in short, everything that belongs to human history has been made by human beings and can in principle be understood by human beings.

To see what difference this makes we can use Galileo's experiments with freely falling bodies as an illustration. Galileo wanted to discover the law governing falling bodies. He measured distance and time and found a mathematical relationship between the two magnitudes. But let us imagine that instead of investigating falling bodies, Galileo wants to find out how the clouds move. One day when he is out watching the motions of the clouds, he suddenly observes some smoke from a bonfire. The formations of the smoke look like clouds, and their motions may be worth studying. Galileo observes that the "smoke clouds" appear at different intervals, so he measures the time of those intervals and tries to find some mathematical law. The task of finding such mathematical relations corresponds to the task of finding the law of freely falling bodies. But if he suddenly realizes that the clouds of smoke are *signals,* the whole situation will change. If they are signals and he wants to *understand* them, their possible mathematical relations will not be so interesting any more.

When clouds of smoke are used for making signals, they are no longer only natural phenomena but objects of language as well. They are still subject to the laws of physics, and they can still be investigated as physical phenomena, but as communication they cannot be reduced to physical phenomena any more than this text can be reduced to a physical phenomenon. We can understand linguistic expressions because they make sense.

Language is the very paradigm of the kind of phenomena that the humanistic tradition has dealt with. That is our reason for taking a closer look at what it really means to understand linguistic expressions. In everyday life we ordinarily have no problems understanding each other. However, if there is a distance between the participants in a conversation, or between the author and a reader of a text, due to difference in social and cultural background, one may have a *problem of interpretation.* The science of interpretation is *hermeneutics.* This designation came into ordinary use during the 17th century, but already the Greeks were engaged in interpreting texts, especially the works of Homer. During the Renaissance hermeneutics became important due to the problems related to interpreting the Bible. In the 19th century the German philosopher Wilhelm Dilthey developed a theory of hermeneutics as the principal method of the humanities. In our century, hermeneutical theory has been further developed by, among others, Martin Heidegger and Hans-Georg Gadamer.

The tradition of Vico and Dilthey has also been carried on by the Frankfurt School. Max Horkheimer, Theodor Adorno, Herbert Marcuse, and Jürgen Habermas are important names in this tradition, which has contributed to the development of the humanities and social science. This school has emphasized that the goal of the humanities and social sciences should primarily be "under-standing," in contrast to the natural sciences, whose goal is to "explain." (In German this is the distinction between "verstehen" and "erklären.")

The assertion that the study of human beings must aim at "understanding," in contrast to natural science's "explaining" implies taking the "spiritual" part of human beings into consideration, in contrast to the material part. On the basis of the humanistic tradition, it is possible to maintain that a science of nursing must take the following as a starting point: (a) a human being is not only a body but a "spiritual" being; (b) the spiritual part of human beings can be studied scientifically by means of a method that recognizes the peculiarity of the subject.

This view represents progress over the scientistic tradition. The spiritual part is what distinguishes man from animals, and a science of nursing must take this fundamental fact as its starting point. Good practical nursing takes the spiritual part of the human being into consideration as well as the bodily part.

To stress that human beings are spiritual beings means stressing that they are beings with a language. This assertion has some important consequences. First, language is something we share with our fellow human beings. We belong to a linguistic and cultural community. One indication of the impor-tance of language for a community is the intensity of the struggle of some ethnic minorities to preserve their language. If the language is lost, the culture itself is easily lost.

To see the essential features of a science of nursing constructed on these assumptions we have to return to the fundamental significance attributed to language in the hermeneutic tradition. Let us take reading a text as an example. When we read a text and we understand it, we grasp the meaning of the text. This meaning is present in every sentence of the text, and every sentence is composed of words. The author of the text has put his message into the words of the text, which he tries to transfer to the reader. However, one complicating factor is that the meaning of a word may depend on the *context*. This can be illustrated by an example. Let us take the two sentences "Peter always pursues his own interests" and "Peter had to pay interest on the loan."

Both sentences contain the word *interest*. But in the first sentence the word means something like "to his own advantage," whereas in the second sen-tence it means that he has to pay a certain fraction of the amount loaned, expressed as a percentage per unit time (day, month, or year). Hence the same word has a different meaning in two different contexts. This is the case more or less on all levels. Words are parts of sentences, sentences are normally parts of a text, and a text is situated in a social, cultural, and historical context. It is important to bear this in mind, especially when reading texts that have been written in another epoch or in another culture. The larger the distance between writer and reader in time, social background, and culture, the greater the problems of interpretation. Much of the disagreement concerning the correct interpretation of the Bible arises from the fact that it consists of texts written about 2,000 years ago, in circumstances very different from ours.

We understand that wholeness and context are important in hermeneutics, and for understanding in general. From a physical point of view, a patient may be regarded as lying isolated in bed. But if we are to understand the patient as a spiritual being, we have to regard him or her as part of a larger context. If the nurse and the patient have approximately the same social background and belong to the same culture, it may be easy for them to understand each other. However, the greater the distance, the greater the problem of mutual understanding.

Another aspect of the hermeneutic approach is very well illustrated in Thomas Kuhn's preface to *The Essential Tension*. There he describes how he struggled to understand Aristotle's theory of motion. At that time it was taken for granted that Aristotle's theory could be interpreted into the frame of Newtonian mechanics. However, what Aristotle said about motion was not only wrong but to a large extent absurd. In contrast, Aristotle's observations in other fields, such as biology and politics, were often penetrating and deep. How could this discrepancy be explained?

Kuhn suddenly discovered that Aristotle's text could be read in an alternative way that made sense of the apparent absurdities. Later he used to give the following advice to his students:

> When reading the works of an important thinker, look first for the apparent absurdities in the text and ask yourself how a sensible person could have written them. When you find an answer, I continue, when those passages make sense, then you may find that more central passages, ones you previously thought you understood, have changed their meaning. (Kuhn, 1977, xi-xii)

This advice is based on another important hermeneutic principle: You are to presuppose that the writer is rational and that the text makes good sense. This principle is valid not only for texts but for actions in general. Basically we shall assume that people are rational. Only when it is impossible to maintain this assumption can we have recourse to causal explanations. This point is often illustrated by an example from chess. Two people are playing chess. We follow every move of the game, and we can understand each action because we know the rules of chess and know that both players want to win.

But suddenly one of the players makes an incomprehensible move. At first we think that the move is rational and that we have not understood the strategy behind it. But if it turns out that the move was not smart, but rather stupid, we will try to find a causal explanation. One possible cause may be that the player has been poisoned. Another may be that he has had a nervous breakdown.

Utilizing a traditional terminology, we may say that using hermeneutics in nursing implies treating patients as subjects and not as objects. This may be an important correction in practice, in which there has been—at least in the past—a tendency not to look at patients as rational beings even if they acted completely rationally.

Psychiatrists, for instance, have routinely interpreted all expressions as symptoms, even when these contained highly justified criticism of the conditions in the unit. Most of us also know the expression "difficult patient." When we think about it, we know that some of the patients who have received this designation may be among the most rational. They are asking critical questions and want to know what is wrong; in short, they want to participate. By branding a patient as "difficult," it is easier not to take him or her seriously.

All this is important, but the hermeneutic tradition is, as far as we can see, not sufficient for founding a nursing science. Even if it is both important and right to emphasize that human beings are spiritual beings, the problem that the spiritual and the physical are separated still remains unsolved. We have not escaped the dualism of Descartes, in which body and soul belong to two different worlds. It is easy to see this dualism in the former example with the chess player. Either he is acting rationally, or we have to explain his acts by causes. But in reality body and soul are related in a completely different way, for we have a continuum from what is completely rational to what is completely explainable in physical or biological terms. Especially when dealing with patients, who are ill, this continuum is important. A science of nursing has to solve the problems of Cartesian dualism.

Phenomenology

One philosophical tradition that has tried to make a radical departure from Cartesian dualism is phenomenology. The founder of this tradition was the German philosopher Edmund Husserl (1859-1938). In his last work, *The Crisis of the European Sciences and Transcendental Phenomenology* (1936/1970)[1] he addresses Cartesian dualism and its fundamental assumptions.

Descartes had turned his philosophy against the dominating tradition of his time, scholasticism. By means of his "methodical doubt," he wanted to start from scratch without any assumptions. But Husserl argues that Descartes' conclusions follow from his hidden premises. Galileo had already laid down the fundamental premises of modern philosophy. He had founded a mathematical natural science and argued that only that which could be described mathematically had an objective existence. Galileo's world was a "world of mathematical bodies." Husserl called this basic point of view *objectivism* and claimed that it is the foundation of most of the problems in modern philosophy.

Even Kant, whose ingenious theory of knowledge developed in *Critique of Pure Reason* is an attempt to make a synthesis between empiricism and rationalism, remains within this framework. Kant also presupposed a world of pure material bodies, a world that at his time had apparently been given its final description in Newton's *Principia*. When Kant claimed that all knowledge comes from experience, given in time and space, he did not have in mind what phenomenologists call "lived space" or "lived time" but rather the mathematical space and time of newtonian mechanics. On the whole it is reasonable to argue that Kant's project consists of justifying Newton's mechanics.

Husserl's important point is that all philosophy after Descartes has taken a scientific world view as its starting point. This can be illustrated by the way we traditionally have dealt with perception. Imagine that I see a house. According to traditional scientific theory, the process goes as follows. Light of different wavelengths is reflected from the house. Some light rays that reach the lens of my eye are refracted and make a picture on my retina. This picture is upside down and two-dimensional. Then light-sensitive rods and cones in my retina convert the elements of this image into nerve impulses, which, after preliminary processing in the retina, pass into the brain. I see one house instead of two, right side up instead of upside down, because of the corrections in my brain.

This scientific description of vision is different from our subjective experience. According to the scientific explanation, the process of vision starts with the object, continues via the retina, and ends up in the brain. Consequently it makes sense to say that the picture we see is some place in our brain. But we do not experience what we are looking at as being in our brain. On the contrary, we catch sight of the house "out there," in almost the same way that we grasp for an object.

According to Galileo and Descartes, the first description is objective and the second only subjective. It is, in a sense, this subjective world that phenomenology describes. One might think that phenomenology is concerned only with subjective experiences and leaves the objective world to the sciences. But that would be a misunderstanding. To show why, we shall use the "moon illusion" as an example.

We know that the moon looks smaller when it is high in the sky than when it is near the horizon, although the picture on the retina is the same size. Laboratory experiments using shining discs have demonstrated that a disc that is close to the horizon must be reduced as much as 50% to be perceived as having the same size as a disc that is directly overhead. The explanation of this illusion is that we in general estimate vertical distance as longer than horizontal distances. A vertical distance of 10 yards will be estimated as longer than a horizontal distance of 10 yards, although the picture on the retina is exactly the same in the two cases.

How can this phenomenon be explained? The well-known Gestalt psychologist K. Koffka gave the following explanation. Because human beings normally move horizontally, it is easier for us to traverse a horizontal distance of 10 yards than a vertical distance of the same geometrical length. Consequently we also estimate vertical distance as longer than horizontal distance. Koffka indicates that this difference is not due to experience but is "imprinted" on our nervous system by the process of natural selection. If Koffka's explanation is true, animals that move as easily vertically as horizontally—monkeys, for instance—will judge the distances as equal. This hypothesis was tested, and the results were seemingly verified (Koffka, 1963, p. 279). (However, Koffka points to the fact that such an experiment carried out with animals involves many uncertainties.)

But are our different judgments of horizontal and vertical distances just an illusion? Galileo and Descartes would argue that the two distances are objectively the same, although it seems to us subjectively that the vertical distance is longer than the horizontal. But Husserl would disagree. He did not accept the traditional dualism between subjective and objective. He insisted that the mechanistic world view was wrong and that we had to rethink the foundation of the natural sciences. To illustrate what Husserl had in mind, we may go back to the example of distance. How can we say that geometrical length is objective and that the length we perceive is just subjective? According to Galileo and Descartes, objectivity was related to things that exist independently of human beings. Such things will still be there even if people no longer exist. Of course, Galileo and Descartes would have to admit that the unit of measurement, the yardstick, has been constructed by us. Consequently, it is a contingent fact that the distances are 10 yards. Another unit of measurement would produce a different magnitude, and if there were no units of measurement there would be no magnitudes at all. Nevertheless, they would insist that the two distances are equal, independently of units of measurement, because objective space is Euclidean.

The perceived distances are subjective in the sense that they exist only in our consciousness and would disappear if we disappeared.

But, Husserl asks, is it really true that geometrical lengths exist independently of us? How is it possible to speak about geometrical lengths at all? For instance, why is it possible to say that the vertical and the horizontal distance is 10 yards? The practical prerequisite is that we need measuring rods and must be able to carry out measuring operations. In principle it is only possible to measure the two distances if we can move the measuring rod along the distances we want to measure. Certainly, we do not usually climb up 10 yards to measure the height of 10 yards. We can carry out measurements indirectly, for instance by optical methods, but at last resort we return to the measuring rods.

Husserl's important point is that even the mathematical natural sciences are founded on practical activities. They presuppose that we can move around and that we can produce and use equipment, such as measuring rods. The "truths" that are discovered in the sciences depend on these presuppositions. Of course, this does not interfere with the fact that geometrical objects are objective in the sense of always giving the same result. The sum of the angles in a triangle is always equal to two right angles regardless of the place in the world, and a right line and a plane surface are the same whether we are in China or in Norway. Standardization and unambiguity are the main aspects of geometry. If there were no human beings, the universe would, of course, have existed. But that is all we can say. Geometrical magnitudes are as much dependent on human beings as colors and smell.

According to Husserl, the mathematical natural sciences presuppose the life world (*Lebenswelt*). Because we always take our life world for granted, it is easy to forget that it is a fundamental presupposition. Husserl is the first philosopher who tried to give a systematic description of the structure of the life world.

The Life World

Husserl's work was carried on by Heidegger, primarily in his main work *Being and Time* (1927/1962),[2] in which he describes the basic structure of the life world. We shall not try to give a detailed exposition of Heidegger's work, which is far from easy to understand, but shall restrict ourselves to stressing some of the points that are important in this context.

One of the most fundamental aspects of the life world is its spatiality: that things are close or remote. When we want to put a measure on remoteness, it cannot be reduced to geometrical distance. It must be measured in what is required to overcome the remoteness. In more everyday language we may say that distance in the life world is what separates one place from another. Distances can be reported in practical measures, such as "a good walk," "a stone's throw," "as long as it takes to smoke a pipe," and so on. Such practical measures do not intend to be objective in a physical sense, but for those familiar with the concepts, these measures are useful. Because of the prevalence of the scientific world view, there has been a tendency to regard such measures as "merely subjective." But Heidegger argues that such measures have nothing to do with subjective arbitrariness. On the contrary, what they describe is the real world.

Now we can easily see that Heidegger's notion of distance in the life world—a matter of obstacles separating one place from another that have to be overcome—corresponds to what has been said previously about the difference between vertical and horizontal distances. It is more difficult for a human being to climb 10 yards than to walk 10 yards on the ground, whereas there is little difference for a monkey.

Perhaps the most important difference between the life world and the world of physics is that the former has meaning, whereas the latter does not. This fundamental aspect of the life world becomes clear in Heidegger's analysis of the concept of a thing. Heidegger asks, Is it not an obvious starting point to claim that the world consists of things? His answer is "No."

According to Heidegger, the entities of the world of science are the result of theoretical attitude. However, this way of looking at things is not primary but secondary. Primarily we use and regard things as articles for everyday use. A hammer (to take one of Heidegger's favorite examples) is primarily an article that we use for driving nails and only secondarily a physical thing. Hence the hammer has a meaning: it refers to what tasks it can be used to perform. To understand the meaning of a hammer is to know what it can be used for and how to use it. Heidegger points out that the meaning of articles is not an addition to their being physical objects. On the contrary, to regard something as a physical object presupposes an assumption of it as a tool. The experimental physicist normally uses more complicated equipment than hammers, but measuring instruments are nevertheless tools. To make experiments he has to handle those instruments in a competent manner, and he needs good instruments. If he is incompetent or his tools are bad, the measurements will be bad as well. But how can we decide if an instrument, for instance a watch, is a good one? Regarded as a physical object it can be neither good nor bad. But regarded as a tool, its quality can be assessed, and it is assessed in relation to the function it was constructed to perform.

What makes it easy to overlook the life world is the fact that we take it for granted in our everyday life. I know what a hammer looks like, and I know how to use it. Consequently I do not need to think more about it. The most fundamental skills we learn without any theory. Children learn to walk and ride a bike without first having to learn mechanics. They learn to speak without first having to learn grammar. Our primary activities, such as walking, speaking, and handling things, are not only pretheoretical; they are not even conscious. When I am walking, I do not need to think of every movement. My consciousness is directed towards other things. Of course, I may think of the way I am walking or decide to walk in a special way. But that is not always a success. If, for instance, one concentrates intensively on walking in a relaxed and unaffected way, one often obtains the opposite.

Much of our knowledge of the life world is not articulated. If someone asks us how we are able to walk or ride a bike, we usually are at a loss for an answer. Such knowledge is often called *unarticulated* or *tacit* knowledge.

In our description of the life world up to this point, we have talked about how to move from one place to another, how to use tools, and so forth. All the time we have presupposed that human beings are bodily beings. But now we return to the problem of an objective and a subjective description of the body, the very problem we raised in connection with vision. From the agent's point of view, the body is a subject. For instance, I decide to go home, so I rise from the chair where I have been sitting, pick up my handbag, and leave. But at the same time my body can be an object of a biological investigation. According to a reductionist biology, the biological description of the body can at last resort be reduced to physics and chemistry. The only way to unify those two descriptions is to introduce a dualism, as Descartes did, dividing the human being into two parts, *res cogitans* and *res extensa,* consciousness and body, psyche and soma. We have previously mentioned that the expressed goal of phenomenology is to break down Cartesian dualism. In philosophical terminology we can say that phenomenology has taken into consideration that the human being is a bodily subject.

Maurice Merleau-Ponty is the philosopher of the phenomenological tradition who has paid most attention to the body. One of the examples he uses to demonstrate the impossibility of maintaining a strict division between body and mind is the following. A girl whose mother has forbidden her to meet the boy she is in love with becomes sleepless, gets a poor appetite, and at last loses her voice. She has lost her voice twice on earlier occasions. The first time she lost her voice as a child after an earthquake. The second time it happened after she had been scared. A somewhat simplified version of Merleau-Ponty's explanation is that of all the bodily functions, the ability to talk is most strongly attached to relationship with other people. Losing the voice can be interpreted as breaking off this relationship. But it is not a rational and conscious action. In this case, the girl did not simply refuse to speak. She lost her voice. On the other hand, losing the voice was in this case not due to a somatic illness. Even though it is not an action, it is still a bodily phenomenon that has *meaning,* expressing a withdrawal from the relationship with others. The lack of appetite has a meaning as well. It means that the girl has cut herself off from life. When she receives psychological treatment and is again allowed to see her boyfriend, she gets both her voice and her appetite back (Merleau-Ponty, 1962, pp. 160-163).

If one maintains the view that human phenomena either are rational and have to be explained by reasons or are nonrational and must be explained by causes, as in the case with the chess player, we miss all the intermediate phenomena that are particularly important to medicine and nursing. Merleau-Ponty showed in his works that there is an area between what is purely biological and what is conscious and rational.

Consequences for Nursing

Let us start with the last point we stressed, that bodily phenomena may have a meaning, as in the case with the girl who lost her voice. It is worth pointing out that bodily phenomena *may* have a meaning but do not necessarily have one. It is possible to lose one's voice due to somatic causes. That is why bodily phenomena are ambiguous, and skill is required to decide if a phenomenon is of one or the other kind or a mixture. But it is only possible to decide if bodily phenomena have a meaning by setting them into context, in relation to the patient's life world. If one does not take into consideration that the girl in the example lost her voice on earlier occasions in dramatic situations, and that she had a boyfriend whom she was forbidden to see, one cannot see the meaning of the loss of voice. We have here a "hermeneutics" with the same structure as ordinary hermeneutics. The most important thing is to see the current situation of the patient in light of her previous encounters and experiences. This applies to bodily and other phenomena.

An everyday example will illustrate this point. In a unit for patients with senile dementia it was usual to take the patients out for a drive on nice days to give them some entertainment. They were usually taken in a dark van. Most of the patients appreciated the ride. However, one of the patients always resisted when the nurses helped him into the van. He was more or less taken into the car by force, and this was justified by the fact that he really enjoyed the ride. After a while the unit hired a new nurse who came from the same district as the patient. She could tell that the patient, who in the past had been a heavy drinker, had often been arrested by the police in his home because of violent behavior. After this was known, he was no longer forced into the van. Instead they allowed him to ride in a private car, and the problem was solved.

Second, bodily changes due to aging, illness, or injury will also change one's life world. To illustrate this point we can take one more example. We have previously said that distance in the life world is an obstacle that has to be overcome. To climb 10 yards is much more difficult that to walk 10 yards on the ground, and therefore the vertical distance is longer than the horizontal. But 10 yards on the ground may also be longer for an old person with weak legs than for a young and healthy person. Old people will perceive distances differently because the distances in their life world are different. For instance, many old people who do not walk very well are reluctant to move as pedestrians in heavy city traffic. For one thing, they are afraid of not being able to cross the street on a green light. People who have bad hearing, are hunchbacked, have weak eyesight, or are disabled in another way may have similar experiences. Just standing in line in a public office where there are no chairs may be a serious burden for a person with back pain, and a person with weak eyesight may be totally lost if steps are not properly marked.

To understand the situation of a person who, for instance, has trouble walking is a matter not primarily of psychology but of understanding the person's life world. When we are able to understand the situation of other people, it is not because we are able to look deeply into their souls but because we are able to imagine their life world. As we have stressed previously, a person's life world is not something subjective in the sense of Descartes. Of course, if we take all individual features into consideration, a person's life world remains private. But a great deal is common. Indeed, we have just described some of the fundamental features of the life world that are common to all human beings. These features can be described more or less concretely. The descriptions of Husserl and Heidegger are very abstract. But we could describe the life world of all types of disabled people—of those who are poor at walking or who have bad eyesight. Such descriptions would again be rather abstract, but they could incorporate specific features of the experiences of people with each type of disability. If we considered everything, we could have a hierarchy of descriptions from the most abstract to the most concrete. According to our knowledge, little research has been carried out in this area.

We take our life world, including the bodily subject, for granted as long as everything works well. When I walk, I do not think of walking but of other things. But just a blister is enough to draw attention to my foot. If I have a severe toothache, all my attention will concentrate on my tooth. The more ill I am, the more I concentrate on my body. The parts of the body that are affected are changed to "objects." The more a patient's body is changed to an object, the more limited is his or her life world. In extreme cases the life world can be restricted to the patient's body (Plügge, 1967, p. 13).

Ethics

We have argued that the most important factor in good nursing is under-standing the life world of the patient. However, we have previously said that good nursing also depends on what is morally right. Hence to relate to the patient is a question not only of understanding but of ethics.

The connection between science and ethics is complicated, and we shall not attempt to address all aspects of the problem. We shall restrict ourselves to dealing with a problem typical of those sciences that have human beings and society as their object of inquiry. Their object is in itself in possession of norms and values, and in this respect they differ from the natural sciences. Is it possible to study these objects without applying one's own values and norms, that is, without making a judgment on the values and norms of the objects? Anthropologists have studied cannibalism in New Guinea, the burning of widows in India, and the effects of colonialism, to take a few examples. Is it possible to give a morally neutral description of these phenomena?

The thesis that the scientist can and should be morally neutral is often attributed to the German sociologist Max Weber. However, it is far from clear what the thesis entails and what kind of neutrality is argued for. The example of the anthropologist may illustrate some of the problems involved. First, the anthropologist who investigates a society is for a time a member of this society. Hence his own presence influences the society, at least to a certain degree. Second, the knowledge produced may influence the society. Third, both the society investigated and the anthropologist are parts of a larger whole. The anthropologist may represent a colonial power interested in obtaining knowledge of the society for the purpose of ruling it smoothly and maintaining its political and economic dependence.

When the larger context is taken into consideration, scientists are hardly neutral. However, a modest interpretation of Weber's thesis says that the scientist, qua scientist, should distinguish between facts on the one side and values and norms on the other, and that in particular he should keep his own private values outside science. It is easy to agree with this modest version of the thesis.

This interpretation does not necessarily imply that facts are independent of values. It may well be that the production of facts presupposes values. As far back as the 1940s, Popper, an advocate of the unity of science, argued that his own philosophy of science was based on a fundamental decision, "a moral decision" (Popper, 1957, p. 232).

That facts cannot be completely separated from moral values can be seen in hermeneutics. We have previously mentioned that one of the fundamental norms of the hermeneutic approach to the study of human beings is the primary assumption that people are rational. The norm "You shall assume that persons act rationally until there are strong indications that they do not" is clearly a moral norm. The hermeneutic approach presupposes a fundamental *recognition* of the object investigated. It can be argued that the recognition of other human beings as rational agents is the very foundation of Kant's categorical imperative and consequently his moral theory. It is also the foundation of the principle of autonomy, which plays an important part in modern medical ethics.

According to some of the advocates of the approach, this is the Archimedean point of moral theory. From this starting point one can allegedly construct a universally valid moral theory in the Kantian tradition (see Apel, 1973). Although we have recognized the importance of the hermeneutic approach, we have also pointed to some of its shortcomings. The previous objections apply to a Kantian moral theory as well. Kantians have always had problems in dealing with agents who cannot be regarded as fully rational: children, the mentally retarded, unconscious people. Today problems concerning the status of the embryo are being highlighted, and a Kantian moral theory has little to say about this.

However, there are no alternative moral theories that do not have serious shortcomings. In view of this situation, one might argue that moral theories are not useful at all. This position was maintained by one of the prominent philosophers in the phenomenological tradition, Jean-Paul Sartre. In the well-known essay *Existentialism and Humanism* he uses an example to demonstrate that moral theory is of no use in practical situations. During the Second World War one of his own pupils came to him and asked for advice on a moral dilemma. His father had left his mother and collaborated with the Germans, and his oldest brother had been killed when Germany invaded France. Sartre's pupil wanted to avenge the death of his brother by joining the French resistance movement in Algeria. But he lived with his mother, and he was well aware that he was her only comfort after her husband had left her and her oldest son had been killed. If he left her to fight against the Germans, it would drive her to desperation. The question he asked Sartre was, Should he stay with his mother or join the resistance movement in Algeria?

Can moral theories help? Sartre deals with various moral theories, in particular Christian and Kantian ethics. However, his conclusion is that none can be of any help, and his answer to the student is:

"I have only one answer: You are free, choose yourself, that is, do something! No universal moral can tell you what to do" (Sartre, 1978).

But even if Sartre points to the important problem of application of theories, his conclusion is not justified, for at least two reasons. First, his

treatise on various moral theories is rather sloppy. Second, like many exis-
tentialists he chooses rather special examples. Several of his important books
were written during and just after the Second World War, and his examples
often addressed problems of one's own life and death. Such choices are of
course very personal, and moral theories are probably not very useful. But
most of our everyday moral problems are, luckily, of a less dramatic sort. It
is not justified to conclude, from the fact that moral theory cannot be used
to deduce simple answers in any possible concrete case, that all moral theory
is superfluous.

An important task of nursing ethics should be to analyze typical cases—for
instance, moral dilemmas that may arise in nursing practice. In this work the
nursing theorist may utilize any moral theory that is relevant.

The following is a typical example of a moral problem facing the practical
nurse. It was experienced by one of the present authors 10 years ago. The
nurse was on afternoon shift in an intensive care unit. One hour before the
end of the working day an old woman with a serious lung disease was
admitted to the unit. The patient had for years been suffering from bronchial
asthma, which also had resulted in considerable heart failure. Full medical
treatment started but seemed to have no effect. The only possibility for
getting the patient through the crisis seemed to be respirator treatment,
although this also was uncertain. The nurse discussed the problem with the
physician on duty, and, of course, with the patient herself. Despite her
breathlessness the patient was calm. She insisted on not being treated by
mechanical ventilation and gave the following reason: "I have had a long and
good life. My current life is mostly suffering. I have once been in a respirator,
and I would rather not have that experience again. As a matter of fact I want
to die." She also asked the nurse and doctor to send for her husband and a
priest. This was done, and her husband said that he respected his wife's
choice. When the nurse went home that night she felt that they had done what
was right, even if they would lose the patient. The woman was still alive
when the nurse came to the unit the next morning, but her state had worsened.
Her difficulty in breathing had increased, and she now showed clear signs of
anxiety. The death process had started, but she still insisted on not being
treated on a ventilator.

However, there was another physician on duty this morning, and he wanted
to treat the patient. He said that the aim of an intensive care unit was to treat
patients and that he had no choice. The nurse told him what had been decided
the day before and said that the patient really wanted to die. But the physician
was not willing to have more discussion with her. Instead he tried to persuade
the patient and her husband that she had to be treated. At last she gave in.
The physician, making it clear that he was responsible, ordered the nurse to

prepare for respirator treatment, and she obeyed. During the preparations the patient several times begged them to leave her alone. But now there was no time to take notice of her begging. She was intubated and put on the respirator.

She died the following day, still on the respirator. The nurse was later blamed by her nursing colleagues for not having been strong enough in arguing against the physician and for not having acted as the patient's advocate.

Moral theory is relevant to this case for at least two reasons. First, although the dilemma, to treat or to let die, is an old one and hardly depends on advanced technology, the power of modern technology has made the problem urgent. Rapid advances in medical science and technology have created numerous new problems without legal and ethical precedents. Unfortunately, technical development is ahead of legal and ethical development.

Second, one might argue that the nurse, who was a novice in the intensive care unit, should have relied on tradition, doing what experienced nurses would have done. But a few decades ago discussing the treatment with the patient might well have been out of the question. After all, medicine has until recently been dominated by the Hippocratic tradition, where it was up to the health professionals, primarily the doctors, to decide what was in the interest of the patient (Pellegrino, 1987, pp. 47-48). The physician in this case relied on tradition. But his view, that it is the unconditional duty of the staff to save life at any cost, was based on an obsolete ethics, not adequate to address problems in modern medicine. Although relying on tradition is in itself a moral choice, especially when this tradition is being challenged, a moral problem arises when one cannot, or does not want to, rely on tradition.

Although practicing nurses might wish the theoretician to develop a moral system containing a set of rules that could be applied in each particular case, we think this is an impossible task. Moral practice is complex, and the types of situations that health professionals may have to deal with are numerous. Therefore the conditions of the particular situation must determine which theory or rule should have priority. To learn moral rules or moral theories is only one part of moral education. But it is nevertheless an important part, and it should be an integrated part of a nursing science. However, the next stage in a moral education is to learn which theory or rule should have priority in particular cases. According to Aristotle, to judge in each case requires prudence (*phronesis*). But prudence can be obtained only through long experience.

This can be seen in the example above. The nurse was blamed for not having been a good advocate of the patient. Although she was convinced that the patient in this case really wanted to die, to find out what patients really want is normally hardly straightforward. Patients are often in existential crisis, they may be on medication, and one cannot expect them to express their opinions in a calculated and rational way. Hence it requires years of experience to understand what the patients' real opinions and decisions are.

This brings us back to the general problem of the relation between theory and practice. Theory, both scientific and moral, can improve practice. But what Aristotle says about moral practice in *Nichomachean Ethics* applies to the relation between theory and practice in general:

> While young men become geometricians and mathematicians and wise in matters like these, it is thought that a young man of practical wisdom cannot be found. The cause is that such wisdom is concerned not only with universal but with particular cases, which become familiar from experience, but a young man has no experience, for it is length of time that gives experience. (1990, 1142a, 10-15)

Notes

1. The main text was written in 1935-1936, but was first published in 1962. The parts of special interest here are §10-25. We want to emphasize that when we refer to Husserl as a philosopher who has transcended Cartesian dualism, we have the later Husserl in mind. The earlier Husserl has rightly been accused of remaining inside Cartesianism.

2. Heidegger's analysis of the spatiality of the life world is in §23. His analysis of tools and their ontological priority is in §§15-18.

References

Apel, K.-O. (1973). Das Apriori der Kommunikationsgemeinschaft und die Grundlagen der Ethik. In K.-O. Apel, (Ed.), *Transformation der Philosophie*. Frankfurt am Main: Suhrkamp.

Aristotle. (1990). *Nicomachean ethics*. In J. Adler (Ed.), *Great books of the Western world* (Vol. 8, pp.). Chicago: Encyclopedia Britannica.

Benner, P., & Wrubel, J. (1989). *The primacy of caring: Stress and coping in health and illness*. Reading, MA: Addison-Wesley.

Böhme, G., Daele, W., & Krohn, W. (1978). Die Verwissenschaftlichung von Technologie. In G. Böhme, W. Daele, R. Hohlfeld, W. Krohn, W. Schäfer, & T. Spengler (Eds.), *Starnberger Studien 1. Die gesellschaftliche Orientierung des wissenschaftlichen Fortschritts*. Frankfurt am Main: Suhrkamp.

Heidegger, M. (1962). *Being and time* (J. Macquarrie & E. Robinson, Trans.). New York: Harper & Row. (Original work published 1927)

Husserl, E. (1970). The crisis of the European sciences and transcendental phenomenology (D. Carr, Trans.). Evanston, IL: Northwestern University Press. (Original work published 1936)

Koffka, K. (1963). *Principles of Gestalt psychology*. New York: Harcourt, Brace & World.

Koyré, A. (1978). *Galileo studies*. London: Harvester.

Kuhn, T. S. (1977). *The essential tension.* Chicago: University of Chicago Press.

Merleau-Ponty, M. (1962). *The phenomenology of perception* (C. Smith, Trans.). London: Routledge & Kegan Paul.

Pellegrino, E. (1987). Toward an expanded medical ethics: The Hippocratic ethic revised. In R. J. Bulger (Ed.), *In search of the modern Hippocrates.* Iowa City: University of Iowa Press.

Plügge, H. (1967). *Der Mensch und sein Leib.* Tübingen: Max Neimeyer.

Popper, K. R. (1957). *The open society and its enemies* (Vol. 2, 3rd rev. ed.). London: Routledge & Kegan Paul.

Sartre, J. P. (1978). *Existentialism and humanism.* London: Methuen.

2

❖

Is a Science of Caring Possible?

MARGARET J. DUNLOP

> Man's love is of man's life a thing apart
> 'Tis woman's whole existence.
> *(Byron, Don Juan, Canto 1, 194)*

Today, under the influence of the feminist movement, we may be more inclined to see Byron's poetic statement as representative of the material life conditions of 19th-century middle-class women rather than as expressing an eternal truth about female nature. We might also be inclined to tie the denuding of male existence—the separation of "love" from "life"—to the mode of commodity production and its "rational" division of labor that relegated "love" to the place of a leisure-time activity outside the ambit of "life," which was equated with work.

If we look at the so-called leisure of middle-class Victorian women and its dependence on the presence of the supporting male(s), it becomes clear that "love" was indeed women's work, that is, it was their means of securing their livelihood. Any direct acknowledgment of this, however, threatened the moral division between prostitution and marriage. Thus women were seen as embedded in a life of love rather than work, where relationships were based on the "gentler" emotions, of which women became custodians as middle-class norms were promulgated as the "right" way of living.

The emergent usage of the word *caring* seems to involve a form of love. Recent nursing literature has picked up the word *caring* and the idea that nursing is a science of caring is gaining popularity (Leininger, 1978; University of California, San Francisco, 1983; Watson, 1979). Exploration of "caring" is also taking place outside of nursing (Gilligan, 1982; Meyeroff, 1971; Noddings, 1984). In this paper, I intend therefore to explore the idea of caring and pose the question of its compatibility with science.

Caring as an Emergent Construct

I have referred to the emergent sense of caring because there is little evidence that "caring" in the sense that it is now being used is a longstanding meaning of the word. Bevis offers Rollo May's 1969 definition: "It is a feeling denoting a relationship of concern, when the other's existence matters to you; a relationship of dedication, taking the ultimate terms, to suffer for the other" (cited in Bevis, 1981, p. 50). This is a decided elaboration, amounting to a shift in meaning of the term compared to the meanings given by the Oxford English Dictionary (OED), even as amended by its 1966 supplement. Of the four meanings examined, the one that seems to come closest is the third meaning, namely, "to care for," meaning "to take thought for, provide for, look after, or take care of," but this meaning does not have the high emotional component that is central to May's definition.

The OED gives a fourth meaning, which it sees as being used largely negatively and conditionally. In this construction, "not to care" passes from the notion of not to trouble oneself to that of "not to mind, not to regard or pay any deference or attention, to pay no respect, to be indifferent." The emergent meaning of *care* and *caring* as exemplified by May could thus perhaps be better understood as the negation of the negation in the fourth meaning.

Citing Partridge, Bevis (1981) claims a common origin for *care* and *cure*, but the OED carefully distinguishes their separate origins. *Care* comes from the Old English *carian,* denoting in the verbal form "to trouble oneself," whereas *cure* comes from the Latin via French (a *curé* in France is still a priest). This is an important distinction because, with the Norman conquest of England, Anglo-Saxon became the language of the conquered, French the language of the conqueror. As the languages came together, many Anglo-Saxon terms retained their "vulgar" or "lower-order" associations. Thus the conquered Anglo-Saxons looked after pigs or swine (Old English), which became pork (from the French *porc,* similarly meaning pig) when slaughtered and placed on the lord's table. The different origins of *care* and *cure* are thus suggestive of an original class difference in the terms—that the higher orders "cured" while the lower orders "cared." Although the meanings of the terms have developed in their separate ways, the relationship to power seems to have remained, with *cure* continuing to express a more direct relationship of power and control.

The purpose of this excursion into etymology is to suggest that "caring" as a concept for ordering human emotions is in the process of being invented or constructed. At the same time, the term brings its complex past with it, including its negative and lower-order associations, which may prove hard to shift because they are so embedded in the background meanings. It seems to be no accident, in other words, that *cure* is associated with a high-status, predominantly male occupation that jealously guards access to the term, whereas *care* is relegated to women (and, particularly in relation to things, to low-status males as well as females).

We might see the emergent construction of caring as a response to problems of "people-work" as it has emerged from the private domain of the home in the forms of health, education, and welfare (Stacey, 1981). Within the private domain, care in the old sense had taken place within the context of love—of personalized affection. The vast literature on the effects of depersonalization in health, education, and welfare can be seen as a public acknowledgment of the problems of separating "care" from "love," and the enriched meaning of caring that is emerging can be seen as a way of attempting to solve the problems. Because care of people in the old sense has been the traditional concern of women, the proposed solution carries the implication that the problems are the result of female deficiencies and should therefore be solved by women. This must seem additionally appropriate because the vast majority of people-workers are women, although they rarely occupy positions of power and control within the health, education, and welfare systems.

The deficiencies of the system are thus to be remedied from below by the relatively powerless, who are to be charged with humanizing the systems through "caring" in its new sense. Meanwhile, the structures themselves remain above the strife, and deficiencies are located in "uncaring" individuals. The stability of the structures, their immunity from criticism, can thus be seen to depend on the development of a particularistic and individualized caring ethic. That this particular package is being bought speaks volumes for the continuing strength of female socialization into both "care" as it used to be and "love," which Byron saw as "woman's whole existence."

This is not to denigrate the emergent concept of caring, which is an attempt to come to terms with real problems. Indeed, I would argue that a central task nursing took upon itself was the translation of "love" into the public domain. But an unexamined adoption of the rhetoric of caring may blind us to its limitations, as suggested above.

With this in mind, let us turn to look more specifically at nursing and its attempts to develop what has most recently been termed *a science of caring*. In this discussion, it will become clearer why I speak of an emergent meaning of caring.

Nursing as Caring

Dean and Bolton (1980) argue that in 19th-century philanthropic thought, care was "the means by which the conditions likely to produce danger [were] constantly monitored and kept under control" (p. 82). The business of the nurse was thus seen as "'caring' for the sick, preventing all conditions detrimental to the health of the individual and family, thereby offering a guarantee of the well-being of the population." Nursing was thus the individualized arm of the public health movement and can be seen as extending care in the old sense into the public domain.

But in the private domain "care" had been linked with "love" in the pattern of female socialization, particularly in the middle-class home, with its heightening of emotional sensibility, and it was probably difficult for females socialized in this way to separate them. In Nightingale's (1860/1969) *Notes on Nursing,* for example, particularly in the sections on "Noise" and "Variety," Nightingale asks her readers to put themselves imaginatively in the place of the invalid in order to consider the effects of the behavior of others and themselves upon him. She is thus demanding of those who nurse the sick something of the quality that is now called empathy—the ability to place oneself imaginatively and sensitively in the world of the other. Such a demand requires a measure of caring in the emergent sense, although Nightingale uses the word *care* itself in the old sense, very much in line with its philanthropic meaning as discussed by Dean and Bolton (1980).

The 1936 nurse cited by Melosh (1982) claimed that she always asked herself how the person who loved the patient the most would work out the solution to the problem she was confronting as a nurse. Thus she continued to link "care" and "love," although the love had become indirect—she acted as if she were the one who greatly loved the patient.

The "as if" is important in marking a transition from the "love" of the private domain to the "caring" (in the emergent sense) of the public domain. It is also suggestive of the way that nursing retained the linkage of the private domain between "care" and "love"—a linkage that is still apparent when nurses talk about their practice. In her recent study, Benner (1984) found that nurses "identified with their patients by imagining themselves or their family members in the same predicament, and they reminded themselves of the otherness of the patient when such identification distorted their caring" (p. 209). From the context, it is clear that "distortion of caring" refers to the use of power to dominate, coerce, and control—in other words, to act as if one were indeed the patient or close relative. Thus the "as if" provides both linkage and separation.

Nursing Education

It is within this context that the apparently contradictory messages of nursing education make sense. Benner (1984) recalls being warned in nursing courses against becoming too involved. I too can recall being repeatedly told this on another continent and in a hospital-based program with little theoretical input. But at the same time I can recall numerous occasions when I was asked, "How would you feel if it was your mother, father, sister, brother, etc.?" Thus, in a very theoretical way, nursing sought to teach me to maintain both separation and linkage in my practice: separation—"you must remember that the other is a stranger"—and linkage—"you must think and act as if he were not." Thus one achieves something like "caring" in its emergent sense as it is applied in the public world—a combination of closeness and distance that always runs the risk of tipping either way.

Within this context, the tendency to claim caring in its emergent sense as central to nursing is understandable, even more understandable in view of its earlier and continuing more physical meaning, because care of the sick or disabled human body has long been the province of nursing. The collapsing of these two meanings of *care* seems to provide the basis for the truth-claim that nursing is caring. In other words, the longstanding involvement of nurses in physical care is being used to claim caring in its emergent sense as in some way unique to nursing, which is quite clearly false. The situation is particularly ironic in light of the increasing tendency with nursing theory developed in the United States to ignore the body and its associated physical care.

In 1964, Wiedenbach introduced her book on nursing as a helping art by declaring, "People may differ in their concept of nursing, but few would disagree that nursing is nurturing or caring for someone in a motherly fashion" (p. 1). Thus the "as if" model that is being used is that of the mother and is one that allows a large place for physical care.

Lydia Hall, in 1966, placed considerable emphasis on the nurse's role in care of the body. It was this physical care, she claimed, that provided the access that allowed the nurse to be an effective teacher and nurturer (Hall, 1966). Although physical care was thus subordinated, in a sense, to the goal of promoting psychological growth, Hall unashamedly saw care of the body as central to nursing. By contrast, Watson, writing in 1979, etherealizes the body by concentrating her attention on the psychosocial correlates of basic physiological needs—"logocentric caring" as my fellow Australian Judith Parker puts it (which I have sometimes characterized as "a tendency to lose the bedpan"). Watson (1979) introduces her section on food and fluid needs, for example, in this way: "Although the food and fluid need is categorized as a lower order biophysical need essential for survival, its satisfaction establishes a vital foundation for a person's higher order needs related to personality and social development" (p. 113).

Although we would be hard put to disagree with this statement, we find it sets the tone for the whole section. After reading the section, one could be pardoned for believing that the only problems with ingestion of food and fluids are psychosocial in origin! Indeed, her whole chapter on biophysical needs is really about their psychosocial correlates—elimination, for example, being largely caught up in a discussion of Freudian theory.

Watson (1979) is instructive, for she titles her book *Nursing: The Philosophy and Science of Caring,* thus implying that nursing *is* caring. Yet it is obviously a disembodied caring she has in mind, the type that one would be hard put to distinguish from that of other "caring professions." Watson is not a solitary example. Almost anywhere within the vast corpus of writings on nursing, whether theory or research, the same dematerializing tendency can be seen. O'Connell & Duffey (1978), for example, in a 5-year review of research published in *Nursing Research* (1970-1975), noted the relative paucity of studies dealing in the physical aspects of care in any way—only 11 such within the period examined.

In some ways the emphasis on the psychosocial aspects of care can be seen as a praiseworthy attempt to redress the perceived imbalance of an excessively physical orientation on the part of nurses. But it can also be seen as on a par with the progressive devaluing of physical care as it has been increasingly delegated to the lower orders of the nursing hierarchy.

The irony thus becomes evident. Nursing has justified its access to caring in the emergent sense at least implicitly, and in Hall (1966) explicitly, on the grounds of its old physical care base, which it has been attempting to shed. In practice, of course, it cannot be shed as easily as in theory, although delegation to the less educated is a partial answer. In a pinch, though, and sometimes through choice, nursing remains embroiled in physical care, which involves contact with the mess and dirt of bodily life, even while it is aspiring to the "cleaner" caring that deals with people's minds and emotions.

But to the extent that it is able to shed physical care, nursing becomes increasingly hard to distinguish from other occupations in which people make their living and justify their involvement by recourse to caring in its emergent sense.

Although an excessive concentration on physical care may have sometimes led to the ideologically denigrated nursing practice of equating patients with the state of their bodies—"the appendectomy in bed 10," for example—care of the physical body remains an important part of nursing practice. Even when delegated to others, it remains within the registered nurse's purview and control. Reduction of the person to a body may be seen as one of the recurrent temptations of nursing, but there are more positive ways of dealing with temptation than by flight. Earlier, we have seen how nurses imaginatively place themselves in the position of the patient or his or her close relatives. This can be seen as a positive way to resist "the temptation of the flesh." At a more theoretical level, a better integration could conceivably be achieved by exploration of the "lived-body" experience, to which Polyani (1958) and Dreyfus (1979), among others, have directed our attention.

In her excellent account of motherhood as a discipline, Ruddick (1984) discusses the temptations of motherhood in the light of its goals. This seems a useful way of looking at the two problems of that specific form of caring we call nursing that have so far been identified. In caring for sick people, many aspects of whose being-in-the-world become problematic rather than taken for granted, there is a temptation to concentrate on either the troubled body or the troubled psyche in order to simplify nursing work, yet what the nursing community agrees is good nursing is neither purely physical nor purely psychosocial. The nurse must thus find her way between the twin temptations of physicality and disembodiment. Nursing theory in the United States seems to have yielded more to the latter temptation than the former, perhaps because it is a "cleaner" form of caring. But yielding to the temptation of disembodiment may also be seen as a result of the association of physicality with medicine, and nursing's desire to cut itself off cleanly from this world in order to support its claim that it is an independent profession.

The second temptation, already dealt with earlier, is, in fact, the twin temptations of overinvolvement and excessive distancing. Both represent failure in terms of the nursing community's consensus on what good nursing is and are guarded against by messages or maxims that, if decontextualized, appear contradictory.

In speaking of the consensus of the nursing community, I do not mean to imply that nurses everywhere agree in some transhistorical and transcultural way. I am merely indicating the widespread agreement that exists among nurses of a particular time and place as to what constitutes good nursing. Following Heidegger (1927/1962), I believe that it is not possible to ever fully spell out the bases of such judgments, for they are part of the deep background of the nursing world. They are, moreover, contextual judgments rather than ones made on the basis of some explicit, decontextualized nursing theory. Indeed, Benner's (1984) work rests heavily on the assumption that good nursing practice is readily apparent if one provides the event and its context, and this assumption seems to be a sound one.

Although it seems possible to claim that nursing is *a* form of caring, it seems much less reasonable to claim it as *the* form of caring. Such a claim does scant justice to other "people-workers" who are endeavoring to overcome the problems caused by the movement of "people-work" into the public domain through caring in its emergent sense. It can reasonably be claimed, however, that there is a particular combination of caring in its old sense and caring in its emergent sense that is recognizable as good nursing, although (as I have indicated) I am skeptical about the possibility of ever spelling this out in detail, as universalistic nursing theories have attempted to do.

Can There Be a Science of Caring?

There does seem to be a basic contradiction between caring in its emergent sense and science as it is usually understood. To clear the ground a little, let me first suggest that a science or sciences *for* caring involve no problems greater than those of science generally, for one is simply applying the findings of science to achieve the ends determined by caring. Thus nurses, for example, can research areas of knowledge that are likely to be useful to them in caring, following patterns that have been laid down in public health, epidemiology, physiology, biology, psychology, and social psychology, to mention those disciplines that seem most central to their focus. Nursing-caring may determine the questions, but conceptualization and methodologies are borrowed from the established disciplines.

Some problems arise when attempts are made to combine the findings from different fields in other than a mechanical way because each field has its own focus of interest and its own conceptual tools. Thus there has been considerable interest in building what is seen as a specifically nursing approach that treats human beings "holistically." But even if such a science proved possible, as suggested by Martha Rogers (1970), it would still be in an important sense science *for* caring, in this case, a nursing science *for* nursing-caring. In other words, science would provide tools for the enterprise without encompassing the enterprise as such.

This is not to denigrate such approaches, provided other sources of knowledge useful in caring are not excluded. Well-informed caring, on the face of it, seems preferable to poorly informed caring, and there is enormous scope for improving the quality of information available to nursing. But a science *of* caring has different implications.

Within the traditional view of science, a science of caring implies that caring can be operationalized in some way as a set of behaviors that can be observed, counted, or measured. This is the approach adopted by Watson (1979) in her listing of 10 primary carative factors, which are then individually examined. It is also the approach of Leininger (1981) in her development of a taxonomy of caring constructs (28 to date). These can be characterized as attempts to describe caring in terms of a set of context-free variables. The difficulties of this approach can be seen by simply examining the carative factors listed by Watson (1979) and the taxonomy of Leininger (1981), for these are no more context-free than the caring they seek to operationalize. It is by no means obvious, for example, that comfort, compassion, and concern (to take the first three on Leininger's list) are any easier to establish than caring itself. Although it is probably true that what counts as comfort, compassion, or concern also counts as caring, we still have the problem of delineating what counts as comfort, compassion, and concern, which are, I would argue, highly dependent on context.

Fundamental Problems

Dreyfus (1986) argues that a fundamental problem arises in the human sciences because it is not possible to describe human capacities in terms of context-free features, abstracted from everyday contexts, as the natural sciences have done. Although in principle it is possible to develop a science of human capacities using features other than those used in everyday practice, Dreyfus (1986) notes that "we have no precedent for such a theory, no reason to believe the abstract features it would require exist, and no way to find them if they did." The truth of the findings of the human sciences is always vulnerable to changes in the practices from which the supposedly context-free features are drawn.

Although Leininger (1978) is hopeful of finding transhistorical and transcultural aspects of caring, it seems likely that such a project will run into the same difficulties as structuralist accounts of, say, language (Chomsky) and culture (Lévi-Strauss). What counts as caring is highly context-dependent, as Leininger herself points out. I have suggested that even within Western society, the term *caring* has developed its meaning in a historical context.

This does not prevent the claim from being made that something to which the term *caring* is now applied exists as a transhistorical and transcultural reality, and this seems to be what Leininger is hoping. But, as Dreyfus argues, it is not at all clear how such an entity, if it existed, could be designated or described.

Philosophically, Noddings (1984) attempts such an undertaking, by grounding caring in the universal memory of being cared for. In order to survive, the human infant requires care, and to become a human being it needs human care. She thus traces one root of human caring to "the longing to maintain, recapture or enhance our most caring and tender moments" (Noddings, 1984, p. 101), although if, why, and how we separate these from the primitive world of pain of the human infant is left unexamined. The other root of caring she sees as lying in "the natural sympathy human beings feel for each other" that enables them to feel "the pain and joy of others" (Noddings, 1984, p. 104). She thus seems to be suggesting both a nature and a nurture source for caring. This could perhaps be seen as analogous to language, for the capacity to develop speech can be seen as innate (in a certain arrangement of mouth, nose, vocal cords, and brain), but the particular forms that speech takes are learned socially. The apparatus that provides the capacity for caring, however, is much less clear-cut (or so it seems).

Bevis (1981. p.50) draws attention to the fact that Heidegger speaks of care as the source of the will. Superficially, this may seem to provide some support for Noddings' claim that caring is, in some way, innate. But Heidegger is using *care* (German: *sorge*) in a more general sense to speak of the deep involvement in the world that he sees as necessary to any human activity. In some sense, *sorge* is a human-centered version of Dante's conclusion of *The Divine Comedy*.

> My will and my desire were turned by love
> The love that moves the sun and other stars.
> (Dorothy Sayers' translation)

Sorge, as the source of the will, is what connects us to the world. It is neither positive nor negative in the usual moral sense, but simply *is*. This is why being-in-the-world (*Dasein*) in an important sense *is* care (*sorge*) (Dreyfus, 1991). But we can obviously care about such things as the purity of the Aryan race, as Hitler did, and such caring will structure the world in particular ways.

Heidegger does, however, distinguish two kinds of care—care for things (concern) and care for other *Daseins* (solicitude). According to Dreyfus, Heidegger sees solicitude as a type of care that reveals certain other beings, not as ready-to-hand or present-to-hand (i.e., like an object) but as there with us in the world (Dreyfus, 1991). This suggests both a specificity of focus (*certain* other beings) and a type of caring that recognizes the "beingness" of the other.

But Heidegger's "solicitude" offers little comfort to those who would seek to develop a science of caring, at least in the traditional sense of science (and probably in any conceivable sense). Because it is a part of the source of all-there-is for human beings, to examine it using tools such as science that are part of its product is to involve oneself in absurdity. To operationalize it is to operationalize all-there-is, and even if this were possible, *sorge* would still escape us because it provides the grounds that make operationalization possible. Thus there is something incongruous between the use Bevis (1981) makes of Heidegger and her development of a four-stage hierarchical model of caring (attachment, assiduity, intimacy, and confirmation—each stage being attained by successfully completing the tasks necessary to each stage).

But it is possible, still following Heidegger, to see caring as a certain mode that being-in-the-world can adopt, as a particular expression of *sorge*. As such, it can be retrieved from the background and subjected to examination, which is basically what those who examine caring as a moral activity do.

Conceptualization Problems

The question that then arises is how best caring can be examined. In deciding this question, we are in fact deciding the form that caring will take. But our conceptualization of caring will also guide our decision as to how it can best be examined. If we conceptualize caring as a finite set of caring behaviors, then caring can be examined in the traditional scientific way. But, equally, if we operationalize caring in terms of context-free variables (despite the difficulties examined by Dreyfus), we are likely to end up with something different from what we now recognize as caring. (The trick has been performed before, perhaps most notably in the case of intelligence.)

Although Noddings claims caring as a universal basis of morality, she sees a basic incompatibility between caring and universal rules.

> Caring involves stepping out of one's own personal frame of reference into the other's. When we care, we consider the other's point of view, his objective needs and what he expects of us. Our attention, our mental engrossment is on the cared-for, not ourselves. . . . To care is to act not by fixed rule but by affection and regard. . . . Variation is to be expected if the one claiming to care really cares. . . . Rule-bound responses in the name of caring lead us to suspect that the claimant wants most to be credited with caring. (Noddings, 1984, pp. 30-78)

Although it can be argued that Noddings is accepting and using a particular historico-cultural concept of caring, it is recognizably what I have previously termed the emergent concept of caring in our own historicocultural context. (One might note, for example, its highly individualized nature as a mark of its roots in a highly individuated society. It is possible that it is in just such a society that caring becomes problematical enough to be noticed or even named.) It is also the concept that Bevis (1981) is picking up in the context of nursing, although unlike Noddings, Bevis seems to believe that it can be cost-free to the carer. Benner (1984) is more realistic when she says, "The demands of nursing are large ones. The pains, risks and dangers encountered are sometimes great and cannot be experienced without personal cost" (p. 208). But for Noddings, to count the cost is to place oneself in the unethical position of not caring. Caring is thus seen not to reside in a set of practices, but in a thinking-feeling (thoughtful in its fullest sense) mode of being that gives rise to activity (including the activity of refraining from activity).

How can such an entity be examined? We have seen how it cannot be subjected to traditional scientific inquiry without distorting it past recognition. There are two problems with developing a science of caring along traditional scientific lines. The first relates to its historical and cultural specificity, and this problem it shares with other concepts investigated by the human sciences. The second lies in its negation of universality—if it could be captured by rules, it would not be caring (and this seems intuitively reasonable). In this, too, it is not unique. If, for example, we consider language, we can see that our culture provides us with a vocabulary of words and patterns for their use, but to simply use set words and follow set patterns is, in an important sense, not to really speak the language. Similarly, our society can be seen as providing us with examples of caring, but to simply copy these is to lay oneself open to the charge that one does not *really* care.

Dreyfus (1984) cites the case of Socrates' asking the prophet Euthyphro for a definition of piety. In reply, Euthyphro appeals to examples and his own special intuition, a reply that Socrates' angrily rejects, for he is looking for a universally applicable definition. (He wants the concept operationalized.) In arguing for the use of paradigm cases (examples) in the human sciences rather than universalizing theory, Dreyfus (1986) concludes:

> After 2000 years it seems clear we must give credit to Socrates and Plato for the vision of theory which has flourished in the natural sciences, but in the human sciences it might turn out that Euthyphro, who kept trying to give Socrates paradigm cases rather than abstract rules, was a true prophet after all. (p. 21)

It seems unreasonable to dismiss out of hand the knowledge obtainable by the human sciences in following the natural science model, although it seems entirely reasonable to dismiss its worst excesses. This knowledge does need to be recognized as knowledge that is historically and culturally specific, for the reasons argued by Dreyfus. Moreover, even within the same historico-cultural time frame, it is limited to statistical prediction and could only be otherwise within a completely homogeneous culture of genetically identical individuals.

But the problem of explicating caring seems to have much in common with explicating piety. This suggests that if nursing really wants to have a science of caring (as distinct from a science for caring) then it will have to take a hermeneutical form, as Dreyfus (1986) suggests. This is the approach that Benner (1984) adopts to uncover the knowledge embedded in clinical nursing practice. As she does this, she is also uncovering the nursing-caring with which it is intertwined. This is extremely useful in elucidating nursing-caring and demonstrating the sort of possibilities for caring that nursing presents. But it does not provide us with any universal truths about caring in general or nursing-caring in particular—indeed, it does not make any such pretension. Even less does it provide us with predictability, and even less does it intend to do so. What it does do is say, "these are the sorts of skilled things that nurses do, these are the sorts of ways they work out their caring in practice." As in nursing theory, the focus is on good nursing rather than on the bad or indifferent, which, one can be sure, also abounds in the real world.

Also missing is the point of view of the cared for (to use Noddings' term). We might well ask what patients experience as caring, and this is a potentially fruitful line of investigation that could be pursued. The line pursued so far tends to assume a congruence between nurses' and patients' views of caring that may not be warranted. But this is by way of showing that there are other possibilities within the approach that Benner has opened up.

Conclusion

If a science of caring is possible and we wish to maintain the emergent meaning of caring, it must take a form that in many ways does violence to our traditional ideas of science (which are in considerable upheaval anyway). A science that neither explains nor predicts in the usual sense is profoundly unsettling. Yet, looked at in another way, it is also profoundly comforting.

For if caring were the sort of entity that could be analyzed into its component parts and spelled out in universal rules, it would mean that, at least in principle, it could be computerized and nurses would become obsolete. This seems to be true also of caring in the older sense. This is not the place to pursue the argument, but care of the physical body seems to require that the carer have a physical body, at the most mundane and emotionally detached level of care imaginable.

The possibility also opens up of developing science in ways that will better encompass the traditional concerns of women. Fox Keller (1984) argues, following Simmel, that science, in its actual historical configuration, has been masculine throughout, in ways that painting and writing (also performed largely by men) have never been. The sharp separation of subject and object that underlies our ideas of science she sees as having its psychic origin in the radical separation of the male child from the mother (as in Chodorow's 1978 account). The female child separates less radically because she is unable to define herself as so radically "other." As Fox Keller (1984) argues,

> The recognition of the independent reality of both self and other is a necessary pre-condition both for science and love. It may not, however, be sufficient—for either. Certainly the capacity for love, for empathy, for artistic creativity requires more than a simple dichotomy of subject and object. Autonomy too sharply defined, reality too rigidly defined, cannot encompass the emotional and creative experiences which give life its fullest and richest depth. (p. 195)

A science of caring thus challenges the male hegemony of science in a way that science for caring does not.

This is not to suggest that the hermeneutic approach is a feminine one—after all, it was developed by males, as was the concept of equality on which women based their arguments for equal rights. But it *is* to suggest the need to explore all the possibilities our intellectual tradition affords us so that we can articulate women's traditional concerns in language that the dominant male culture can understand. In such a struggle, which has a strong intellectual component, nursing and feminism can be fruitfully allied, for recognition of nursing skills, knowledge, and values is part of the broader struggle for recognition of women as thinking (as well as feeling) beings who operate intelligently in the world.

I end on a note of caution that arises out of the introduction. There is a need to develop concurrently with consideration of caring itself a critical evaluation of the structures in which people are expected to care. A more powerful and public statement of caring can be of assistance but is not in itself sufficient. There is little reason to doubt that caring is profoundly shaped by the social structures of the institutions of care. Harding (1980), for example, explores the way altruism is "cooled out" and subverted in nursing.

In this enterprise, too, nursing can be fruitfully allied with feminism, and in particular with those feminists who are concerned that the qualities that have been nurtured in the traditional world of women should not be lost. This amounts to more than the demand that men should share the caring, although as Chodorow (1978) points out, if this were practiced on a wide scale, it could do much to change the psychological structures of both males and females. It is a vision of a different sort of society, perfused by caring, that would be more flexible and attuned to the meeting of human needs. Although such a society might reduce the need for nursing, it is a vision that feminism and nursing can share.

References

Benner, P. (1984). *From novice to expert: Excellence and power in clinical nursing practice.* Reading, MA: Addison-Wesley.

Bevis, E. O. (1981). Caring: A life force. In M. Leininger (Ed.), *Caring: An essential human need.* Thorofare, NJ: Charles B. Slack.

Chodorow, N. (1978). *The reproduction of mothering: Psychoanalysis and the sociology of gender.* Berkeley: University of California Press.

Dean, M., & Bolton, G. (1980). The administration of poverty and the development of nursing practice in nineteenth century England. In C. Davies (Ed.), *Rewriting nursing history* (pp. 76-101). Totowa, NJ: Croom Helm.

Dreyfus, H. L. (1979). *What computers can't do: The limits of artificial intelligence* (rev. ed.). New York: Harper & Row.

Dreyfus, H. L. (1986). Why studies of human capacities modeled on ideal natural science can never achieve their goal. In M. Margolis, M. Krausy, & R. M. Burain (Eds.), *Rationality, relativism, and the human sciences* (pp. 3-22). Dordrecht, Netherlands: Martinus Niijoff.

Dreyfus, H. (1991). *Being-in-the-world: A commentary on Heidegger's "Being and time," Division I.* Cambridge: MIT Press.

Fox Keller, E. (1984). Gender and science. In S. Harding & M. Hintikka (Eds.), *Discovering reality: Feminist perspectives on epistemology, metaphysics, methodology and philosophy of science* (pp. 187-205). Dordrecht, Netherlands: D. Reidel.

Gilligan, C. (1982). *In a different voice: Psychological theory and women's development.* Cambridge, MA: Harvard University Press.

Hall, L. (1966). Another view of nursing care and quality. In K. Straub & K. Parker (Eds.), *Continuity of patient care: The role of nursing* (pp. 47-60). Washington, DC: Catholic University Press.

Harding, S. (1980). Value-laden technologies and the politics of nursing. In S. Spicker & X. Gadow (Eds.), *Nursing: Images and ideals* (pp. 49-75). New York: Springer.

Heidegger, M. (1962). *Being and time* (J. Macquarrie & E. Robinson, Trans.). New York: Harper & Row. (Original work published 1927)

Leininger, M. (1978). *Transcultural nursing: Concepts, theories and practices.* New York: John Wiley.

Leininger, M. (1981). The phenomenon of caring: Importance, research questions and theoretical considerations. In M. Leininger (Ed.), *Curing: An essential human need.* Thorofare, NJ: Charles B. Slack.

Melosh, B. (1982). *"The physician's hand": Work culture and conflict in American nursing.* Philadelphia: Temple University Press.

Meyeroff, M. (1971). *On caring.* New York: Harper & Row.

Nightingale, F. (1969). *Notes on nursing: What it is and what it is not.* New York: Dover. (Original work published 1860)

Noddings, M. (1984). *Caring: A feminine approach to ethics and moral education.* Berkeley: University of California Press.

O'Connell, K., & Duffey, M. (1978). Research in nursing practice: Its present scope. In N. Chaska (Ed.), *The nursing profession: Views through the mist* (pp. 161-174). New York: McGraw-Hill.

Polyani, M. (1958). *Personal knowledge.* Chicago: University of Chicago Press.

Rogers, M. (1970). *An introduction to the theoretical basis of nursing.* Philadelphia: F. A. Davis.

Ruddick, S. (1984). Maternal thinking. In J. Trebilcot (Ed.), *Mothering: Essays in feminist theory* (pp. 213-230). Totowa, NJ: Rowman & Allanheld.

Stacey, M. (1981). The division of labour revisited or overcoming the two Adams: The special problems of people-work. In P. Abrams, R. Deem, J. Finch, & P. Rock (Eds.), *Practice and progress: British sociology 1950-1980* (pp. 172-204). London: Allen & Unwin.

University of California, San Francisco. (1983). *The science of caring: Nursing at the University of California, San Francisco.* University of California, San Francisco.

Watson, J. (1979). *Nursing: The philosophy and science of caring.* Boston: Little, Brown.

Wiedenbach, E. (1964). *Clinical nursing: A helping art.* Springer, New York.

3

❖

A Heideggerian Phenomenological
Perspective on the Concept of Person

VICTORIA W. LEONARD

Much recent debate in nursing research centers on the relative merits of quantitative versus qualitative research methods. Insight into current philosophical thinking affords us an alternative to this endless, currently irresolvable controversy. Much of the debate in nursing research concerning method resolves along the battle lines drawn by 17th-century science: the controversy over how the private mind apprehends the external world through a mechanically driven and unreliable body. In sum, how do we know what we know; how do we know that what we know is "true"? Must we choose between the subjective, relative truth of the private subject and the "objective" truth of the "brute" data? A review of recent trends in philosophy suggests that there are other ways of framing the problem that yield fruitful insights into the problem of how we study human beings.

Much of the current thinking in philosophy that attempts to get beyond the objectivism/relativism debate stems from the work of Martin Heidegger. It was Heidegger's shift from considering problems of epistemology to considering the problem of ontology, that is, of what it is to be a human being, that radically altered modern debates on the nature of science and of knowing. Nursing could well profit from considering the question of what it is to be a person, of ontology, prior to considering questions of epistemology.

Once fundamental notions of what it is to be a person are clarified, the at times acrimonious debate concerning methodology will resolve. For, as Laudan (1977) argues, a research tradition includes methodological and ontological commitments, and these are inextricably linked.

To illustrate this point, I first briefly discuss the Cartesian view of the person. Then I present a Heideggerian phenomenological view of person and outline the hermeneutical method. Hermeneutics is a method for studying human beings that flows out of the Heideggerian view of person and is consistent with it. It is critical, however, to consider the Heideggerian notion of person prior to considering any notions of methodology, for to consider hermeneutics as a methodology in the absence of an ontological commitment to a view of persons is to beg the question. The issue is not what methodology is "best" or even necessarily what method is right for the question being asked because method acts as a theoretical screen and often determines the types of questions that are asked. Rather, the issue is, first, what it means to be a person; then, in light of our answer, how we ask our research questions; and finally, how we answer the questions we pose. Too often, researchers facilely seize on a method without considering the more profoundly important philosophical assumptions that undergird the method and whether those assumptions are consistent with the researcher's own view of what it means to be a human being.

The Modern Cartesian View of the Person

As a consequence of taking up the world according to the canons of Cartesianism, we are preoccupied, in nursing, with a notion of person as an assemblage of traits or variables, such as anxiety, control, and self-esteem. These are viewed as context-free elements to be combined according to formal laws that can be discovered through the scientific method, the goal of which is prediction and control. Such a notion of person flows out of an implicit acceptance of 17th-century Cartesian notions of the self. This self is viewed as subject, an uninvolved self passively contemplating the external world of things via representations that are held in the mind. This self *possesses* a body and, by extension, traits or attributes such as anxiety or self-esteem. The self is always seen as subject and the world or environment as object. The world is understood as representable via ideas, beliefs, and so forth that are cognitively developed and held in the mind. Meaning is therefore grounded in the actions of individual subjects.

This Cartesian view of person led inevitably to 300 years of debate over whether knowledge is real (i.e., an accurate representation of an external reality) or ideal (a subjective idea or private view of the world that is idiosyncratic and can never really be fully shared or communicated). We are still experiencing modern versions of this debate in nursing today. In other words, the focus from within the Cartesian position is epistemological: it asks what counts as knowledge and what our criteria are for evaluating truth claims. The assumption has been that if the criteria for evaluating truth claims could be determined, knowledge would have a foundation that placed it outside history and culture.

The Heideggerian Phenomenological
View of the Person

Heideggerian phenomenology criticizes both the objective and subjective positions of Cartesianism for not pushing the question back from an epistemological one (i.e., how we know what we know) to an ontological one (i.e., what it means to *be* a person and how the world is intelligible to us at all). For in asking what it means to be a person, we come to understand more clearly how we know the world. Further, by coming to grips with the ontological question, nurses, particularly those doing research, can move away from the imperialist belief in science and the scientific method, variously referred to as *scientism* or *the received view,* to embrace a multiplicity of methods, including the scientific method, that do not violate phenomenological notions of what it is to be a person (i.e., in cellular-level or epidemiological studies). For phenomenology does not argue for the abolition of traditional science, but rather for its appropriate use: that is, for its use in levels of study in which participants' meanings and interpretations do not figure—for instance, the study of the effects of maternal hyperglycemia on idiopathic neonatal hypoglycemia or the rate of prenatal complications in pregnant women employed in jobs requiring strenuous work. There is no question but that traditional science has accomplished astonishing results in the past two centuries, particularly with regard to disease. But, as Baron points out, "these accomplishments are not great in and of themselves. They derive their significance from what they mean for human beings and what effect they have on suffering and individual capability" (1985, p. 608).

Heideggerian phenomenologists argue that traditional science is itself a theory screen that constrains our ability to understand human agency (that is, intentionality in human action constituted or shaped by concerns, purposes, goals, and commitments), limits our imaginative ability to generate questions, and, further, limits the answers we can generate for those questions that we do manage to pose.

The view of person here presented derives primarily from the writings of Martin Heidegger (1927/1962, 1975). The author is also indebted to the contributions made by Charles Taylor (1985a, 1985b) and Hubert Dreyfus (1991).

The view of person described in Heideggerian phenomenology derives fundamentally from Heidegger's shift of emphasis from epistemological concerns centering on issues of the relation of the knower to the known to the more fundamental concern with ontology: what does it mean to *be* a person and how is the world intelligible to us at all?

> The proximal goal of *Being and Time* is to develop a descriptive metaphysics. Heidegger is not interested in fanciful speculation about Being. He is concerned with what Being means to us, and this requires at the outset an understanding of the being of that entity which understands what it is to be namely, Dasein. . . . Dasein in the course of its everyday activities and practices is characterized as 'Being-in-the-world.' (Guignon, 1983, p. 69)[1]

The Person as Having a World

From a phenomenological viewpoint, the first essential facet of a person centers on the relationship of the person to the world. *World,* in the phenomenological sense, has a fundamentally different meaning from our common understanding of world as environment, or nature, or the sum total of all the "things" in our world. *World* is the meaningful set of relationships, practices, and language that we have by virtue of being born into a culture. For example, the common expression "the world of science" reflects the set of relationships, questions, skills, and practices related to science. World, as Heidegger (1975) describes it,

> comes not afterward but beforehand, in the strict sense of the word. Beforehand: that which is unveiled and understood already in advance in every existent Dasein before any apprehending of this or that being. The world as already unveiled in advance is such that we do not in fact specifically occupy ourselves with it, or apprehend it, but instead it is so self-evident, so much a matter of course, that we are completely oblivious to it. (p. 165)

World, according to Heidegger, is a priori. It is given in our cultural and linguistic practices and in our history. Language, in particular, sets up a world; it both articulates and makes things show up for us. "For Heidegger, a vocabulary, or the kinds of metaphors one uses can name things into being and change the sensibility of an age" (Dreyfus, 1987, p. 274). Language creates the possibility for particular ways of feeling and of relating that make sense within a culture. World is the shared skills and practices on which we depend for meaning and intelligibility.

> World cannot be described by trying to enumerate the entities within it; in this process world would be passed over, for world is just what is presupposed in every act of knowing an entity. Every entity in the world is grasped as an entity *in terms of* world, which is always already there. The entities that comprise man's physical world are not themselves world but in a world. Only man has a world. (Palmer, 1969, pp. 132-133)

World is both constituted by and constitutive of the self. This notion of the self as *constituted* by world is fundamentally different from the Cartesian notion of self as possession. The world is constitutive in that the self is raised up in the world and shaped by it in a process that is not the causal interaction of self and world as objects, but rather the nonreflective taking up of the meanings, linguistic skills, cultural practices, and family traditions by which we become persons and can have things show up for us at all. The self of possession is the modern subject: autonomous, disengaged, disembodied, rationally choosing his actions based on explicit, cognitively held principles and values. The self of possession has a body and traits or characteristics that belong to it. As Sandel (1982) puts it, they are *mine* but not *me*. Thus these traits can come and go without altering the self in any constitutive way, that is, without becoming part of who the self is and shaping how that self knows itself. As Ricoeur (1986) has commented, this is a self robbed of the health of sameness. Along with this goes a view of the self as a radically free, autonomous agent, "the human subject as a sovereign agent of choice, whose ends are chosen rather than given" (Sandel, 1982, p. 22). Heidegger argues that the only way one can arrive at this view of the self is by passing over the world, by not seeing that it is world that circumscribes our choices and creates our possibilities.

Heidegger uses the term *thrownness* to express his view of the person as *always already situated*, as being-in-the-world and therefore, as Benner (1985, p. 5) says, "not a radically free arbiter of meaning." Human existence is involved in the working out of the possibilities that exist for us by virtue of our being "thrown" into a particular cultural, historical, and familial world. Heidegger's is also a teleological view of a self inconceivable apart from and prior to its ends and purposes, whereas for the radically free self of Cartesianism, values and purposes are the products of choice, "the possessions of a self given prior to its ends" (Sandel, 1982, p. 176). Freedom, in the Heideggerian view, is *situated* freedom (Taylor, 1991). Thus although the self also constitutes her world, she is constrained in the possible ways she can constitute the world by her language, culture, and history, by her (constitutive) purposes and values. In other words, world sets up possibilities for who a person can become and who she cannot become. As Hoy (1986) has commented, "personal identity is not a matter of ownership."

Taylor (1985a) argues that part of the attraction of traditional science for the Western world has been that it *does* include this view of the self as radically free. Such a view of self, suggests Taylor, is profoundly appealing to us because it coincides with our modern notions of freedom and liberation. It is thought that by getting clear about values, purposes, and choices, the radically free self can gain enlightened control over his or her life. It is the pervasive appeal in the West of this modern identity of the radically free, autonomous self standing over and against the world that causes us to overlook the essential inability of 17th-century science to afford us an understanding of human agency and causes us to privilege detached theorizing over practical activity.

World is *not* a purely intentional cognitive set of beliefs, a definition that falls back into the Cartesian notion of the conscious subject. Nor is it the "environment" as described by science as "object." Rather, because world is constituted by our common language and culture and is requisite for anything to show up for us at all, the subjective-objective Cartesian dualism that necessarily forces us into idealism/subjectivism or realism/objectivism can be replaced by understanding the person as in the world. World is neither held in the mind nor "out there" to be apprehended. Although we may each constitute our world in the sense of taking up in a personal way the common meanings given in our language and culture, we nevertheless have some aspects of world in common with all other members who share our language and culture. For instance, the American notion of upward mobility, though taken up in many ways within our society, makes sense only within our cultural context, in which class lines are supposedly fluid and opportunities supposedly exist for self-improvement. Such a notion makes little sense in a culture in which class lines are fixed and opportunities for self-improvement are not available to most people. Further, the notion of upward mobility is not something we are taught but rather something we are born into and become constituted by.

Heidegger argues that the detached, reflective mode of knowing the world exemplified by Descartes is *dependent on* the a priori existence of world in which the meaning given in our language and culture is what makes things show up for us at all. The taken-for-granted, involved skills and practices of what Heidegger calls the ready-to-hand mode are presupposed by the abstract, theoretical, reflective knowledge that Heidegger calls the present-at-hand mode, which is what we more commonly know as theoretical knowing.

World is so all-pervasive as to be overlooked by persons; it only appears to us in a conscious way in breakdown. For instance, Heidegger gives us the example of the hammer. In using a hammer we do not think of it and its purpose in an abstract theoretical way. We use it in an assumed, taken-for-granted way until such a time as it breaks or fails to serve the purpose we intend it to have. By appreciating what it *is not* doing we derive a sense of what "hammer" in the taken-for-granted, ready-to-hand mode is like. A notion of "hammer" in the present-at-hand, abstract, theoretical mode (as, for example, weighing 22 ounces, measuring 14 inches in length, and having certain proportions) will give us a notion of "hammer" that excludes hammering in the taken-for-granted, lived experience of hammering. Heidegger's example of the hammer exemplifies the phenomenological objection to our emphasis in Western culture on the primacy of the abstract, present-at-hand mode: it passes over the world, the taken-for-granted, lived experience of our everydayness, and, concomitantly, it misses the meaning that is made intelligible through the linguistic and cultural skills and practices given by world.

The Person as a Being for Whom
Things Have Significance and Value

A second essential facet of person from a phenomenological perspective is that a person is a being for whom things have significance and value.

> [Dasein] *finds itself* primarily and constantly *in things* because, tending them, distressed by them, it always in some way or other rests in things. Each one of us is what he pursues and cares for. In everyday terms we understand ourselves and our existence by way of the activities we pursue and the things we take care of. (Heidegger, 1975, p. 158)

Dreyfus (1987) points out that it is a "basic characteristic of Dasein that things show up as mattering—as threatening, or attractive, or stubborn, or useful, and so forth" (p. 264), and this mattering is the background for more reflective desiring or evaluating. Another aspect of Heidegger's account of significance is the way in which our activity is directed in a transparent, taken-for-granted, nonmental way towards the future, the "for-the-sake-of."

Borgman (1984) further expands Heidegger's notion of the things we care for and traces the modern fate of things in the face of technology. Things are inseparable from Heidegger's view of world and from our engagement with them via practices that guard things and protect them from the technological disruption that reduces them to means and ends. The practice of preparing a good meal protects the meal from being reduced to a microwaved frozen dinner. Things are contrasted by Borgman with devices, in which means are, as much as possible, invisible and anonymous. In the microwaved meal example, the preparation of the food is minimized; only the end, the meal, is important. The practices (means) essential to things are irrelevant to devices, the sole purpose or end of which is the facile production of commodities for private consumption. The practices that gather us together in human community and give richness and meaning wither into empty and meaningless rituals in the face of technology. An example of Borgman's thesis is found in some modern parents' attitudes toward childrearing. The whole enterprise is reduced to the efficient production of a perfect "product" that embodies certain external goods: physically well formed, well educated, well mannered, employable, attractive. The practices that embody the means for childrearing are considered irrelevant to this project or, worse, disdained. The everyday, practical routines of feeding, bathing, entertaining, supervising, and cleaning up after small children that gather parents and children together and formed the substance of family life in the past are now left to parental substitutes.

Persons, in the phenomenological view, have not only a world in which things have significance and value but qualitatively different concerns based on their culture, language, and individual situations. Taylor (1985a) suggests that the scientific rejection of "secondary" properties—those properties, qualities, or feelings that cannot be "intersubjectively univocal," that are not beyond interpretation (for instance, "feeling blue")—is one of the factors that make traditional science inappropriate for the human sciences. It gives no weight, says Taylor, to motives such as shame, guilt, or love that cannot be given a significance-free account:

> These are the ones, therefore, where the variables occur between human cultures, that is, between different ways of shaping and interpreting that significance. So that what is a matter of shame or guilt or dignity, of moral goodness, is notoriously different and often hard to understand from culture to culture: whereas the conditions of medical health are far more uniform. (Taylor, 1985a, p. 111)

Because there can be no significance-free account of desires, feelings, and emotions, our understanding of these types of terms necessarily moves in the hermeneutical circle: we understand the term *shame* by referring to the situation that is shameful and to the purpose of covering up the shameful act or saving face. The act, the feeling, and the purpose all refer to each other. Nowhere can one step out of the circle to get a significance-free "brute datum" to ground the account (Taylor, 1985b).

Thus to understand a person's behavior or expressions one has to study the person *in context*. For it is only in context that what a person values and finds significant shows up. Understanding the relational and configurational context allows for a more appropriate interpretation of what significance things have for a person. For example, anxiety is a variable often considered in pregnancy as a possible "predictor" of events in labor and delivery. Here we see the traditional treatment of variables as context-free elements that the researcher attempts to relate in some law-like way. To obtain an "intersubjectively univocal" measure of anxiety, a tool such as the Spielberger State-Trait Anxiety Inventory is used to measure anxiety. Problems arise, however, because the meaning of pregnancy and the meaning of parenthood vary widely, so that the meaning of the anxiety also varies widely. Assuming in advance that anxiety is a trait that is not fundamentally shaped by the meaning of the situation can cause the researcher or the clinician to miss the essential piece of the situation required to understand what is going on. Certain events may be predicted, but at the cost of sacrificing an understanding of the transactional process going on between person and world. For instance, for older women with established careers and marriages, pregnancy interrupts long-established rhythms of work and love, and anxiety can be interpreted as the realistic anticipatory working through of the problems and issues that the infant will bring. This kind of anxiety is potentially desirable and means that the woman is looking ahead and planning realistically how she will handle the situation of motherhood. In other cases, the pregnancy is not wanted and motherhood not valued. The anxiety focuses on despair how and foreclosing possibilities and should raise a red flag to the clinician providing prenatal care.

Thus we can see how 0an appreciation for the fact that persons are beings for whom things have significance and that this significance may change with context and can reveal a different kind of understanding. It matters to the clinician what meaning a pregnant woman's anxiety has because by understanding the *world and meanings* of the pregnant woman, the clinician is far more able to determine whether to intervene to help the woman to see new possibilities in her situation that will have meaning for her, *given her world*. For her world provides the only access to what is possible *for her*. Her world can be expanded only in relation to existing concerns and possibilities. This point has significant import for nurses practicing in clinical settings.

The Person as Self-Interpreting

Another critical piece in the Heideggerian phenomenological view of person is that being is self-interpreting, but, importantly, in a nontheoretical, noncognitive way. We are beings who are engaged in and constituted by our interpretive understanding. Contrary to Husserl, who claims that these interpretations are a product of individual consciousness, of subjects, Heidegger claims that these interpretations are not generated in individual consciousness as subjects related to objects but rather are given in our linguistic and cultural traditions and make sense only against a background of significance. An example of this is Caudill and Weinstein's (1969) study of Japanese and American babies, which found that by the age of 4 months the babies studied had become distinctly Japanese or American. Thus by the age of 4 months, human beings are already interpreting themselves in light of their background as either Japanese or American: all those hidden skills and practices and linguistic meanings that are so all-pervasive as to be unnoticed and yet that make the world intelligible for us create our possibilities and the conditions for our actions. In the phenomenological view, then, persons can never perceive "brute facts" out there in the world. Nothing can be encountered independent of our background understanding. Every encounter is an interpretation based on our background. "What appears from the 'object' is what one allows to appear and what the thematization of the world at work in his understanding will bring to light" (Palmer, 1969, p. 136).

The Person as Embodied

The phenomenological notion of person includes a view of the body that is fundamentally different from the Cartesian notion of the body as object of possession. The Cartesian body is mere *res extensa,* "a machine driven by mechanical causality . . . extrinsic to the essential self" (Leder, 1984, p. 30), exhibiting no intelligence or power to respond to the world. In the phenomenological view, rather than *having* a body we *are* embodied. It is assumed that our common practices are based on shared embodied perceptual capacities (Benner, 1985). Our bodies provide the possibility for the concrete action of self in the world. It is the body that first grasps the world and moves with intention in that meaningful world. Merleau-Ponty (1962) calls this bodily intelligence. "Viewed as intentional, bodily functioning can express affective, cognitional influences in a way perhaps inexplicable within the Cartesian model" (Leder, 1984, p. 38). Those researchers and clinicians who have an implicit understanding of the intentional body but frame their research and clinical problems from a Cartesian body position find themselves articulating multicausal notions of disease but are incapable of ever satisfactorily explaining the Cartesian mind-body problem: how the physical and mental relate. "The paradigm of the lived-body, wherein subjectivity is always corporeally expressed, avoids these problems" (Leder, 1984, p. 39).

Baron (1985) points out that health is the state of "unselfconscious being that illness shatters" (p. 609). Our everyday lived experience in which the embodied self is taken for granted breaks down in illness. Our ready-to-hand understanding of ourselves as embodied doesn't work for us anymore. Thus it is in this state of "breakdown" that we develop insight into the taken-for-granted understanding of health: the unity of self and healthy body. "That the body is not a mere extrinsic machine but our living center from which radiates all existential possibilities is brought home with a vengeance in illness, suffering, and disability" (Leder, 1984, p. 34). This position affords the clinician a new position from which to understand the patient's experience of illness. Rather than viewing the problem as one of breakdown in an objective machine, one approaches illness as a rupture in the patient's ability to negotiate the world. It is one's embodiment that is the problem, not one's objective machine body (Baron, 1985).

This author would argue that Baron's position pertains even more accurately to nursing than to medicine. It is nursing, more than medicine, that seeks to help the patient reclaim that sense of embodiment that allows for their taken-for-granted, unselfconscious transactions with the world.

The Person in Time

Finally, the Heideggerian phenomenological notion of person includes a view of person or being-in-time that differs radically from more traditional Western notions of time. Our traditional view of linear time is of an endless succession of nows: "the common conception thinks of the nows as free-floating, relationless, intrinsically patched on to one another and intrinsically successive" (Heidegger, 1975, p. 263). This "snapshot" view of time presents us with the problem of conceiving continuity or transition. It also leads, in the scientific research tradition, to a system of formal laws that are supposed to be atemporal. It gives us a notion of things existing as static, atemporal entities. For example, Sandel's (1982) self of possession *has* traits that may come and go but that do not fundamentally alter the self. Temporality, in this view, is the accrual of events: that is, I "had" anxiety, but then X occurred, and I no longer "had" anxiety. The "I" doesn't change, in this view, in the sense of having been constituted by anxiety, because it merely "had" the anxiety. In this view, time is not a constituent of human events.

In the Heideggerian phenomenological view, temporality is *constitutive* of being. For instance, Heidegger describes the past as "having-been-ness":

> The Dasein can as little get rid of its bygoneness as escape its death. In every sense and in every case everything we have been is an essential determination

of our existence. Even if in some way, by some manipulation, I may be able to keep my bygoneness far from myself, nevertheless, forgetting, repressing, suppressing are modes in which I myself am my own having-been-ness. (1975, p. 265)

Temporality is thus the term Heidegger uses to describe a notion of time that is prior to or more original than our common sense of time as a linear succession of nows. Linear time creates the problem of relating past and future to the now, but temporality, according to Heidegger, is directional and relational and applies only to being, not to physical objects. "The not-yet and no longer are not patched onto the now as foreign but belong to its very content. Because of this *dimensional content*, the *now* has within itself the *character of a transition*" (Heidegger, 1975, p. 249). Rather than being empty, something (like space) to be filled up, time is "*essentially* content: it *exists as* activity, such as concernful dealing and attention" (Faulconer & Williams, 1985, p. 1184). Thus, the Cartesian self of possession is not constituted by time, and traits or attributes can be studied without considering their order or meaning in relation to each other; they are context-free elements. Being-in-time, on the other hand, cannot be studied except within the context of its having-been-ness and being-expectant, its past and future, by which it is constituted. To return to the example of anxiety in pregnancy, the older pregnant woman with career commitments has a having-been-ness that includes, perhaps, insisting on doing things with great precision and care. Her having-been-ness has also included much rumination on whether an infant can be left in the care of a nonparent while the parents both return to work full time. Her being-expectant includes an awareness that her company expects her to return to work full time as an equally functioning member of the "team." Her anxiety in pregnancy, then, can be seen as being constituted by her past and future.

Related to Heidegger's notion of temporality is his account of the essential structure of human being that he describes as care: "Earlier than any presupposition which Dasein makes, or any of its ways of behaving, is the '*a priori*' character of its state of being as one whose kind of Being is care" (1927/1962, p. 249). Care, in Heidegger's sense, is having our being be an issue for us. We exist existentially in terms of the things that we care about, the for-the-sake-of-which. Temporally, the not-yet belongs to the now because we exist in terms of what matters to us. A further structure of being is Heidegger's notion of *thrownness*: we always already find ourselves in a particular nexus of cultural, familial, and situational practices and meanings and out of this thrownness we have to take a stand on ourselves (the structure of care).

Having outlined the essential aspects of a Heideggerian phenomenological view of person, I now turn to the implications of this view for research.

Hermeneutics as a Method Appropriate to the Heideggerian Phenomenological Study of Human Beings

A being who exists only in self-interpretation cannot be understood absolutely; and one who can only be understood against the background of distinctions of worth cannot be captured by a scientific language that essentially aspires to neutrality. Our personhood cannot be treated scientifically in exactly the same way we approach our organic being. What it is to possess a liver or heart is something I can define quite independently of the space of questions in which I exist for myself, but not what it is to have a self or be a person. (Taylor, 1985a, pp. 3-4)

Appreciating the implications for research of a phenomenological view of person involves going beyond the qualitative-quantitative, objectivism-relativism debate. It involves a fundamental shift in orientation away from traditional notions of objectivity as unitizing and generalizing, with the goal of prediction and control. This notion of objectivity strips human actions of their context and assumes the possibility of an Archimedean point from which a foundational knowledge can be discovered based on "judgments which could be anchored in a certainty beyond subjective intuition" (Taylor, 1987, p. 37). Heideggerian phenomenologists, on the other hand, propose that there is no Archimedean point, no privileged position for "objective" knowing and that all knowledge emanates from persons who are already in the world, seeking to understand persons who are also already in the world. One is always within the hermeneutical circle of interpretation. Researcher and research participant are viewed as sharing common practices, skills, interpretations, and everyday practical understanding by virtue of their common culture and language. Also, because human beings are constituted by temporality, all knowledge, in this view, is temporal. Atemporal, ahistorical transcendent knowledge of human behavior is impossible. "The human sciences, because they are engaged in temporal investigation, are not designed to arrive at an atemporal causal certainty. Instead, their investigations have as their object the rendering of life and the world continually understandable" (Faulconer & Williams, 1985, p. 1186). Further, because persons are fundamentally self-interpreting beings for whom things have significance, understanding human action always involves an interpretation, by the researcher, of the interpretations being made by those persons being studied. This interpretive approach is called *hermeneutics*.

Hermeneutics is an ancient discipline that can be traced back to the early Greeks. Early Greek root words of *hermeneutics* suggest the idea of bringing to understanding, particularly where this process involves language. That is, something foreign, strange, or separated in time, space, or experience is revealed so as to seem familiar and comprehensible (Palmer, 1969, p. 13).

In modern times, hermeneutics has had two separate foci. The first is the rules, methods, or theory governing exegesis of linguistic texts. Biblical exegesis is the most well-known example and dates from the 17th century. Legal discourse and literary criticism also draw on hermeneutics. The second focus of hermeneutics has been the philosophical exploration of the character and requisite conditions for understanding. In the early 19th century, Schleiermacher redefined hermeneutics as the study of understanding itself. He was followed by Dilthey, who saw hermeneutics as the core discipline or foundation for all the humanities and social sciences (i.e., those disciplines that interpret expressions of the inner life of human beings) (Palmer, 1969).

In the early 20th century, Heidegger's analysis of being suggested that interpretation is a foundational mode of man's being. *Being and Time* (1927/1962) is referred to as "a hermeneutic of *Dasein*," an interpretive effort through which light is shed on the meaning of being. Thus the relevance of hermeneutics to the human sciences today derives primarily from Heidegger's writings. Currently, the hermeneutic approach is being taken up by researchers in diverse human science fields, including nursing, who are concerned with understanding human beings.

The goal of a hermeneutic, or interpretive, account is to understand everyday skills, practices, and experiences; to find commonalities in meanings, skills, practices, and embodied experiences; and "to find exemplars or paradigm cases that embody the meanings of everyday practices . . . in such a way that they are not destroyed, distorted, decontextualized, trivialized, or sentimentalized" (Benner, 1985, pp. 5-6). Paradigm cases and exemplars are strong instances of a particular pattern of meanings; they are effective strategies for depicting the person in the situation and for preserving meanings and context. The access to everyday lived experience opens up a new understanding of the person and the possibility for overcoming the subject-object split of Cartesianism.

Further, rather than looking for deterministic or mechanistic notions of causality, hermeneutics seeks to develop explanations and understanding that are based on concerns, commitments, practices, and meanings. This understanding is such that it "will focus on sufficient conditions and make statements such as, all other things being equal, one expects such and such to occur. Such a statement leaves room for transformations in meanings and changes in human concerns" (Benner, 1985, p. 3).

Hermeneutics as an approach makes several assumptions based on the Heideggerian phenomenological view of person. First, it is assumed, based on common background meanings given in our culture and language, that the researcher has a preliminary understanding of the human action being studied. It is by virtue of our world that we, as researchers, have the questions we have, and that we see the possibilities we see. Thus we approach our interpretive project with some preunderstanding, or, as Heidegger called it, a forestructure of understanding, into which by virtue of the structure of being (care), we are thrust or projected. This forestructure has three aspects. We are first of all given a taken-for-granted sense of "the totality of relations that *constitutes* the phenomena" (Packer & Richardson, 1991, pp. 343-344) under investigation: the *fore-having*. Next, we approach our research question with a point of view, from the perspective of a particular interpretive lens (the *fore-sight*) that orients us globally toward the phenomena in a particular way and is therefore critically important to the study. This is what is meant by entering the hermeneutic circle "in the right way" (Dreyfus, 1991, p. 201). This conceptual orientation to the phenomena functions as a vehicle for gaining access to the phenomena and is open to revision as the analysis proceeds and new meanings and understandings are revealed by the study. The final aspect of the forestructure is the *fore-conception:* there is always a preliminary sense of what counts as a question and what would count as an answer.

The interpretive process is necessarily circular, moving back and forth between part and whole, and between the initial forestructure and what is being revealed in the data of the inquiry. There is the constant mandate to go beyond existing, available, publicly authorized interpretations of things, to follow a more authentic and deeper analysis that is projected in the possibilities available to the project through the forestructure. This demands a deep and enduring commitment (and existential presence) on the part of the researcher to stay true to the text and to honor the lived experience of the research participants. Through systematic analysis of the whole, we gain new perspective and depth of understanding. We use this understanding to examine the *parts* of the whole, and then we reexamine the whole in light of the insight we have gained from the parts. The interpretive process follows this part-whole strategy until the researcher is satisfied with the depth of his or her understanding. Thus the interpretive process has no clear termination.

Another assumption made in hermeneutics is that there is no Archimedean point from which one can have a "privileged," foundational view of the world that is atemporal and ahistorical. The researcher has a world and exists in historical time just as the subject does. In order to have an "objectively valid" interpretation, one would have to understand from a position outside of history, which is impossible, given the phenomenological view. Objectivity, then, is no longer a process of decontextualization, of securing abstract, eternal truths that correspond to "things as they are," but rather of finding what can show up in agreement in our local cultural clearings (Benner, 1985). Skills, practices, and meanings are "objective" in the sense of being shared and therefore verifiable with both research participants and colleagues. They are not objective in the sense of being ahistorical, atemporal, or acontextual, or of corresponding to things as they really are. Taylor (1985a, p. 7) argues that plausibility is the ultimate criterion for any hermeneutic explanation.

It should be emphasized, however, that although individuals may take up common background meanings in a personal way, these personal meanings are not infinitely variable or completely relative. They are bounded by the cultural and linguistic meanings that we all share. Thus, although I may aspire to be a hero in labor and delivery, it is not within my background meanings to go off and deliver alone, unattended. My options for giving birth are narrowed by my Western cultural tradition and by my own history. Within that bounded set of meanings I find my possibilities for being a hero. And because the background meanings that create those possibilities for me are commonly shared, consensual validation of a hermeneutic interpretation of my heroic behavior is possible. Private, idiosyncratic meanings are not the data of hermeneutic inquiry.

In hermeneutics, the role of theory is to show up meanings that arise out of the lived experience, to create new possibilities for understanding, and, as van Manen (1990) suggests, to have a more tactful and thoughtful practical engagement with the phenomenon under investigation. Phenomenology mandates a new account of what constitutes adequate theory. No formal theoretical assumptions or predictions are made. Formal theory (in the sense of having formal propositions, causal mechanisms, and structures) is not to be used as a grid or screen through which all data are filtered. Nor is the goal of research to be the development of formal theory defined as propositional statements that seek to outline in a predictive way the law-like relationships of atomistic elements in a static structure. The theory that results from hermeneutics involves the presentations of revealed, or "unfolded" (Caputo, 1987, p. 81) meanings, skills, and practices, the practical knowledge that is so hidden from traditional empirical research.

Data Collection in a Hermeneutic Inquiry

In hermeneutics, the primary source of knowledge is everyday practical activity. Human behavior becomes a text analogue that is studied and interpreted in order to discover the hidden or obscured meaning. This meaning is hidden because it is so pervasive and taken for granted that it goes unnoticed. The data for the text analogues can come from interviews, participant observation, diaries, and samples of human behavior (Benner,

1985). Because our everyday lived experience is so taken for granted as to   ✳·
go unnoticed, it is often through breakdown that the researcher achieves
flashes of insight into the lived world, although it is important to note that
the taken-for-granted, everyday lived world can never be made completely
explicit.

Interpretive Analysis

Transcribed interviews, observational notes, diaries, and samples of human action are treated as text analogues for interpretive analysis. The data
analysis in a hermeneutic study is carried out in three interrelated processes:
thematic analysis, analysis of exemplars, and the search for paradigm cases.

In the thematic analysis, each case (all interviews, field notes, etc.) is read
several times in order to arrive at a global analysis. When several cases have
been read in this way, lines of inquiry are then identified from the
theoretical background that grounds the study and from themes consistently emerging in the data. From this, an interpretive plan emerges. Each
interview is then read from the perspective of the interpretive plan. As this
microanalysis is carried out, additional lines of inquiry may emerge from the
data and are added to the interpretive plan. All whole cases are then subjected
to the additional interpretive analysis. The interpretive effort culminates in
the identification of general categories that form the basis of the study's
findings.

The second aspect of the interpretive process involves the analysis of
specific episodes or incidents: all aspects of a particular situation and the
participant's responses to it are analyzed together. The analyzed event
encompasses the individual's situation—her concerns, actions, and practices—and not her opinions, analyses, or ideology. From this analysis come
"exemplars": stories or vignettes that capture the meaning in a situation in
such a way that the meaning can then be recognized in another situation that
might have very different objective circumstances. An exemplar is "a strong
instance of a particularly meaningful transaction, intention, or capacity"
(Benner, 1985, p. 10).

The last aspect of the interpretive analysis involves the identification of
paradigm cases: strong instances of particular patterns of meaning. Paradigm
cases embody the rich descriptive information necessary for understanding
how an individual's actions and understandings emerge from his or her
situational context: their concerns, practices and background meanings.
They are not reducible to formal theory—to abstract variables used to predict
and control. Rather, what are recognized are "family resemblances" between
a paradigm case and a particular clinical situation that one is trying to
understand and explain (Chesla, 1988, p. 53).

> All three interpretive strategies . . . work both as discovery and presentation
> strategies. They all allow for the presentation of context and meanings. In in-
> terpretive research, unlike in grounded theory, the goal is not to extract theo-
> retical terms or concepts at a higher level of abstraction. The goal is to
> discover meaning and to achieve understanding. (Benner, 1985, p. 10)

The presentation of a study's findings involves distilling the data down to
their most essential terms while still providing the reader with enough
evidence for the reader to participate in the validation of the findings
(Benner, 1985).

Evaluation of an Interpretive Account

The fundamental point to be grasped in evaluating interpretive accounts
is that there is no such thing as an interpretation-free, objectively "true"
account of "things in themselves" (the traditional positivist definition of the
correspondence theory of truth), and that there is no technical procedure for
"validating" that an account corresponds to this timeless, objective "truth."
Although it is beyond the scope of this paper to critique the correspondence
theory of truth as it is applied in the natural sciences, I think it can be reliably
claimed that even there the idea of a timeless, interpretation-free account has
been discredited. Although technical procedures for "validating" interpretive
accounts are impossible, there remain effective tools for evaluation. As
Packer and Addison (1989) suggest, what must be made explicit is the *type* of
evaluation these tools provide. Criteria such as coherence, consistency, and
plausibility do not help us to determine the degree of correspondence between an account and the way things "really are." Rather, they help us to
determine how well an account serves to answer the original concern or
breakdown that initiated the line of inquiry leading to the research in the first
place. Interpretive inquiry always begins from practical, concernful engagement. Interpretive inquiry never seeks to simply describe a phenomenon but
is always concerned with some kind of breakdown in human affairs. Thus
the ultimate criterion for evaluating the adequacy of an interpretive account
is the degree to which it resolves the breakdown and opens up new possibilities for engaging the problem. For instance, in the example of the clinician
working with pregnant women, a study undertaken on the effects of anxiety
on pregnancy outcomes would be evaluated by how effectively the clinician
was able to refocus her care of these patients in the service of mitigating
anxiety, based on her new understanding of anxiety as revealed by the study.
What does the account make available to the clinician that did not exist
before except as concealed and baffling? What kind of new access do the
study's findings give her to the clinical phenomenon of anxiety in pregnant

women? Do the findings increase her thoughtfulness and ethical comportment in her practice and, by extension, the range of alternative ways of coping available to pregnant women themselves?

Disputes in hermeneutic interpretation resolve based on the plausibility of alternative interpretations, and the plausibility of an interpretation, cannot be reduced to a-priori-derived, cut-and-dried criteria. As Bernstein (1986) recently commented, "a fundamental ontological motif of modernity has been variations on the theme of fundamental indeterminism. Our being-in-the-world is fundamentally indeterminate. Wisdom requires learning to live with this." Thus although we must live with a plurality of interpretations of meaning, we can narrow things down. And, importantly, living with a plurality of meanings, or indeterminacy, doesn't mean we don't understand each other. It is a tenet of this kind of research that there can always be another, deeper and perhaps more persuasive, interpretation of a phenomenon. The forestructure of the study may be quite different from one study to the next and will therefore produce quite different accounts of the same phenomenon. Competing accounts do not negate each other. Rather, they set up a conversation. This decreased emphasis on one true account of a phenomenon has a further effect beyond the scope of an individual research project: it encourages the creative exchange of perspectives and ideas in human science research.

Certainly, interpretive researchers agree that there are better and worse interpretive studies. A study can be judged by how carefully the question is framed and the initial interpretive stance laid out, how carefully the data collection is accomplished and documented, and how rigorously the interpretive effort goes beyond publicly available understandings of a problem to reveal new and deeper possibilities for understanding.

In summary, Heideggerian phenomenology offers a view of person that is profoundly different from more traditional Cartesian notions of person. It is a view that has much to offer to nurses who are, in their practice, fundamentally concerned with the lived experiences of health and illness. Hermeneutics is a method that assumes the philosophical tenets of Heideggerian phenomenology. It offers nurse researchers the opportunity for understanding the meaningfully rich and complex lived world of those human beings for whom nurses care.

Note

1. *Dasein* is the term Heidegger uses to designate "the being to whose being an understanding of beings belongs"(1975, p. 312). In discussing what it is to *be*, Heidegger uses *Dasein* to reflect the type of beings we are a priori to the reflective, conscious ego of the

Cartesian tradition. "In German the word 'Dasein' means simply 'existence', as in man's everyday existence. But it also means, if you take it apart, 'being-there.' This conveys that this activity of human beings is an activity of being in the situation in which coping can go on and things can be encountered" (Dreyfus, 1987, p. 263).

References

Baron, R. (1985). An introduction to medical phenomenology: I can't hear you while I'm listening. *Annals of Internal Medicine, 163,* 606-611.

Benner, P. (1985). Quality of life: A phenomenological perspective on explanation, prediction and understanding in nursing science. *Advances in Nursing Science, 8*(1), 1-14.

Bernstein, R. (1986, May). Interpretation and its discontents. *Proceedings of Approaches to Interpretation Conference.* Hayward: California State University.

Borgman, A. (1984). *Technology and the character of contemporary life.* Chicago: University of Chicago Press.

Caputo, J. (1987). *Radical hermeneutics: Repetition, deconstruction and the hermeneutic project.* Bloomington, IN: Indiana University Press.

Caudill, W., & Weinstein, H. (1969). Maternal care and infant behavior in Japan and America. *Psychiatry, 32,* 12-43.

Chesla, C. (1988). *Parents' caring practices and coping with schizophrenic offspring: An interpretive study.* Unpublished doctoral dissertation, University of California, San Francisco.

Dreyfus, H. (1987). Husserl, Heidegger and modern existentialism. In B. Magee (Ed.), *The great philosophers: An introduction to Western philosophy* (pp. 254-277). London: BBC Books.

Dreyfus, H. (1991). *Being-in-the-world: A commentary on Heidegger's "Being and time," Division I.* Cambridge: MIT Press.

Faulconer, J., & Williams, R. (1985). Temporality in human action. *American Psychologist, 40*(11), 1179-1188.

Guignon, C. (1983). *Heidegger and the problem of knowledge.* Indianapolis: Hackett.

Heidegger, M. (1962). *Being and time* (J. Macquarrie & E. Robinson, Trans.). New York: Harper & Row. (Original work published 1927)

Heidegger, M. (1975). *The basic problems of phenomenology (A. Hofstadter, Trans.).* Bloomington: Indiana University Press.

Hoy, D. (1986, May). *Proceedings of Approaches to Interpretation Conference.* California State University, Hayward.

Laudan, L. (1977). *Progress and its problems: Towards a theory of scientific growth.* London: Routledge & Kegan Paul.

Leder, D. (1984). Medicine and paradigms of embodiment. *Journal of Medicine and Philosophy, 9,* 29-43.

Merleau-Ponty, M. (1962). *Phenomenology of perception* (C. Smith, Trans.). London: Routledge & Kegan Paul.

Packer, M., & Addison, R. (1989). Evaluating an interpretive account. In M. Packer & R. Addison (Eds.), *Entering the circle: Hermeneutic investigation in psychology* (pp. 275-292). Albany: State University of New York Press.

Packer, M., & Richardson, E. (1991). Analytic hermeneutics and the study of morality in action. In W. Kurtines & J. Gewirtz (Eds.), *Handbook of moral behavior and development: Theory, research, and application* (pp. 335-371). Hillsdale, NJ: Lawrence Erlbaum.

Palmer, R. (1969). *Hermeneutics.* Evanston, IL: Northwestern University Press.

Ricoeur, P. (1986, May). Self-identity and the interpretation of narrative. *Proceedings of Approaches to Interpretation Conference.* California State University, Hayward.

Sandel, M. (1982). *Liberalism and the limits of justice.* Cambridge, UK: Cambridge University Press.

Taylor, C. (1985a). *Human agency and language: Philosophical papers* (Vol. 1). Cambridge, UK: Cambridge University Press.

Taylor, C. (1985b). *Philosophy and the human sciences: Philosophical papers* (Vol. 2). Cambridge, UK: Cambridge University Press.

Taylor, C. (1987). Interpretation and the sciences of man. In P. Rabinow & W. Sullivan (Eds.), *Interpretive social science: A second look* (pp. 33-81). Berkeley: University of California Press.

Taylor, C. (1991). *The ethics of authenticity.* Cambridge, MA: Harvard University Press.

van Manen, M. (1990). *Researching lived experience: Human science for an action sensitive pedagogy.* Ontario, Canada: Althouse.

4

❖

Hermeneutic Phenomenology

A Methodology for Family Health and Health Promotion Study in Nursing

KAREN A. PLAGER

The question asked and the self-understanding held are crucial issues in how a research project is approached. This was essentially the claim made by Martin Heidegger when he set out on his philosophical investigation of the "question of the meaning of Being" (Heidegger, 1927/1962, p. 1). He proposed to ask the question anew because philosophers from the ancient Greeks to Descartes and Kant and up to the 20th-century philosophers, such as Husserl, trivialized the question by removing it from its temporal and historical context to a pure presentness, that is, as an independent, objective entity with absolute properties. In *Being and Time*, Heidegger developed hermeneutic phenomenology as a philosophical methodology to uncover the meaning of being of human beings, the significance of which he claimed had been covered over by past philosophical approaches that were reductionistic and objectifying. Further, he claimed that we are so culturally and socially embedded in familiarity with our practices and skills that we lose sight of our being from existing within this familiarity (Dreyfus, 1991; Heidegger, 1927/1962).

For Heidegger, hermeneutic phenomenology provided a philosophical investigation to interpret the being of human beings; to determine the conditions for the possibility of ontological investigations, that is, to uncover the phenomena for investigation; and to provide an analysis for the structures of existence. It was a method, he contended, that would accomplish what traditional (e.g., empirical and rational) philosophical approaches had missed (Heidegger, 1927/1962). Heidegger's philosophical investigation using hermeneutic phenomenology also opens up a fourth methodological possibility: it provides nursing with a theoretical basis for conducting research projects that does not reduce issues of human beings' concerns to mere characteristics, absolute properties, or brute data (Taylor, 1987). The hermeneutic methodology fills gaps in understanding that are often left by empirical science research approaches when these are used in nursing. This chapter explicates hermeneutic phenomenology as a methodology for nursing to study health and health promotion in families.

As nursing is increasingly involved in the delivery of primary health care for families and their individual members, it needs to ask critical questions about the delivery of health promotion care. For instance, what are the circumstances in success or failure of health promotion interventions? How congruent is delivery of health promotion care with families' understanding of health and their health activities and practices? Health beliefs, attitudes, values, activities, and practices are learned largely in early life in the context of family, and family continues to be a major influence on health throughout life. Yet nursing studies have scarcely addressed this aspect of health promotion. This chapter suggests that an interpretive methodology may be the best means of accessing and beginning to uncover an understanding of health and health activities and practices in families, and of the implications this may have for primary health care delivery of health promotion care.

The Questions

Two general questions are proposed to guide a hermeneutic inquiry into family health and health promotion:

1. What is the family's perspective on the significance of health and well-being of their family and its members?
2. What are the situated possibilities, health and caring activities and practices, and lived experiential meanings that constitute and are constitutive of the family's perspective on its health and well-being?

These questions will form the basis for the discussion that follows.

In support of hermeneutic phenomenology as a significant method for these questions, several basic assumptions of the Cartesian mode of inquiry as they are used in the natural science model and applied to family health and health promotion research are critiqued. In addition some of Heidegger's philosophical underpinnings and several assumptions of the methodology are laid out. These are followed by a discussion of some basic philosophical and methodological issues of hermeneutic phenomenology.

What Existing Research Does

The vast majority of the research on health and health promotion in the family and in nurse practitioner practice characterizes health and health promotion and providers and receivers of care by sets of dimensions, correlates, concepts, and independent and dependent variables that are or can be fitted into models and theories of health and health promotion. These also might be reduced to numbers expressed as descriptive and inferential statistics. These approaches remove subjects from the context of the situation and attempt to characterize them by a set of objective properties. The meaning of the person's or family's life world, their lived experience, their situatedness, their concerns, and what matters to them are left out of the picture. These contextual issues constitute significance in families' lives and in how they participate in health care situations.

It is no surprise that the majority of existing family health research studies are conducted in this decontextualizing framework. Like the world we live in, research is deeply entrenched in a world view, a heritage in our Western culture that is embedded in our practices and skills and has been articulated by a long line of philosophers (Heidegger, 1977). Part of this heritage is expressed in the Cartesian model of inquiry on which most of modern science and research is based. It is this model that Heidegger criticizes in *Being and Time*. The model has two basic assumptions that Guignon (1983) summarizes in his analysis and critique of Heidegger's philosophical writings. The first is the Cartesian mind-body dualism, according to which we picture "ourselves as subjects distinct from a world of objects about which we come to have beliefs" (p. 30). The second assumption is that entities can be broken down into "discrete, isolable units" (unitized) and generalized "to find regular, orderly relations among the units . . . in order to show how they are combined into the organized whole of nature" (p. 35). The presupposition of the Cartesian method of abstraction and generalization is "that we will be able to decontextualize entities from their places in specific situations in order to grasp them as interchangeable bits that can occur in a wide variety of law-governed situations" (Guignon, 1983, p. 37). This is the heritage referred to when Taylor (1985) writes about the appeal of the natural science model. It is in our background practices, he states, that we are "capable of achieving a kind of disengagement from our world by objectifying it" (p. 4). Similarly, Kirmayer (1988) writes that the mind-body dualism is so much a part of what it is to be human beings in our culture that it is totalizing of our practices even in the practice of health care (Kirmayer specifically refers to Western medicine, but the case can be applied to all of Western health care). Further, Gordon (1988) elaborates on the assumptions in biomedicine that are so tenacious because of this very social embeddedness, the "embodiment in practices, which thus entails ways of being and not just explicit beliefs" (p. 23).

This brief look at the Cartesian model that has long been in use in the natural sciences and has been the standard for much of the human sciences suggests the difficulties in giving up the model even in nursing health promotion and family health research. It is deeply embedded in our practices as a way of being in the world of academe and research and indeed in Western society in general. Yet to continue solely within the Cartesian mode of inquiry holds dangers for nursing research on health promotion, family health, and family primary care practice and for implications and applications of research in practice. It leaves out the contexts of the family's narrative, which holds significant meanings for the family regarding health, health practices, and how health-related activities come about in the family (Stein, 1989). The person's or family's narrative can fill in many gaps in understanding that our traditional empirical science mode of inquiry leaves out. Oliver Sacks (1970) related this poignantly when telling a story of a young woman, Rebecca, who was born with many physical and neurological defects:

> Our tests, our approaches, I thought, as I watched her on the bench—enjoying not just a simple but a sacred view of nature— . . . are ridiculously inadequate. They only show us deficits, they do not show us powers, they only show us puzzles and schemata, when we need to see music, narrative, play, a being conducting itself [sic] spontaneously in its own natural way. Rebecca, I felt, was complete and intact as "narrative" being, in conditions that allowed her to organize herself in a narrative way; and this was something very important to know, for it allowed one to see her, and her potential, in a quite different fashion from that imposed by the schematic mode. (pp. 181-182)

Taking a look at self-understanding as laid out by Martin Heidegger in *Being and Time* helps us understand how we can become so embedded in one way of understanding the world. It also puts forth a very different vantage point from which to pursue family health studies in nursing.

Heidegger's Phenomenological Perspective

In laying out his philosophy, Heidegger (1927/1962) dealt extensively with the situatedness of human being-in-the-world. It is a world of shared background practices and familiarity. We get all of our possibilities and potentialities from this shared background. Our skills and practices are acquired from being-in-the-world of our cultures and societies. The intelligibility of how we use things (equipment) and relate to others in the world is all part of our understanding of being in our world of shared background practices and familiarity. It is because of this shared understanding that we are able to be involved with things, relations, and situations in our world, to cope smoothly and skillfully in our everyday life, and to take a stand on what it is to be human beings in our world. As human beings we are engaged and involved in the world in a concernful way with practical activities (Benner & Wrubel, 1989; Dreyfus, 1991).

This shared background familiarity that discloses our shared world and makes it possible for us to have shared and individual interpretations of our world Heidegger called "the clearing": "To say that [human being] is 'illuminated' means that as being-in-the-world it is cleared in itself . . . in such a way it is itself the clearing" (Heidegger, 1927/1962, p. 171).

World-disclosing, or the clearing, was the one basic idea throughout Heidegger's philosophy that he never changed. His perspective on the clearing, however, changed through his career and is important to note in this discussion of hermeneutic phenomenology. In *Being and Time*, he described the general clearing that is acultural and ahistorical (i.e., not specific to a particular culture or historical period), that makes it possible for our general understanding of what it means to be human beings and therefore allows us to interpret our human activities. In later philosophical work, Heidegger explicated the clearing as it pertains to Western civilization and has evolved throughout its history. This is a cultural and historical understanding of being.

In his later works, Heidegger (1971) discussed focal, local clearings that are specific for individuals or groups (such as families or friends). These focal, local clearings are special events, practices, or things in our lives that may gather special significance for us from time to time. For example, a clearing might occur on special occasions when a family gets together (such as a celebratory feast), or when I am riding my bicycle along a country road.

The main point in this brief explanation of Heidegger's work on local clearings is that a person or a group may have an individual clearing but that clearing is an interpretation or understanding that is possible only because of our shared background understanding. That is, we are not atomistic, monological beings (or even families) disengaged from others in our practices but dialogical beings engaged in our world through a shared, community understanding that is for the most part unarticulated (Taylor, 1991).

There is another important distinction to make about our understanding of being. We have understanding because we are always already in the familiarity of our cultures and societies. We grow up in this familiarity. Understanding makes it possible to uncover things in our world, that is, it discloses the world. Living in an already meaningful world allows us to make sense of what we are doing, makes it possible to do the activities we are doing, and allows possibilities for activities we have not yet done. The other side of this familiarity is that we may lose sight of the understanding that is in our everyday activity. Certain aspects get covered over just because of their taken-for-granted nature. For example, health and what constitutes it in the life of families and their members often goes unnoticed until illness or some disorganizing event occurs to bring the meaning of health to the forefront for them. What is of concern in hermeneutic phenomenology is this practical engaged activity of our everyday lives and the description and interpretation of what gets disclosed and what might have got covered over in the process of our being-in-the-world.

To summarize according to Dreyfus (1984), Heidegger maintains three theses throughout his career that are crucial to his philosophical stance and to hermeneutic phenomenology as research methodology:

1. Human being is a self-interpreting activity. This is the hermeneutic relation.
2. This activity involves an understanding of what being means, and it is this understanding that opens a clearing [for human beings' encounters]. All members of society share a preontological understanding of this interpretation.
3. Everyday practices and everyday awareness take place inside this clearing that governs what everyday human activity takes for granted. These practices embody specific cultural ways . . . all of which adds up to an understanding of what counts as real for us. (p. 73)

The idea of the clearing is central to each of these three theses.

Assumptions and Basic Philosophical Issues
of Hermeneutic Phenomenology

The preceding discussion of Heidegger's philosophy lets us now put forth several assumptions of hermeneutic phenomenology. These assumptions, it will be noted, differ greatly from the disengaged, monological, subject-object stance of the Cartesian assumptions that were looked at earlier.

Assumptions

1. Human beings are social, dialogical beings.
2. Understanding is always before us in the shared background practices; it is in the human community of societies and cultures, in the language, in our skills and activities, and in our intersubjective and common meanings.
3. We are always already in a hermeneutic circle of understanding.
4. Interpretation presupposes a shared understanding and therefore has a three-fold forestructure of understanding.
5. Interpretation involves the interpreter and the interpreted in a dialogical relationship. (Heidegger, 1927/1962; Taylor, 1987, 1991; Ten Have & Kimsma, 1990)

Basic Issues: Forestructure of Understanding, Interpretation, the Hermeneutic Circle, and Modes of Involvement

These assumptions allow us to examine more specifically several basic issues that Heidegger addresses in *Being and Time* and that are essential aspects for hermeneutic phenomenology as a methodology. These include the forestructure of understanding, the relationship of interpretation and understanding, and the hermeneutic circle. A fourth issue is the modes of involvement that humans have in different situations. These modes are important for two reasons: (a) they situate our involvement in an interpretive study, and (b) they situate the participants of a study in their engagement in everyday activities and in their self-interpretations. This will be clarified shortly.

The shared public world of background familiarity that makes life intelligible for human beings was previously discussed. Only because of this understanding that is always before us is interpretation possible. Heidegger (1927/1962) spelled this out when he wrote: "This thing in question already has an involvement that is disclosed in our understanding of the world, and this involvement is one that gets laid out by the interpretation" (p. 191). Heidegger explicates, as "the essential foundations for everyday circumspective interpretation" (p. 191), a threefold forestructure of understanding upon which all interpretation is grounded. It consists of:

1. A *fore-having*: we come to a situation with a practical familiarity, that is, with background practices from our world that make an interpretation possible.
2. A *fore-sight*: because of our background we have a point of view from which we make an interpretation.
3. A *fore-conception*: because of our background we have some expectations of what we might anticipate in an interpretation.

The forestructure links understanding with interpretation. Heidegger (1927/1962) calls it "that which [is] taken for granted" (p. 192). We all have everyday circumspective interpretations, as in transparent coping in day-to-day life, in which the taken for granted remains in the background. This is true for the investigator and participant alike. However, in interpretation as a method of inquiry, two senses of the forestructure need to be brought forward more explicitly. First, as part of the credibility of the project, the investigator lays out preconceptions, biases, past experiences, and perhaps even hypotheses that make the project significant for the investigator and that may affect how the interpretation takes shape. Second, the investigator may bring forth the forestructure of understanding for the study participants. This may be part of the narrative that the investigator elicits in the study in order to make sense of the participants' situation.

Human beings as circular beings are always in the world in a way that presupposes understanding. Our world is always already meaningful and intelligible, and our activities are constituted by and make sense in the world. We are in what Heidegger (1927/1962) calls the "circle in understanding" (p. 195). In the circle we understand and *interpret something as something* because we have this background of shared human practices. Understanding allows us to be involved in our daily activities as meaningful events, that is, we are *involved with something as something*. Interpretation is a derivative of understanding and allows us to bring out something as something; thus it enriches our understanding by "the working out of possibilities projected in understanding" (Dreyfus, 1991, p. 195; Heidegger, 1927/1962, p. 189). Being in the circle is not a matter of choice, for without understanding meaning would crumble. Without the familiarity of the shared background of our world, all would be rendered meaningless and unintelligible. All of our possibilities and potentialities in our various life situations are possible because of personal and cultural history (Packer & Addison, 1989). And so it is that all of human life, including research, takes place within this ontological circle.

Heidegger (1927/1962) described three interrelated modes of involvement or engagement with equipment or practical activity that we have in day-to-day life. He referred to these as *ready-to-hand, unready-to-hand,* and *pre-*

sent-to-hand. Within these modes are also situated the research activities of the natural and human sciences.

In the *ready-to-hand* mode of engagement, equipment and practical activities function smoothly and transparently. The person is involved in an absorbed manner so that the equipment is for the most part unnoticed. For example, when a family is healthy and life is going along well, smooth relating in the family occurs in a spontaneous and transparent fashion. This mode discloses "the most primordial and direct access to human phenomena" (Packer, 1985, p. 1084) in that it is where practical activity of everyday life is primarily focused. Hermeneutic interpretation focuses on this mode of engagement and also on the next mode.

In the *unready-to-hand* mode, some sort of breakdown occurs in the smooth functioning of equipment or activities. Here the equipment and its functioning become conspicuous to the user. For example, if one of the parents in the family loses his or her job or gets temporarily laid off, usual family activities may be disrupted and conflicts may arise in the family. It is in this mode that aspects of equipment or practical activity often become more noticed. For this reason investigators may focus on this mode of engagement. However, reading back from this mode to the ready-to-hand may not provide an accurate interpretive account (Benner & Wrubel, 1989). For instance, to study unhealthy families to learn about family health and well being may provide a misunderstanding rather than an understanding of positive health in the family.

The final mode is the *present-to-hand*. In this mode, practical everyday activity ceases, and the person stands back and observes or reflects on the situation. Equipment is seen as objects with isolable properties and characteristics. Human actions are explained by strict characterizations. It is in this mode of activity where skilled scientific activity, theoretical reflection, and observation and experimentation take place (Dreyfus, 1991). Heidegger (1927/1962) referred to the present-to-hand as "a deficient mode of concern" (p. 103). Here is where investigations in the Cartesian mode of inquiry take place. This brings us to the question of the suitability of the natural science model for the human sciences.

The Natural Science Model

Why won't the natural science model work to study issues and concerns of human beings and specifically to study them in the context of health in families? Heidegger (1977) maintains that the human sciences, in contrast to the natural sciences, "must necessarily be inexact just in order to remain rigorous" (p. 120). But isn't being inexact in order to be rigorous a contradiction in terms?

By the natural science model, the answer is certainly yes. Natural science relies on exact measurement and precise representation of natural or manmade scientific phenomena. These can then be represented in covering laws, rules, and theories that can be used for prediction and explanation of the phenomena. The natural science method attempts to establish and maintain correspondence between laws, rules, and theories and the phenomena studied from the detached and objective standpoint of the scientist (Packer & Addison, 1989).

Benner and Wrubel (1989) point out that major strides in the 20th century in science and technology, and especially those related to understanding human physiology and disease processes, are attributable to the "technological view that grew out of the Enlightenment" (p. 51). But this detached, objectifying approach that reduces phenomena to such techniques as cause and effect modeling and independent and dependent variables that can be statistically correlated cannot account for everyday human experiences that are historical and temporal and based on participating in language and cultural practices (Benner, 1985). Dreyfus (1986) maintains that theory and prediction failures are always possible in the human sciences and that imprecision is inevitable. This, he explains, is because "the meaning of the situation plays an essential role in determining what counts as an event [in everyday human activity], and it is precisely this contextual meaning that theory must ignore" (p. 15).

Taylor (1987) explains that prediction is not possible in the human science of interpretation for three reasons. First, human life is an open system not amenable to prediction. Second, in a science based on practical activity, the fine exactitude of a science based on brute data cannot be achieved. Third, prediction is impossible because human beings are self-defining animals.

Where to Begin?

If not with observable facts and brute data, the prescribed starting points for the Cartesian model and natural science, where does one begin in studying issues of human concern in nursing? In laying out his philosophical investigation, Heidegger critiqued Cartesianism and science as being "derived from and dependent on everyday being-in-the-world" (Guignon, 1983, p. 244). Nursing research based on the natural science model is in this sense a privative mode of understanding: that is, it is deprived of and disengaged from the understanding that presupposes it. So instead Heidegger situated his investigation in the everyday situations of being-in-the-world, a shared public world, in order to access a more primordial way of being than that uncovered by theoretical reflection or pure contemplation. This is also where hermeneutic phenomenological study of family health and health activities and practices commences. It begins in the everyday practical activity of family life, in the transactions that are both person(s) and situation constituted and that form a web of relations in our everyday involvements (Benner, 1985; Guignon, 1983). In the research process, family life is accessed through the investigator's establishing a dialogue with the family, a dialogue that may occur through conversation (interview) and participation (participant observation) with the family. This dialogue brings forth the family's stories or narrative about actual events or episodes, which then becomes the text or text analogue. The text is what gets interpreted in the hermeneutic study, with the aim being "to bring to light an underlying coherence or sense" (Taylor, 1985, p. 33). According to Taylor (1985), there are three interrelated and inseparable conditions involved in interpretation: (a) there is an object or field of objects (the text) about which we want to make some sense; (b) there are meanings in the text that can be distinguished from the expression of the meanings, that is, how they are expressed or embodied in the everyday practices; and (c) there must be a person or persons (e.g., family) for which these meanings and expressions are significant. When approached in this manner, the family and its health and health activities are viewed as a coherent whole inseparable from the temporality and contextuality of the family's situated life, their possibilities and potentialities. From this vantage point, the Cartesian subject-object distinction falls away "as superfluous and pointless" (Guignon, 1983, p. 243). Instead the hermeneutic study discloses what is at stake for the family, their issues and concerns in their everyday activities, and an understanding of these issues and concerns.

Methodological Rigor

The natural science research model is well known for its methodological rigor. There are theoretical and practical procedures and rules and routines to follow. Standards exist for drawing a sample population that is representative and unbiased. Instruments are designed to be objective and standardized for repeated reliable and valid use. Research projects are aimed at producing research procedures and results that are repeatable and generalizable. A further aim of research is that it will provide explanatory, predictive, and even prescriptive guidelines (in the form of theories and conceptual and theoretical frameworks) for future events. These are standards and aims that many have tried to apply to the human sciences, and it has been argued that the rigor of the method will not work in the human sciences in a truly law-governed way. At least it will not work if the aim is to have disclosed what counts as an event in the everyday world of a person or family and is meaningful in their world (Dreyfus, 1984). Human beings can be reduced to objects and studied as in the natural science mode, but something essential will elude the investigator, and that is the "human self-interpretation essential to an understanding of human beings" (Dreyfus, 1984, p. 7). Predictions may be correct, but they will be reliable only insofar as they happen to coincide with what is selected and related in the daily activities of the person (or family) (Dreyfus, 1984).

So apparently we are left with an inevitable imprecision and inexactitude for hermeneutic phenomenology in the human sciences. Does this mean that method is laissez-faire or absent? Not according to Heidegger (1977), who maintains it is "much more difficult of an execution than is the achieving of rigor in the exact sciences" (p. 120). This can be understood for several reasons. First, the human sciences are inevitably retrospective and historical. One can reflect on lived experience only after it has happened (Taylor, 1987; van Manen, 1990). One might question how this can be so in, for instance, the case of participant observation. Although the investigator and partici-pants are present during the event, it is only after the event is fixed as text that it is interpreted. Also the intelligibility of the event as it occurs is possible only because of the understanding that is in the tacit background practices, and these are by nature historical. The forestructure of understanding gives some anticipation of the event but does not permit exact prediction. Everyday practical activities are bound up in a web of relations that require careful and sensitive engagement with the study participants and then with the resulting text analogue.

A second reason is that to access everyday practical activity, especially in family life, it is necessary to be present where the activity takes place. This requires involvement with the study participants (e.g., families in their natural settings). A pen and paper instrument, standardized interview, or laboratory exercise will not disclose being-in-the-world, though it may fit predictive models that Dreyfus referred to. This can be a time-consuming process in that one visit with the family may be inadequate to uncover their lived experience, complete with the possibilities and potentialities that their situation might offer. Benner (1985) notes that multiple interviews and observations help to reveal conflicts, contradictions, or surprises that might not have been present in earlier visits. Also redundancy that can occur over multiple visits not only allows for emergence of patterns and themes in the family's experience but also provides confidence in the interpretation.

A third and final, though not exhaustive, reason that I will address here is the actual interpretation. Multiple visits with multiple families make for large amounts of narrative text. These must be attended to in a sensitive and involved way. The investigator must be attuned not only to the text as narrative but to her or his own narrative, which is the forestructure of understanding discussed earlier. This is a dialogical process that requires openness, sensitivity, and scrutiny so that the world disclosed in the interpretation provides an understanding and not a misunderstanding of the families' lived experiences. Whereas in Husserlian phenomenology the preconceptions are supposed to be bracketed out of the interpretation (Denzin, 1989), in Heideggerian phenomenology the forestructure is integral to interpretation and should be acknowledged for any possible influence it has on the process of interpreting the text.

The interpretative process is unavoidably a writing and rewriting process (van Manen, 1990) that requires remaining close enough to the text to preserve the temporality and contextuality of the situations for the families but also an ability to move back and forth in the hermeneutic circle to be able to uncover understanding that might have gotten covered over by everyday familiarity. The interpreter must always be receptive to new interpretation that crops up because human activities are by nature transient and contextual. Guignon (1983) captures the "measure of truth" that an interpretive account should provide:

> The measure of truth of Heidegger's phenomenology is not whether it offers us a correct representation of who and what we are; [rather it] lies in the way our lives are enriched and deepened through these descriptions. . . . At the deepest level, prior to the correspondence of statements to facts in the world, truth is envisaged as the emergence of a clearing or opening that releases entities from hiddenness. . . . The description is measured not by criteria of correctness, but by criteria pertaining to its consequences for our lives. (p. 250)

In summary, three factors contribute to the rigor of hermeneutic phenomenology: the inevitable retrospective and historical nature of interpretive work, the involved and time-consuming need for studying participants in their everyday situatedness, and the arduous commitment involved in interpreting the text.

Some Interpretive Research Guidelines

Several scholar/practitioners of hermeneutic phenomenology have offered some principles and activities to guide interpretive research. In a recent publication on hermeneutic phenomenology for education and other human sciences, van Manen (1990) offers an in-depth discussion of six research activities that he sees as dynamically interrelated in interpretive research. He lists these in the first chapter as follows:

1. turning to a phenomenon, which seriously interests us and commits us to the world;
2. investigating experience as we live it rather than as we conceptualize it;
3. reflecting on the essential themes, which characterize the phenomenon;
4. describing the phenomenon through the art of writing and rewriting;
5. maintaining a strong and oriented pedagogical relation to the phenomenon;
6. balancing the research context by considering parts and whole. (pp. 30-31)

He elaborates on these in the balance of the book, maintaining that they are practical approaches and not mechanistic cookbook techniques. Although he tends to meld Husserlian and Heideggerian philosophical underpinnings, these activities provide salient guidelines, especially for the beginning interpreter or for those interested in learning about hermeneutic phenomenology. What must be kept in mind is that as one gains skill and alacrity in interpretative work, the need for models (and rules) falls away; indeed, as Dreyfus (1991) contends, models and rules would not even work to capture the know-how of skilled involvement in the world that Heidegger calls the ready-to-hand mode of engagement, that is, the smooth functioning of expertise or understanding.

Validation, both internal and external, is the standard for critiquing the worth of research under the natural science model. Five criteria form the standard: reliability, validity, objectivity (neutrality), generalizability, and repeatability (Sandelowski, 1986). But this standard throws us right back into the Cartesian model for research that claims interpretation-free validation. Both Madison (1988) and Packer and Addison (1989) argue that interpretive accounts are evaluated rather than tested and validated.

Packer and Addison (1989) offer a rather unique interpretation of the hermeneutic circle as being constituted by a forward arc of projection and a return arc of uncovering, thus constituting a constant dialogical process of interpretation and evaluation. The forward arc of the circle is the understanding that is the projecting of possibilities. They refer to this as the researcher's perspective or point of view that makes understanding possible. The reverse arc of uncovering "provides the possibility for evaluating an interpretive account" (p. 275). This interpretation of the hermeneutic circle provides philosophical underpinning for evaluation in interpretive research.

However, in using this interpretation, one must take care not to misinterpret Heidegger (1927/1962). For "projecting has nothing to do with comporting oneself towards a plan that has already been thought out" (p. 185); rather, it is what is always already understood in the background practices that makes our pressing into possibilities possible—that is, our possibilities in any given situation are shaped by the person or family's background history, culture, society, and language. Projecting is not a mental intentionality involving plans, purposes, and goals (Dreyfus, 1991). The point of view, recall, is the fore-sight, part of the threefold forestructure of understanding in which the question we have will structure the possible answers. This brings to light one of the challenges in using hermeneutic phenomenology—to remain in tune with the philosophical underpinnings.

Packer and Addison (1989) consider four evaluation approaches, including "requiring that an interpretive account be coherent; examining its relationship to external evidence; seeking consensus among various groups [including participants' interpretations]; and assessing the account's relationship to future events" (pp. 279-280). They emphasize that these are not ways to validate but ways to "consider whether what has been uncovered in an interpretive inquiry answers the practical, concernful question that directed [the] inquiry" (p. 289). Interpretive accounts will not be true for all persons (families) at all times because concerns and issues are different depending on the situations and possibilities of the person/family.

Madison (1988) offers nine principles for evaluation, which he maintains are "appropriate to, or derivable from, a phenomenological hermeneutics" (p. 29). These include

1. *Coherence*: the account presents a unified picture including letting contradictions show up and making as much sense of them as the text will allow.
2. *Comprehensiveness*: the account must give a sense of the whole that is the context (situatedness) and temporality for the participants.
3. *Penetration*: the account "attempts to resolve a central problematic" (p. 29).
4. *Thoroughness*: the account deals with all the questions posed.
5. *Appropriateness*: the questions must be those raised by the text itself.
6. *Contextuality*: the historical and contextual nature of the text must be preserved.
7. *Agreement*: the account must agree with what the text says (not attempt a hermeneutic of suspicion) but should reserve room for reinterpretation by showing where previous interpretations were deficient.
8. *Suggestiveness*: a good understanding in the interpretive account will raise questions to stimulate further interpretive research.

9. *Potential*: the ultimate evaluation of the account "lies in the future" in that it "is capable of being extended" (p. 30): that is, insights, tact, and critical discussion are revealed and possibilities uncovered that can be illuminating for future events.

The principles for evaluation posed by Madison (1988) are based on practical reason as a model for interpretation. Practical reason, he argues, unlike theoretical reason, which aims at "insight into what simply is" independent of the subject, "is concerned with all those situations where one must make a choice, produce something, or decide on a course of action, the outcome of which is contingent in that it depends, precisely, on the subject oneself [sic]" (p. 34).

Madison's list is comprehensive and appears to be consistent with the philosophical underpinnings of Heidegger. His guidelines incorporate two of Packer and Addison's (1989) approaches (coherence and implications for future events). Unlike those of Packer and Addison, his suggested principles deal with issues that are primarily internal to the text.

Limitations

As with any research methodology, there are limits to which one can take it. Hermeneutic phenomenology is best suited for answering questions about human issues and concerns. These are primarily the "what" and "how" questions.

Hermeneutic phenomenology will not aid in prediction. However, gaining a better understanding of what are the issues and concerns may help to anticipate future events for a person or family and aid in an understanding of the significance the person or family gives them.

Not all persons, whether potential investigators or participants, are willing or able to participate in this type of research. Such an undertaking requires commitment and plenty of time and can even be expensive to conduct.

The forestructure of understanding, including one's preconceptions and biases, must be acknowledged as clearly as possible. Some have criticized interpretive work for being biased toward the investigator's knowledge and experience and for not being true to the participant's lived experience (Tripp-Reimer & Cohen, 1987). Getting too far out on the hermeneutic circle can decontextualize the interpretation from the original text. This risk of biasing exists in all human sciences. Hermeneutic phenomenology tries to address this risk by remaining close to the original text and by uncovering biases for scrutiny.

A final limitation to hermeneutic phenomenology addressed here was one addressed by Heidegger (1927/1962) in *Being and Time*:

> Whenever a phenomenological concept is drawn from primordial sources, there is a possibility that it may degenerate if communicated in the form of an assertion. It gets understood in an empty way and is passed on, losing its indigenous character and becoming a free-floating thesis. . . . The difficulty of this kind of research lies in making it self-critical in a positive sense. (pp. 60-61)

This point is particularly salient to hermeneutic phenomenology and is driven home by several scholars of Heidegger and hermeneutic inquiry (Dreyfus, 1991; Guignon, 1983; Packer & Addison, 1989). When an interpretive account loses its contextuality and temporality and operates beyond its original context, it may be reduced to what Dreyfus (1991) refers to as "leveling to banality" and then become mere assertion. This, according to Dreyfus, is equivalent to sliding "from the truth of primordial pointing out to the untruth of mere correspondence" (p. 276), thus reverting to the present-to-hand or Cartesian mode of inquiry.

Conclusion

Heideggerian hermeneutic phenomenology, then, is a nursing research methodology well suited to studying health and health promotion practices and activities in families. Hermeneutics is an appropriate methodology because it aims to understand the significance of practical activities in our everyday lives. The underlying assumption is that it is in the everyday practical activities of families and their members that the significance of health for the family can be uncovered and thus understood. This question of significance of health and health activities and practices for families is important in the delivery of health care. A primordial understanding of what constitutes and is constitutive of health and well-being for families has far-reaching implications in terms of educational programs for nurses, other health care professionals, and families, and for research, health policy, and delivery of primary health care.

The philosophical underpinnings of hermeneutic phenomenology as worked out by Martin Heidegger in his early philosophical work have been summarized. It is important for the reader to realize that Heidegger's work on the fundamental ontology of the meaning of being is much more extensive than what has been presented here. This chapter has primarily addressed one aspect, understanding, of a complicated existential structure. For Heidegger maintained that "disclosedness is constituted by affectivity, understanding, and telling, and pertains equiprimordially to the world, to being-in, and to the self" (Dreyfus's translation, Dreyfus, 1991, p. 240; for same passage see also Heidegger, 1927/1962, p. 263).

In addition, the assumptions of hermeneutic phenomenology have been contrasted with those of the natural science model, and basic philosophical and methodological issues have been discussed. This chapter has not addressed some concrete issues, such as how one selects the study participants for a hermeneutic study and methods for collecting and analyzing the narrative text. These issues, although essential to the overall project of an interpretive study, are beyond this chapter's intended scope.

References

Benner, P. (1985). Quality of life: Phenomenological perspective on explanation, prediction, and understanding in nursing science. *Advances in Nursing Science, 8*(1), 1-14.

Benner, P., & Wrubel, J. (1989). *The primacy of caring.* Reading, MA: Addison-Wesley.

Denzin, N. K. (1989). *Interpretive interactionism.* Applied social science research methods series, No. 16. Newbury Park, CA: Sage.

Dreyfus, H. L. (1984). Beyond hermeneutics: Interpretation in late Heidegger and recent Foucault. In G. Shapior & A. Sica (Eds.), *Hermeneutics: Questions and prospects* (pp. 66-83). Amherst: University of Massachusetts Press.

Dreyfus, H. L. (1986). Why studies of human capacities modeled on ideal natural science can never achieve their goal. In M. Margolis, M. Krausy, & R. M. Burain (Eds.), *Rationality, relativism, and the human sciences* (pp. 3-22). Dordrecht, Netherlands: Martinus Nijhoff.

Dreyfus, H. L. (1991). *Being-in-the-world. A commentary on Heidegger's "Being and time," Division I.* Cambridge: MIT Press.

Gordon, D. (1988). Tenacious assumptions in Western medicine. In M. Lock & D. Gordon (Eds.), *Biomedicine examined* (pp. 19-56). Boston: Kluwer Academic Publishers.

Guignon, C. (1983). *Heidegger and the problem of knowledge.* Indianapolis: Hackett.

Heidegger, M. (1962). *Being and time* (J. Macquerrie & E. Robinson, Trans.). New York: Harper & Row. (Original work published 1927)

Heidegger, M. (1971). *Poetry, language, thought* (A. Hofstadter, Trans.). New York: Harper & Row.

Heidegger, M. (1977). *The question concerning technology and other essays* (W. Lovitt, Trans.). New York: Harper & Row.

Kirmayer, L. J. (1988). Mind and body as metaphors: Hidden values in biomedicine. In M. Lock & D. Gordon (Eds.), *Biomedicine examined* (pp. 57-93). Boston: Kluwer Academic Publishers.

Madison, G. B. (1988). *The hermeneutics of postmodernity.* Indianapolis: Indiana University Press.

Packer, M. (1985). Hermeneutic inquiry in the study of human conduct. *American Psychologist, 40*(10), 1081-1093.

Packer, M. J., & Addison, R. B. (1989). Introduction. In M. J. Packer & R. B. Addison (Eds.), *Entering the circle: Hermeneutic investigation in psychology* (pp. 13-36). Albany: State University of New York Press.

Sacks, O. (1970). *The man who mistook his wife for a hat and other clinical tales.* New York: Harper & Row.

Sandelowski, M. (1986). The problem of rigor in qualitative research. *Advances in Nursing Science, 8*(3), 27-37.

Stein, H. G. (1989). Family influences on health behavior: An ethnographic approach. In C. N. Ramsey (Ed.), *Family systems medicine* (pp. 373-394). New York: Guilford.

Taylor, C. (1985). *Human agency and language. Philosophical papers* (Vol. 1). Cambridge, UK: Cambridge University Press.

Taylor, C. (1987). Interpretation and the sciences of man. In P. Rabinow & W. M. Sullivan (Eds.), *Interpretive social sciences: A second look* (pp. 33-81). Berkeley: University of California Press.

Taylor, C. (1991). The dialogical self. In D. R. Hiley, J. F. Bohman, & R. Shusterman (Eds.), *The interpretive turn: Philosophy, science, culture* (pp. 304-314). Ithaca, NY: Cornell University Press.

Ten Have, H., & Kimsma, G. (1991). Changing conceptions of medical ethics. In G. Mooney & U. Jensen (Eds.), *Changing values in medical and health care decision making* (pp. 33-51). Chichester, UK: John Wiley.

Tripp-Reimer, T., & Cohen, M. Z. (1987, April). Using phenomenology in health promotion research. In M. E. Duffy & N. J. Pender (Eds.), *Conceptual issues in health promotion* (pp. 121-127). Report on Proceedings of a Wingspread Conference, Racine, WI. Indianapolis, IN: Sigma Theta Tau.

van Manen, M. (1990). *Researching lived experience: Human science for an action sensitive pedagogy.* Ontario, Canada: Althouse.

5

❖

Toward a New Medical Ethics

Implications for Ethics in Nursing

DAVID C. THOMASMA

As medical ethics matures, so too will the implications for nursing ethics. The two disciplines are parallel. Yet because of specific features that are not common to the two, nursing ethics should be seen as a separate discipline with its own patterns of development.

In this paper I will examine the changes that have taken place in medical ethics. The purpose of this examination is to ferret out the implications of those changes for the parallel discipline of nursing ethics. Because broad strokes are used to sketch the changes in the former, with apologies to historians of medical ethics (Burns, 1977), my comments are necessarily sweeping and elemental. The first section of the chapter is devoted to historical analysis, the second to the relation of a nursing ethic to medical models, and the third to a hermeneutics of models of care. Building on this analysis, I propose a relationship ethics for nursing and draw some conclusions.

Historical Analysis

Dramatic increases in the technological capacity of modern medicine occurred after the Second World War. Ironically, these enhanced interventions took place precisely at the same time the world was first informed of, then repulsed by, the details of how the Nazi party was able, through the instruments of state power, to turn medicine toward evil human ends (Lifton, 1986).

Simultaneously Americans were beginning to express their first uneasiness with technology as a result of being the first nation to use nuclear power to destroy hundreds of thousands of people in Hiroshima and Nagasaki (Mumford, 1964). Recall the science fiction movie genre of the 1950s and 1960s, wherein atomic experiments produce enormous mutant creatures that destroy cities, and in which we see the Einstein look-alike, benign, humanistic scientist. Armies and politicians are powerless against the mutants until the boyfriend of the daughter of the scientist (who does *not* look like Einstein), a practical person such as a reporter or a carpenter, thinks of the way to save the human race.

Thus was born the current version of the ambivalence about science and technology built into Western civilization (earlier versions are the Faust legend and, more exactly for medicine, the story of the Frankenstein monster). This ambivalence in turn expresses the caution about applying medical technology to human beings without attention to primary values. These latter are found not only in the hierarchy of values the patient brings to the encounter with medicine (Pellegrino & Thomasma, 1988) but also in the system of traditional values articulated in the past by health care professionals as part of their discipline. Not only patient but also health professional values were discovered to be at risk.

"Lookey-Here Ethics"

The first step in this discovery can be called "Lookey-Here ethics." Most of the early articles in medical ethics were dominated by rhetorical questions posed after identifying one or another difficult issue: Are we playing God? Who should decide? How should the resolution proceed? What values must be sacrificed? From 1960 to 1970 or so, these issues first were very broadly identified as matters of social concern (Callahan, 1973), just as today we are only beginning to identify the problems involved in allocation of health care (Callahan, 1987, 1990). After the early identifications, specific issues began to emerge in the same way that, for example, the general problems of genetics are now giving way to specific issues in the use of genetic manipulation (gene mapping, altering gene therapy for leukemias, etc.).

"Applied Turn"

The second step of the development in medical ethics was getting genuine, certified philosophical ethicists interested in the issues. In the main this was accomplished by inviting the philosophers over from the liberal arts school to make rounds with physicians. This strategy created friendships and liaisons that endure to this day, producing much of the creative, interactive, interdisciplinary writing in the field. The basis of a deeper analysis was thereby created.

Indeed, this activity has not been confined to philosophers alone. Specialists in literature, sociology, anthropology, law, history of medicine, and other humanities began to enrich and be enriched by medicine and medical education (Pellegrino & McElhinney, 1982). In addition, some physicians began to get a joint degree, embodying in themselves the interaction of ethics and medicine and contributing to the growing discipline of philosophy of medicine (Brody, 1977; Engelhardt, 1986). This activity began in 1969 with the creation of the Department of Medical Humanities at Penn State Medical School at Hershey and vigorously expanded throughout the 1970s.

"Legitimation"

Another important step in the development of the discipline was to interest the "biggies" in ethics in the importance of the field. These established scholars, such as Alasdair MacIntyre (MacIntyre, 1981, 1988), have contributed a true sense of philosophical discipline in their works. H. T. Engelhardt and S. Spicker inaugurated in 1976 and still coedit a series on philosophy of medicine that began this effort (1976); subsequently it gave birth to two journals, *The Journal of Medicine and Philosophy* and *Theoretical Medicine*, which encourage such deeper philosophical analysis of medicine beyond ethical analysis. This effort also helps junior scholars who "leave" their home department for a position in an interdisciplinary medical humanities department but who must still be concerned about obtaining rank and tenure in their research.

The danger of this move is already producing a backlash. It produces an artificial, deductive, rationalistic cast to the discipline because most of the major thinkers do not get involved in the clinical setting. Today scholars are referring to this rationalistic cast as the "Georgetown mantra": principles of autonomy, beneficence, and justice that have dominated much of the public thinking about medical ethics to this date. It also produces monochromatic cultural assumptions that only persons from other cultures are able to identify (Thomasma & Pellegrino, 1981).

"Agreement on Principles"

Major territorial claims for the basic principles just discussed were mapped out during the late 1970s and dominated the discussion of medical ethics during the 1980s. They were first adumbrated in the Belmont Report of 1973, a report of the President's Commission for the Protection of Human Subjects (National Commission, 1979). But the heyday of rationalistic, principled medical ethics really began with the first publication of Beauchamp and Childress's *Principles of Biomedical Ethics*, now in its third edition (Beauchamp & Childress, 1989). The problem of relying overly much on principles in medical ethics is that agreement on principles may not lead to agreement on conclusions, and agreement on conclusions may not imply an agreement on principles (Graber & Thomasma, 1989).

"Hey, Wait a Minute!"

The next step in the natural development of any discipline is a period of adjustment after initial success. This is true for medical ethics as well. Those who "labor in the vineyards" of health care began to protest the essential tidiness of an ethics of principles. This protest centered largely on an overreliance on the principle of autonomy. At one time, James Childress said that autonomy trumps all other values (Childress, 1981). This has been countered by an analysis of the strengths and weaknesses of an autonomy-based medical ethics; at least one of the weaknesses is that it leaves out the essential partner in the medical encounter, the physician (Beauchamp & McCullough, 1984; Pellegrino & Thomasma, 1988). The result of this backlash, if it might be called that, has been a medical ethics that is becoming more sensitive to clinical realities.

"Focus on Method"

Following the protest about overreliance on autonomy has come a more sensitive analysis of the methods used in medical ethics. This methodological turn has assisted medical ethics in becoming more self-reflective (Graber & Thomasma, 1989). It appears that the content of analysis is influenced by the method employed, and vice versa.

"Enrichment"

Meanwhile, constantly developing issues and new technologies enrich and add complexity to the discipline. I have already mentioned the progression in genetics. Other flashpoints today in medical ethics are the withdrawal of fluids and nutrition; direct, voluntary euthanasia; reproductive ethics; justice and access to care; transplantation technology; institutional norms and "consciences"; expectations and codes for professionals; and questions about the nature of the community that might limit care, for example, to the elderly or incompetent patient. Each of these issues, as it is discussed and elaborated for several years, contributes sophisticated nuances in reasoning that simply were not conceivable in earlier stages of the discipline. Further, if questions are raised in some subsets of the discipline, they may or may not be carried over into others. A good example would be the resistance to "single principle" ethics. If methodological concerns betray a resistance to using the principle of autonomy as primary, then corresponding concerns will be carried over in the active, direct euthanasia debate. There, some philosophers such as Margaret Battin argue that the right to voluntary, direct euthanasia is based on the principle of autonomy, whereas others contend that autonomy is not the only value to be protected in this national debate (Thomasma, 1992).

"Clinical Methodology"

Emerging from these debates only in the past five years has been a discussion of casuistry, generally speaking, a clinical and individually tailored ethical methodology (Jonsen & Toulmin, 1988). The idea of casuistry is that ethical resolutions depend on a "fit" of principles and axioms to individual circumstances. That is to say, weights are given differently to different values in different circumstances. I have called this "contextualism" (Thomasma, 1979). Casuistry goes further than this due to its insistence on inductive ethics. According to this tenet, principles and axioms themselves are "induced" from the case, not applied to it. Clearly, though, this more clinical sensitive ethics relates more directly to the method of clinical decision making itself (Graber & Thomasma, 1989, pp. 173-202).

"Philosophy of Medicine"

As mentioned already, the efforts to invite more established scholars to examine medicine and its ethics produced a movement we should call the philosophy of medicine. This is a separate discipline from medical ethics, and it is still in its infancy, despite the journals and books devoted to it already mentioned (Pellegrino & Thomasma, 1981).

At least a portion of the vision that underlies philosophy of medicine is that current medical ethics must be grounded in an epistemology and a philosophical anthropology, even in an ontology, if it is to endure. This is also true of ethics generally. Nevertheless, the movement of this discipline in recent times is toward a more international cultural awareness that will continue as scholars in other countries turn their intellectual beacons on medical practice and theory.

"Inadequacy Awareness"

Finally, implied in the last step and made explicit in the past two years in medical ethics is an awareness of its inadequacy to address primary problems in medical ethics. Philosophical medical ethics has always suffered from this inadequacy, but it has been masked by the sheer energy of trying to mark out the boundaries of the discipline and nurture it to its present state of adolescence. As individuals have spent more and more time in the clinical setting, a decade or more in some instances, it has gradually dawned on them that something much more profound is happening in the encounter of the sick with the healer—something "religious" in an unclear sense. There is a reluctance to define it for fear of being taken as a doddering mystic, much as Elizabeth Kuebler-Ross was accused of becoming as she ventured ever more deeply into her field of death and dying. Pellegrino and I have just completed a manuscript that attempts to dig into this dimension of healing and redefine some essential medical ethics terms as a result.

Nursing Ethics

Though nursing ethics is a discipline different from medical ethics, it is not yet as advanced. It will move through the same steps of development and may be able to skip some of them.

How Can Nursing Ethics Define Itself?

In traditional medical ethics there are actually three subdisciplines. The first can be called "ethics and medicine," in which common themes, such as trust, are examined. Much of phenomenological analysis takes this tack. The second is a form of applied ethics, in which philosophers take their fundamental theories, such as deontologism and utilitarianism, and apply them to issues such as abortion or euthanasia to test the validity of their hypotheses and shed light on the issues themselves. The third I call clinical ethics. This subdiscipline arises out of the clinical realities of health care and is actually a branch of medicine itself.

Pellegrino and I constructed a philosophy of medicine that would undergird the latter sense of medical ethics, arguing that medicine is a relational discipline. It is not what doctors do or what patients do to remain healthy. It is the interactive interplay of values about the body, the life world, and science when individuals become sick and must rely on other human beings for healing (Thomasma & Pellegrino, 1981).

These developments are important for an understanding of nursing ethics. It will not do to claim that nurses ought to be treated the same as physicians in the relationship, because they are not. Thus the ethics cannot be constructed exactly the same. But the insight about relationships is important. Nursing ethics is not about the primary curing relationship. It is ancillary to that relationship, and so are the ethical issues that arise from it from the point of view of nursing as a profession. But nursing ethics is about the primary healing relationship. It is essential for healing, and so are the ethical issues that arise from that task. Thus its fundamental principle is to act toward individuals as they would act toward themselves in an effort to restore them to health. Healing the individual is primary. I will discuss this dimension in more detail later.

Partnership and Educational Models

Nursing ethics can skip over unimportant steps in the development of a discipline if it goes for a partnership in the clinical setting first. If the focus of nursing is on healing, then the specific modalities that can bring that about are found in the practice of the discipline. Though it is a simpler matter for a philosopher to target ethical decision making on rounds, it is much more difficult for that person to imagine the healing task that is so often masked in nursing procedures—suctioning the endotracheal tube, taking a temperature, and the like.

It will take some real educational efforts on the part of nurses to enlighten the liberal arts professors they might invite into their clinical realities. This in itself will assist the development of a theory of nursing ethics and an educational structure of training future nurses in the most important tasks they undertake.

I now turn to the problem of overcoming models of rationalistic ethics in favor of an ethics of caring. The purpose of this sketch is to establish how nursing ethics can move beyond such models to developing models of care.

Beyond a Rationalistic Ethics

Essentially rationalistic ethics is geared toward analyzing means and ends. If the ends are consonant with medicine itself (e.g., the restoration to health of a person, or giving comfort to a dying person, and these ends are considered goods, then the means supplying the ends are subject to criticism). This tradition of analysis has dominated medical ethics until the present time. It has been very successful in helping develop a set of public policies about major issues in health care, from experimentation on human beings to the organization of hospital ethics committees.

Lately the modality of applying the four major principles of beneficence, autonomy, nonmaleficence, and justice to individual categories of cases (such as withdrawing fluids and nutrition) has been called into question in favor of more casuistic analyses provided by case-oriented methods such as casuistry itself (Jonsen & Toulmin, 1988), hermeneutical ethics (Graber & Thomasma, 1989, pp. 173-202), and narrative ethics (Benner, 1985, in press). How would such a methodology aid nursing ethics?

Models of care might be divided into interpreting the body, interpreting the spirit (values), and interpreting the relation of the body and spirit, along with interpreting the relationships of the person with his or her support group (family, job, neighborhood), with special attention to the incredibly complex dynamics of these relationships.

Interpreting the Body

Today, touching the patient seems to be a lost art even in nursing. I have observed that nurses, dedicated to enriching their professional abilities, are focused on technology to a greater extent than in the past. Many have left the profession from burnout with overloads of tasks to the detriment of individual caring touch. Others have chosen to go into home health care, where independence of judgment and individualization of care are possible (Feuerstein, 1990).

I am using "touch" in an expanded meaning, but I do want to emphasize the importance of this healing and interpretative modality in the care of individuals. Through touching the patient, trust is built, and comfort is offered. Information is conveyed not only about the illness but, more importantly, about the illness's impact on the patient. Interpreting this fact is the beginning of healing, for it then permits the healer to face the true personal struggle of the patient rather than the abstract, scientific categories of disease automatically promoted by our modern understanding and training. Another way of putting it is that any professional training fits us with tinted glasses through which we interpret reality. That is the whole point of years of study and learning tasks. Yet to heal one must put aside the glasses temporarily to "see" the patient's struggle and to face one's own powers and limitations in that struggle.

The expanded meaning of touching then enters here. To "touch" the patient physically is to touch a body like ours reacting in a unique and personal way to an illness or accident. Through that physical touch an entry into the realm of that suffering person is affected. Interpreting the person begins.

Interpreting the Spirit (Values)

No two individuals are truly alike. This is almost a truism. Even when individuals are emerging newborn from the womb, likes and dislikes have already formed. Over the years, however, individuals continually assess their lives and their actions. As part of that assessment, values are formed and solidified. New challenges to life and limb reestablish those values within the judgments patients make. In effect, every judgment rests upon either explicit or implicit values. The latter rarely change, though attitudes might during one's life.

This means that a hierarchy of values is formed in each clinical encounter. Interpreting the spirit as well as the body requires attention to this hierarchy in decision making (Pellegrino & Thomasma, 1988). There are at least four levels operative in the relation between healer and the sick: the medical, the therapeutic plan, the life plan, and the ultimate value.

The Medical. The realm of medical values includes all procedures that are medically indicated. Usually medical values focus on organ systems. This is the realm of decisions regarding kidney output, blood gases, and the like. For the most part, patients want these values because they wish to recover and return to their life. But these values can be trumped by more important values to follow.

The Therapeutic Plan. The therapeutic plan is the objective of medical treatment. In simplest form, it is a plan to help patients recover and leave the hospital, returning to their life in some improved measure or at best in as good shape as they were before the illness or accident. Often, however, the therapeutic plan involves an adjustment to the patient's own lifestyle, as it might when a person is recovering from a broken leg. What is important to note here, however, is that the therapeutic plan should guide the medical values. Sometimes, in cases of dying patients, there is no articulated therapeutic plan. Health professionals simply concentrate on medical values without asking the difficult questions of the purposes of the targeted treatments.

Life Plans. Patients bring to their hospital and home care experience a set of life plans that express the means to their ultimate value. Many have relationship plans. For example, besides working and providing for a family, buying a retirement home in the south, and so forth, they speak about repairing their relation with their daughter or getting along better at work.

These life plans should guide the therapeutic plan. If an individual wants to get out of the hospital (therapeutic plan) once her hypertension is reduced, it pays to find out what she plans to do when she does get out. What are her life plans toward which we could help by designing a good therapeutic plan?

Ultimate Value. All of the above-mentioned realms of values are ultimately guided by the individual's superior value. For some people this is religious: they wish to go to heaven or be virtuous so they can obtain a reward from God. But all persons, even nonreligious persons, do possess an ultimate value that must be respected at all costs in every clinical relationship. An elderly person may request to go off dialysis and be allowed to die precisely because he wants to "get his reward." Sometimes when persons are ready to die, they are ready in a way the rest of us are not because they see with greater focus how their lives are now moving toward their final end. To obstruct this end by using technology that prolongs life is to destroy the trust implied in the healing encounter (Pellegrino & Thomasma, 1988).

Interpreting Relationships

Given the realms of values that occur in every healing encounter, nurses must learn to interpret the relations of the body, and of the functions that work or are impaired, to the person's values. This is like interpreting the relation of the body and the spirit of the sick person. Further, nurses should be the experts who attend to the relations of persons (who are syntheses of the relation of body and spirit) to their support groups at home, at work, in the neighborhood, and in society. Most importantly, however, the very complex web of interrelationships, the dynamics of this web, can be the special provenance of the nurse.

Relationship Ethics

Now we may see why nursing ethics cannot be the same as the traditional rationalistic ethics employed by many medical ethicists. Analysis of principles is but one part of a very complex picture. Nursing ethics is more complicated than this and often hard to pin down. As Ten Have and Kimsma (1990) note, nursing ethics is not a "technethic."

Hence the essence of nursing ethics is not what patients do or what nurses do but the way the dynamic of the healing relationship unfolds, not only in the hospital or clinic but also back in the home environment.

A relationship is the most elusive of all realities, yet the most important to human beings. Think of all the time we spend on relationships in our daily

life! Witness the breakup of relationships that occurs during a serious illness
or accident:

1. The self may disintegrate into an ego and a body that betrayed the person.
   The body is seen as an object. Reintegration is needed in order for healing to
   take place (Bergsma & Thomasma, 1982).
2. The person may disintegrate into a self and disrupted social relationships.
   This dynamic relationship also requires intense attention during the healing
   process. It is often overlooked in the joy of "getting the kidneys functioning
   again," and the person is whisked out the hospital with little or no follow-up
   care. This is especially true in the age of DRGs.
3. The human being underlying the person and the self is a social animal. The
   disruptions to social relations caused by altered relationships on the other
   levels just adumbrated can create disease long after the person returns home
   from the hospital. The classic example of this is the patient who has recovered
   from a heart attack but whose wife won't let him enjoy normal activities again
   out of worry that he will die.

These brief reflections prompt a reiteration that the goal of health care and
healing is not life preservation per se but assisting individuals in the accomplishment of their life plans (Walter, 1990). Hence when considering the
withholding and withdrawing of any form of medical care, including fluids
and nutrition, the mode of analysis ought not to be solely dependent on
principles of medical ethics. In addition to those, I have suggested, ought to
be employed principles of "caring" as developed above. A conclusion would
be that when the patient can no longer participate in the spiritual and material
relationships sketched and can no longer accomplish the goals of a self, a
person, or a human being, then withholding and withdrawing care could be
permitted.

On a more positive note, for in the main we are successful in curing
patients, healing is that step beyond cure that restores the ability of persons to
develop and nurture their relationships. Nonetheless, as Andrew Jameton points
out, caring is a labor-intensive form of helping persons that is often under-
valued when compared to highly technical interventions:

In dealing with suffering and the cure of disease, nurses encounter a double
stereotype. As *nurses*, they are associated with care over cure, even though
care and cure are integrated processes provided by both nurses and physicians. As *women*, for the most part, they are associated with a humane and
gentle response to suffering. Since skills in caring are labor-intensive—
whether practiced by men or women, physicians or nurses—and have little
economic value to investors, those who engage in caring do not receive

the rewards and respect awarded those with more technologically oriented skills. (Jameton, 1984, p. 224)

Much more needs to be developed on this theory of care, and a number of nurses have already been exploring its ramifications. Sara Fry, for example, is concerned that the ethic of caring cannot survive in nursing in the face of shortages, unsafe staffing, and payment-directed nursing unless nurses themselves insist that caring is central to their role. This means that they must require sufficient time to develop care between themselves and their patients or clients so that it may be realized (Fry, 1988). My modest contribution has been to underscore how this theory of care and healing is important for the kind of nursing ethics that ought to be taught in the basic nursing curriculum. As Curtin (1988) argues, ethics cannot be confined to abstract discussions but must relate directly to the standards of practice in the profession.

Conclusion

I have argued the following points:

1. The curriculum in nursing ethics ought to be constructed in partnership with the clinical practice training program so that the nurses learn on the scene how the ethical questions of their profession arise in their practice.
2. Thus the curriculum would be clinically sensitive, that is, it would arise from and return to the everyday experience of nurses now and in the future.
3. The theory underlying nursing practice suggests that the proper ethic should be a relational ethic, one that targets the problems patients have with their disease, with family, with disruptions in their social and work structure, and in relation to their values, including their ultimate value. This is in contrast to a growing number of families of patients who report that nurses have lately been "uncaring, cruel, rough, thoughtless, mean, indifferent" (Kelly, 1988, p. 17).
4. There ought to be a religious dimension to the training in ethics insofar as all persons have an ultimate value they wish to protect, restore, and nurture during illness and recovery, and during their dying process as well. This would include help for nurses in being critical of their own thinking, self-reflective about their ultimate values, and mature about discussing these with their patients.
5. I would encourage the development of R.N. and Ph.D. degrees with emphases on philosophy, religious studies, ethics, and other areas of the humanities. Persons with these degrees would have an ability from their training to integrate ethics training with the regular curriculum in nursing schools.

6. It is clear that the role of ethics in the nursing curriculum may help shape the future of health care in that the latter will be aimed more and more at prevention and individual control over health risks. Such individual control cries out for encouragement, the kind of encouragement a nurse can provide by promising to help, to be "there," at the junction of a person's life and values.

References

Beauchamp, T., & Childress, J. (1989). *Principles of biomedical ethics* (3rd ed.). New York: Oxford University Press.

Beauchamp, T., & McCullough, L. (1984). *Medical ethics: The moral responsibilities of physicians*. Englewood Cliffs, NJ: Prentice Hall.

Benner, P. (1985). Quality of life: A phenomenological perspective on explanation, prediction and understanding in nursing science. *Advances in Nursing Science, 8,* 1-14.

Benner, P. (in press). Discovering challenges to ethical theory in experience-based narratives and nurses' everyday ethical comportment. In J. Monagle & D. Thomasma (Eds.), *Health care ethics: Critical issues.* Frederick, MD: Aspen.

Bergsma, J., & Thomasma, D. C. (1982). *Health care: Its psychosocial dimensions.* Pittsburgh: Duquesne University Press.

Brody, H. (1977). *Placebos and the philosophy of medicine.* Chicago: University of Chicago Press.

Burns, C. (1977). *Legacies in ethics and medicine.* New York: Neale Watson Academic Publications.

Callahan, D. (1973). *The tyranny of survival.* New York: Macmillan.

Callahan, D. (1987). *Setting limits: Medical goals in an aging society.* New York: Simon & Schuster.

Callahan, D. (1990). *What kind of life: The limits of medical progress.* New York: Simon & Schuster.

Childress, J. (1981). *Priorities in biomedical ethics.* Philadelphia: Westminster.

Curtin, L. L. (1988). Ethics in nursing practice. *Nursing Management, 19,* 7-9.

Engelhardt, H. T., Jr. (1986). *The foundations of bioethics.* New York: Oxford University Press.

Engelhardt, H. T., Jr., & Spicker, S. (Eds.). (1976). *Philosophy and medicine.* Boston: Kluwer Academic Publishers.

Feuerstein, P. (1990, December 30). We get to know patients on a more personal level. *Chicago Tribune Magazine,* sec. 10, p. 29.

Fry, S. (1988). The ethic of caring: Can it survive in nursing? Editorial. *Nursing Outlook, 36,* 48.

Graber, G. C., & Thomasma, D. C. (1989). *Theory and practice in medical ethics.* New York: Continuum.

Jameton, A. (1984). *Nursing practice: The ethical issues.* Englewood Cliffs, NJ: Prentice Hall.

Jonsen, A., & Toulmin, S. (1988). *The abuse of casuistry.* Berkeley: University of California Press.

Kelly, L. S. (1988). The ethic of caring: Has it been discarded? Editorial. *Nursing Outlook, 36,* 17.

Lifton, R. (1986). *The Nazi doctors: Medical killing and the psychology of genocide*. New York: Basic Books.

MacIntyre, A. (1981). *After virtue*. Notre Dame, IN: Notre Dame University Press.

MacIntyre, A. (1988). *Whose justice? Which rationality?* Notre Dame, IN: University of Notre Dame Press.

Mumford, L. (1964). *The myth of the machine: The pentagon of power*. New York: Harcourt, Brace, Jovanovich.

National Commission for the Protection of Human Subjects of Biomedical and Behavioral Research. (1979). *The Belmont Report: Ethical principles and guidelines for the protection of human subjects of research*. Washington, DC: U.S. Government Printing Office.

Pellegrino, E. D., & McElhinney, T. (Eds.). (1982). *Teaching ethics: The humanities and human values in medical schools: A ten-year overview*. Washington, DC: Institute on Human Values in Medicine, Society for Health and Human Values.

Pellegrino, E. D., & Thomasma, D. C. (1981). *A philosophical basis of medical practice*. New York: Oxford University Press.

Pellegrino, E. D., & Thomasma, D. C. (1988). *For the patient's good: The restoration of beneficence in health care*. New York: Oxford University Press.

Ten Have, H., & Kimsma, G. (1990). Changing conceptions of medical ethics. In G. Mooney & U. Jensen (Eds.), *Changing values in medical and health care decision making* (pp. 33-51). Chichester, U.K.: John Wiley.

Thomasma, D. C. (1979). A contextual grid for medical ethics. *AAR Abstracts*. Minnesota: Scholar's Press.

Thomasma, D. C. (1992). Mercy killing of the demented elderly: A counterproposal. In P. Whitehouse, R. Binstock, & S. Post (Eds.), *Dementia and aging: Ethics, values, and policy choices* (pp. 101-117). Baltimore: Johns Hopkins University Press.

Thomasma, D. C., & Pellegrino, E. D. (1981). Philosophy of medicine as the source for medical ethics. *Metamedicine* (now called *Theoretical Medicine*), *2*, 5-11. [Entire volume devoted to responses of philosophers to philosophy of medicine]

Walter, J. P. (1990). The meaning and validity of quality of life judgments in contemporary Roman Catholic medical ethics. In J. P. Walter & T. Shannon (Eds.), *Quality of life: The new medical dilemma* (pp. 78-90). New York: Paulist Press.

6

✛

The Tradition and Skill of Interpretive Phenomenology in Studying Health, Illness, and Caring Practices

PATRICIA BENNER

The phenomenon and its context frame the interpretive project of understanding the world of participants or events. The interpretive researcher creates a dialogue between practical concerns and lived experience through engaged reasoning and imaginative dwelling in the immediacy of the participants' worlds. The goal is to study the phenomenon in its own terms (Husserl, 1964), and this requires being critically reflective on the ways that any one set of prescribed methodological strategies, personal knowledge, and social context create a theoretical and perceptual access that influences understanding. Interpretive phenomenology involves a rigorous scholarly reading of texts—questioning, comparing, and imaginatively dwelling in their situations. The scholarly skills of analysis, synthesis, criticism, and understanding are used to articulate the meanings of the text and generate interpretive commentary (Taylor, 1985a, 1993).

The goal of studying persons, events, and practices in their own terms is to understand world, self, and other. The interpreter moves back and forth between the foreground and background, between situations, and between the practical worlds of the participants. The interpretive assumption is that world can never be spelled out completely (Dreyfus, 1991a; Heidegger, 1927/1962). Human worlds, being historical, contextual, and multifaceted, are only grasped under finite, situated aspects (Benner & Wrubel, 1989; Dreyfus, 1991a). The other is always understood under certain aspects and conditions. Respect for commonalities and differences between the researcher and the researched as embodied member participants and others requires dialogue and listening that allow the voice of the other to be heard or reveal silence. No claims can be made that the other will be understood completely because human beings and worlds are not objects and cannot be frozen in time or explicated fully. Furthermore, the interpreter can never escape his or her own taken-for-granted background or stance that creates the possibility of an interpretive foreground.

Seeing and saying what something is *not* (its absence or opposite) is a form of understanding and may help clarify when an insider's description has been achieved. However, oppositional understanding (describing phenomena in dichotomies or opposites), or defining things in terms of what they are *not*, is an insufficient endpoint for an interpretive project. Naming the silences is a similar form of saying what is not there, but saying what is not there is always privileged by one's own expectations, sets, and world (Hauerwas, 1990). Naming the silences and describing participants and groups in terms of what they are not are critical movements in interpretive phenomenology that cannot stand alone. Defining or describing marginalized groups or other cultures only with respect to their difference from the dominant culture or one's own culture qualifies as cultural imperialism (Taylor, 1991). Feminists have pointed out this problem in the study of women's lives and practices (Fox-Keller, 1985; Gordon, 1991; Keller, 1986; Ruddick, 1989; Tronto, 1993). If the "self" is defined as a self created by individuation and separation, that is, the separatist self of possession (Sandel, 1982; Taylor, 1989), then the ways that all selves are socially constituted by relationship, habits, skills, and cultural practices are excluded and invisible. Defining men, women, and cultural groups in terms of what they are not gives an incoherent and often a denigrating picture of what they are. Likewise, accounts of difference without accounts of commonalities also set up false dichotomies and oppositions.

Levels of Analysis and Voice

The interpreter seeks to hear and understand the voice of the participants. It is expected that this voice is not a privatized, purely subjective voice but rather an embodiment and lived understanding of a world and set of local clearings created by social groups, practices, skills, history, and situated events (see Plager, Chapter 4 of this book; Borgmann, 1984; Dreyfus, 1991a, 1991b). The interpretive researcher strives to accurately present the voice of the participants. After presenting the participants' voice, the interpreter moves to a level of commentary that considers the first level of presentation from various interpretive vantage points (see Chesla, Chapter 9 of this book, p. 163). Interpretive commentary should clarify the meanings of the first level description and articulation.

The goal of interpretative commentary is neither a total systems account nor a single-factor theory. Interpretive commentaries or theories are not considered more "real" or "true" than the text itself. The interpreter seeks to give greater access and understanding of the text in its own terms, allowing the reader to notice meanings and qualitative distinctions within the text. Reducing an interpretive account to terms or models of power, exchange, role negotiation, ego psychology, adaptation, or nursing is not viewed as an advance over understanding of the text in its own terms. These theoretical moves for the sake of interpretive commentary, however, present limited ways of considering the first level of analysis.

The ethical stance of the interpretive researcher is one of respect for the voice and experience described in the text. The guiding ethos is to be true to the text. Throughout the interpretive project the researcher asks, "What do I now know or see that I did not expect or understand before I began reading the text?" If the interpreter's own views have not been challenged, extended, or turned around, the quality of the account is questioned and the danger of just reading in preconceptions must be considered.

At the heart of interpretive phenomenology is engaged reasoning in transitions (Benner, 1994; Taylor, 1993). Understanding is historical and must be understood historically. Thus the researcher keeps track of movements in understanding: "When I understood the text from this aspect, I saw these issues and themes, but when I began to consider conflicting stories and events and to hear certain arguments within the text, I was able to see new issues and new clearings." Typically there are false starts, but a rejected false start is an advance on understanding. Writing is part of the intellectual work of doing interpretation; therefore, interpretation is best served if these false starts are captured in writing. Misunderstanding can illuminate the interpreter's own taken-for-granted background.

Teaching and Learning Interpretive Phenomenology

One might despair of teaching interpretive phenomenology because in this technical age we have come to think of teaching as information and technology transfer, and teaching strategies are thought to consist primarily of breaking things down into separate behaviors and units that can then be applied to a whole range of situations. For example, the problem-solving processes of assessment, planning, intervening, and evaluating are taught as a general way to approach situations. These strategies of "unitizing and generalizing" (Guignon, 1983, p. 34) or representing and intervening (Hacking, 1983), both forms of disengaged reasoning, have become synonymous with "method" and with teaching or "transferring knowledge." But these methods work best in new situations where the person does not have experiential understanding of the situation.

Analysis of a novel situation more closely approximates an artificial intelligence or information-processing approach in that a computer must always build situations up element by element (Dreyfus, 1979; Dreyfus & Dreyfus, 1991). An elemental or criterial analysis of the situation misses experiential gains achieved in moving from situation A to situation B and therefore does not mimic human expertise in engaged reasoning—that is, the ability to approach a situation with a background understanding and to ask questions of the situation from this background, keeping track of the gains and losses in understanding (Dreyfus & Dreyfus, 1986; Taylor, 1993).

Criterial reasoning (artificial intelligence or linear problem solving) cannot account for the capacity to perceive which problems are salient (Benner & Wrubel, 1982) or even the ability to read a situation. By design, traditional rational calculation strategies overlook the ability to understand human worlds, context, and temporality (Benner & Wrubel, 1989; Dreyfus, 1979, 1991a; Dreyfus & Dreyfus, 1986). However, interpretive phenomenology can be taught much like literary criticism. The learner must first learn the philosophical background to interpretive phenomenology (see Chapters 1-4) so that the background assumptions about the primacy of the everyday world of practices, meanings, habits, and skills are seen in new ways based on a critique of traditional epistemology. Common meanings of researchers and participants allow for sensible disagreements as well as understanding (Taylor, 1989). Although complete incommensurability is possible, it is assumed to be a rare occurrence limited to historical eras, cultural traditions, or physical experiences that one has not participated in and cannot imagine (Kuhn, 1991).

Learning the skills of interpretive phenomenology comes much more easily once the ontological concerns are recovered and the researcher is able to shift from questions about what it is to know (epistemology) to questions about why and how we "know" some things and not others and what constitutes our knowing (ontology). The dialogical process of learning to create, understand, and interpret texts begins with preexisting abilities to understand world, read texts for meanings, and extend those everyday capacities with rigor and attentiveness to interpretive research. Although many situated maxims and strategies can be taught in working with specific texts, it is impossible to formalize all the possible areas of learning that a particular student will need in order to develop insightful best-account interpretations of particular texts.

Interpretive phenomenology calls for the ability to do engaged reasoning in particular situations and particular texts. In this sense it is analogous to doing clinical reasoning. Perhaps this is why nursing students can be taught this approach more easily if they are expert clinicians. Expert clinicians understand reasoning in transitions because they are used to comparing directly one practical world with another in their clinical practice. It is not accidental that the study of practical knowledge, like the study of all knowledge development, requires taken-for-granted practical knowledge about understanding and reading human situations. Knowledge from a practice such as nursing, teaching, medicine, or law can create enhanced perceptual recognition skills, as is evident in Doolittle's study (Chapter 11) of recovery from stroke, in which her expertise as a neuroscience clinical nurse specialist creates an interpretive lens, or in Chesla's study (Chapter 9), in which her family therapy and psychiatric nursing expertise locates her lines of inquiry and provides the skills required for being with and interviewing participants with schizophrenia. Nurses often come with superb interviewing skills. They are accustomed to getting the person's story in a wide variety of settings: home, community, and institutions. The researcher's own background practical knowledge is considered as part of the perceptual lens, enabling skills and limits for conducting the study. Thus the starting point for teaching interpretive skills is to extend reasoning skills and increase researchers' ability to be reflective about the impact of their own background on articulating practical, everyday understandings and knowledge of their research participants. At the same time, clinicians must critically reflect on their usual assumptions of clinical expertise that filter the data only through clinical and health related concerns. The clinician, who is accustomed to functioning in the immediacy of the situation, must learn patience with reflection, poring over the same text, considering it from multiple perspectives with no view of action or intervention in mind. This increased reflectiveness involves a profound shift in sense of agency and self-understanding.

Interpreting a text analogue from everyday practices and concerns is more difficult than reading a constructed written piece of literature that has been composed by the author with the intent of communicating a particular world or perspective. The author of a written text has already struggled with the first level of articulation, whereas research participants will tell stories and events and perform in situations in ways about which they may not have thought. For example, an expert clinician is seldom aware of the highly skilled, taken-for-granted areas of practice. A range of situations and narratives may be required to disclose meaningful patterns and repeated concerns. Taylor (1985b, p. 27) calls interpreting these action texts "proto-'interpretation.'"

Commonalities and Differences

The goal of interpretive phenomenology is to uncover commonalities and differences, not private idiosyncratic events or understandings. In rational empirical studies, the strategy for achieving patterns, trends, and common-alities is to decontextualize, that is, to objectify by removing all the histori-cal, timing, and world aspects that will create accurate predictions when circumstances or self-understandings do not change or when learning or transformation does not occur. Increased prediction is achieved with greater levels of abstraction (Taylor, 1964, 1985c). This strategy works well only when taken-for-granted aspects of the world continue to be stable. For example, economists make predictions based upon assumptions of continued cultural patterns, preferences, and concerns. If these change, their predictions of buying and selling and markets change radically (Taylor, 1985c, p. 42). The threats to validity listed in traditional rational-empirical texts, such as maturation, history, and learning, are all aspects of human agency, world, and temporality that form the interpretive phenomenological project, so controlling for them by excluding them makes it impossible to uncover transitions that occur over time (Wrubel, 1985). Nevertheless, interpretive phenomenologists, though interested in distinctions and differences, are also interested in what human conditions and commonalities make these distinc-tions and differences possible. They look for commonalities not in determi-nistic laws or mechanisms but rather in culturally grounded meanings.

Five sources of commonality explored in phenomenology are (Benner & Wrubel, 1989):

1. *Situation.* This includes an understanding of how the person is situated, both historically and currently. Questions related to situation are whether the situation is understood as a situation of smooth social functioning or as a breakdown situation of novelty, error, confusion, or conflict.

2. *Embodiment.* This includes an understanding of embodied knowing that encompasses skillful comportment and perceptual and emotional responses. Phenomenology explores embodied understandings of the situation in highly skilled, taken-for-granted bodily responses such as an early recognition of

impending patient crisis as a result of perceptual acuity and pattern recognition, or anticipatory nausea experienced by a patient approaching a chemotherapy situation (Benner, 1985a, 1985b, 1991; Doolittle, 1990; Kesselring, 1990; Schilder, 1986).

3. *Temporality.* The experience of lived time is the way one projects oneself into the future and understands oneself from the past. Temporality is more than a linear succession of moments. It includes the qualitative, lived experience of time or timelessness (see Leonard, Chapter 3). For example, in a chronic illness, one's sense of time may be radically altered.

4. *Concerns.* Concerns are the way the person is oriented meaningfully in the situation (Benner & Wrubel, 1989; Heidegger, 1927/1962, 1975; Wrubel, 1985). Concerns will dictate what will show up as salient and therefore what will be noticed in the situation. They constitute what matters to the person.

5. *Common meanings.* These are taken-for-granted linguistic and cultural meanings that create what is noticed and what are possible issues, agreements, and disagreements between people. For example, a classroom situation is predicated on certain taken-for-granted meanings about what it is to be a teacher or a student. Even the disagreements about what it is to be a teacher or a student depend upon taken-for-granted understandings that allow meaningful distinctions and disagreements to occur (Dreyfus, 1991a).

Developing Lines of Inquiry and Examining Modes of Engagement

Interpretive questions are explicated along with the reasons for those particular questions (Packer, 1985). Interpretive researchers critically reflect on what their biases and blind spots might be and why they think the questions that they are asking are relevant. They follow this critical reflective exercise by recreating a sense of openness and ability to hear questions and challenges to their questions that they had not even considered prior to encountering the text. This creates a true dialogue and not a monological question-asking and answering exchange. The participants' own practical worlds and concerns must challenge the initial questions. The researcher makes explicit as many assumptions as possible prior to beginning the study and establishes boundaries to the lines of inquiry for the study, but these must be held tentatively and allowed to be challenged, altered, extended, and transformed by what is learned in the field. Interpretive phenomenologists are similar to cultural anthropologists, who try to be clear about their own culture prior to entering another culture but who expect to have their own cultural assumptions made visible and challenged in new ways by actually living in the culture. The ability to have initial questions challenged is an essential discipline of interpretive phenomenology.

Strategies for creating openness to the other and confrontations with differences and similarities are central to good interpretive phenomenology. The design of interpretive research is created by establishing lines of inquiring and considering how to study both smooth functioning and breakdown situations. Studying disease does not explicate the nature of health. Lines of inquiry are critically evaluated for what they allow the researcher to consider and what they exclude. Lines of inquiry, while phrased as questions, should be sufficiently broad and open so that they can be altered, shaped, and reexamined by the dialogue with the actual text. For example, in a study of mid-career men coping with stress at work (Benner, 1984b), I started with the broad lines of inquiry about work stress. As the study progressed, it became apparent that work functioned as a major coping resource in the lives of the men I studied and that this was true even for the men who "hated" their work. Work is such a central source of identity, way of structuring time, and means for all other aspects of life (housing, food, shelter, leisure, social status, and so on) that it serves as a coping resource, an identity anchor, and a source of pride and satisfaction or worthy adversary. I had to reconsider my initial question that assumed work was stressful and a frequent source of alienation and meaninglessness. In fact, the "stress" of the work often gave it added importance for the participants as they heroically faced the aggravation and stress of their work. As long as I was in the stance of examining all the ways that work was stressful, I could not make sense of large portions of text that pointed to work as a major coping resource. Work for my North American participants gave a sense of place and identity, and contrary to the common myth of the home as the "safe haven from the heartless work world," work was often comforting, offering a sense of control, mastery, and predictability that the intense relationships of family life did not necessarily offer. Clearly, the lines of inquiry about work stress shaped the study, but the people's narratives about their private and work lives required me to critically reconsider my questions (Benner, 1984b).

Study Design, Evolution and Dialogue, Capturing Transitions

On the basis of the lines of inquiry, one chooses the sources of text and a sample of situations that may include individual or group interviews, participant observation, videotapes, documents, public writings, media, and many sources of data as illustrated in the studies in Part 2 of this book. Because the goal of interpretive phenomenology is understanding, multiple interviews are preferred in that they give interviewers the opportunity to carefully review the tape prior to the next interview. This allows the researcher and participant a second chance to make sure that understanding has occurred. Often the interviewer will fail to ask an "obvious" question, assuming that he or she understands the participant's story, terms, descriptions, and feelings. Reading the prior interview allows the researcher to clarify initial interpretations and thus to ask crucial descriptive questions overlooked before. Clarifying questions and probes paraphrase and follow up on topics from the prior interview: "When you said in the last interview that you do not like to take medications, how does that influence the way you take your asthma medications?" Additional probes may be asked to move the participant to describing how "not taking medications" actually occurs in everyday practice.

Description is not as easy or straightforward as it might seem. In the early stages of the interviewing process, critique and review from other researchers help uncover blind spots or systematically avoided questions. For example, if the interviewer has high death anxiety, he or she may fail to pursue participants' discussions of dying. Interpretative dialogue begins with the first interview so that data collection, inquiry, and analysis are not separated. This allows the researcher to pursue lines of questioning that are generated by the study itself, ensuring dialogue.

Sample size is limited by the size of the text that will be generated and the number of researchers available to analyze the text. The sample may consist of events or critical incidents as well as individuals or groups of participants. A sample size is projected at the beginning of the study, but this is often adjusted depending on the quality of the text and the way that the lines of inquiry are reshaped by the participants. In considering the sample size, the researcher plans, where possible, for repeated observations or interviews with the same participants. These repeated interviews increase the text and must be considered in planning the sample size. For example, my dissertation sample included 12 interviews each with 23 participants, yielding 276 interviews (Benner, 1984b). Though such a large text required a great deal of reading time, it made the interpretation easier because a great deal of richness and redundancy in the multiple interviews made meanings and coping patterns more visible and increased my confidence about understanding the practical worlds of the participants. A large text that provides redundancy, clarity, and confidence in the text is more plausible and reliable than a small text covering an inadequate range of situations.

The Communicative Context:
Interviewing, Conversing, and Engaging in Dialogue

Because interpretive phenomenologists study everyday practical knowledge and events, the communicative context is set up in naturalistic ways so that the participants do not feel unduly awkward and constrained by the research interview or foreign, abstract language. For example, early in the Lazarus Stress and Coping Project (Benner, 1984b; Lazarus & Folkman, 1984; Schaefer, 1983) we asked our pilot participants about their "emotions," only to find that people don't ordinarily have "emotions," though they feel strongly, or "good" or "bad," about things. By phrasing the question in foreign, academic (abstract) terms, we cut participants off from their everyday language use, thereby cutting them off from their ordinary spontaneous responses. Once we put our questions in more conversational language, people could talk about or deny their feelings in their ordinary patterns. Beginning researchers often have difficulty translating their lines of inquiry into answerable questions with normal conversational language. They must imagine the context of the concerns and events they wish to hear about and develop ordinary language to stimulate narrative accounts. The role of storytelling is central to interpretive phenomenology because when people structure their own narrative accounts, they can tap into their more immediate experiences, and the problem of generating false generalities or ideologies is diminished. But beginning interpretive researchers and participants have to be coached to generate narrative accounts because participants may expect to give only "facts" and "opinions." The interviewer has to learn to listen to the story with as little interruption as possible. And the participant must be instructed that narrative accounts of events, situations, feelings, and actions are wanted.

Establishing a familiar communicative context is also achieved by observing and interviewing participants in the situation of interest. For example, in the study of skill acquisition (Benner, 1984a; Benner, Tanner, & Chesla, 1992), we included informal interviews as well as observations in the workplace because, in the context of the situation, the sights, sounds, smells, and demands experienced become visible in ways that simply do not occur to the participant outside the situation. Much of our knowledge is retrievable only in our situated actions (Suchman, 1987). A level of ordinary engagement is difficult, if not impossible, to create outside the situation. Narrative memory and practical knowledge are solicited by our being in the familiar circumstances of performance.

The small group interview too is an effective way to set up a familiar communicative context and dialogue. The assumption is that any organized social practice, such as nursing, has knowledge and notions of the good internal to it (MacIntyre, 1981). In our studies of nursing practice and skill acquisition (Benner, 1984a; Benner, Tanner, & Chesla, in press) we interviewed nurses who had spent similar amounts of time in their clinical practice and who, by the appraisal of their supervisors, were at a similar skill level. We instructed them to tell their stories directly to one another and coached the participants to be active listeners, asking clarifying questions when they could not understand another's story. We had two researchers in the interview actively listening so that we could maximize our own reflective capacities by "double" listening. What one researcher picked up or missed could be augmented by the other. We specifically asked the nurses to talk to one another as they might do over coffee, trying to establish a familiar context for narrative accounts.

Nurses were asked to talk directly to one another rather than talking down or up to the researchers. We were trying to capture natural language and discourse that would occur between peer clinicians. We were also trying to decrease "performance" anxiety by focusing on the story and allowing one another to discover the socially embedded commonalities and contrasts within the stories. We encouraged other nurses to respond with similar or dissimilar stories that were brought to mind by the story just told.

The whole group interview session becomes a discourse in practical reasoning because one story organized around particular concerns raises either confirming or disconfirming stories. Aristotle called this type of practical moral reasoning *phronesis* (Aristotle, 1985). For example, when several stories were told about heroic treatment that had become futile, prolonging dying rather than promoting recovery, a counter-story would almost always be told about the danger of being too certain that there was no hope of recovery. These counter-stories seemed to function in the clinician's own practice by keeping open rather than foreclosing clinical possibility (Benner, Wrubel, & Phillips, in progress). Thus small group interviews achieve several purposes.

1. They create a natural communicative context for telling stories from practice, allowing peers to talk to one another as they ordinarily talk rather than translating their clinical world for the researchers.
2. They provide a rich basis for active listening when more than one listener is trying to understand the story.
3. Meanings of the stories can be enriched by stories triggered to counter, contrast, or bring up similarities. In our study, the links between stories were often indirect and surprising. What the story reminded another about often revealed aspects of the story and clarified the participant's understanding of the story.

4. The small group simulates a work environment. In our study, hearing other nurses' stories created a forum for thinking and talking about work situations.

Narrative accounts of actual situations differ from questions about opinions, ideology, or even what one does in general because the speaker is engaged in remembering what occurred in the situation. Spoken accounts allow the speaker to give more details and include concerns and considerations that shape the person's experience and perception of the event. A story of an event is remembered in terms of the participant's concerns and understanding of the situation. Therefore narrative accounts are meaningful accounts that point to what is perceived, what is worth noticing, and what concerned the storyteller (Rubin, in press). Narrative accounts of actual situations give a closer access to practice and practical knowledge than do questions about beliefs, ideology, theory, or generalized accounts of what people typically do in practice. Therefore narratives can be used to examine discontinuities between theory and practice. Interviewers listen intently to the story without interrupting the speaker unless they can no longer follow the story at all. Then probes are asked to get the speaker to fill in unclear aspects or details of the story. It is important to allow the storyteller to tell the story in his or her own way without interruption so that the speaker is telling about the event. The interviewer can go back and ask for clarification of the details of the story. He or she can find out what the participant means by common phrases such as "I was really upset" or "I tried not to take it personally" by asking questions such as "What would you have looked like to others if they had seen you upset?" "Did you do anything to express that you were upset?" "How could you have taken it personally?" "What would that have been like for you?" Such questions may feel like asking the "obvious" in the context of the story, but those who ask the most obvious questions get the best descriptions, and often the participant's answers are not what the researcher would have anticipated. Such questions allow the speaker to stay in the situation and expand his or her understanding. If someone talks about being afraid, the researcher must not assume that she or he understands what the participant fears. Staying concrete and descriptive in the interview allows for thick descriptions of significance issues and moral concerns (Geertz, 1973, 1983). Rich accounts of the nature and meaning of emotional responses allow access to moral concerns (Benner, in press; Taylor, 1985, Vol. 1, p. 62).

Multiple interviews are helpful because they allow the interviewer to listen to the interview again or, if they are transcribed, to read them for gaps or blinds spots. Common phrases that are in vogue must be clarified so that the researcher understands the participant's particular meaning of the phrase (Tanner, Benner, Chesla, & Gordon, 1993). Imaginative and pictorial language may help—for example, asking, "How would you think that looked to others?" "Do you think anyone else would have known how you were feeling?" "How would your friend have responded to this situation?" By introducing practical contrasts, participants can often give a much fuller account of their own perspective and practical knowledge. In small group interviews the presence of two researcher-listeners can increase the quality of hearing what is said and left unsaid.

Engaged, active listening leads to probes to clarify whether understanding has occurred. It is good to clarify interpretations with the participant. This can be done by paraphrasing what the speaker has said. This clarification stance puts the researcher at risk for "putting words into the participant's mouth" or asking leading questions. The researcher avoids these errors by staying as close to the participant's account as possible, offering interpretations tentatively, and leaving open and enhancing the participant's ability to disagree. Some common strategies help equalize the power between the participant and researcher and allow the participant to disagree with the researcher. First, the most general, least inferential questions must be asked, and closer paraphrasing or interpretative questions are offered only after the direction of the participant's response is understood. When possible, the researcher gives the participant at least two ways of paraphrasing a situation, offering two naturally occurring alternatives from the situation just heard and keeping the question open for alternative interpretations generated by the participant. Depending on the line of inquiry, the interviewer may move directly into a dialogue with participant. A study conducted by Richard MacIntyre (1993) with HIV-positive gay men who were talking about their decisions about whether to have their T-cells counted demonstrates the power of familiar communicative contexts and dialogue. The dialogue was real, with acknowledgment of the researcher's own position. The participants' own positions showed up more clearly in the dialogue than they would in a hypothetically constructed stance or a more neutral and one-way conversation between the researcher and participants.

Interpretive researchers must confirm that they have understood the participants' stories, responses, and actions. Open listening, allowing the interviewee to shape the telling of the story, and getting a larger contextual story of the person's life and situation limit the interviewer's structuring of participants' responses and assists with understanding parts of the story that follow. The threat that the interviewer will shape what is remembered or considered salient is ever-present. The underlying assumption is that no one precise story exists, but rather multiple stories that are shaped by the particular clearing created by the interview situation. After open listening, the researcher follows up, making sure that he or she has understood what the person has said. This is a form of active listening in which the interviewer paraphrases his or her own understanding of what has been said with a questioning and open voice: "Let me see if I understand what you were saying. . . ." The interviewer's goal is to empower the participant to tell the story in his or her own words. Conveying a genuine interest in understanding the participant, along with the use of natural language and communication contexts, increases the participant's effort and ability to communicate. Participants may be inarticulate and nonreflective, and the goal is to learn even from the most silent participant. However, the researcher does not want to create false silences by ineptitude in speaking the participant's language or setting up a strange communicative context.

Interviewing for interpretive phenomenology requires training and critical reflection on the part of the researcher. For example, in reading the research interview, the researcher critically evaluates his or her own avoidance, silence, or inability to follow up on or hear about certain concerns and meanings. A critique by other researchers can help one identify blind spots and areas of avoidance. Multiple interviews give the interviewer a chance to clarify what was left unexamined in the prior interview.

Narrative and Practical Knowledge

Narrative accounts of everyday skillful comportment allow participants to describe their everyday concerns and practical knowledge, thereby giving access to practical worlds. One analytic strategy would be to identify strategies, structures, and processes in the narrative. This would require theorizing or moving to a theoretical framework, such as conflict processes, power relationships, or role negotiation, for analyzing the narrative, as is often done in Grounded Theory (Corbin & Strauss, 1990; Glaser & Strauss, 1967). Or one might examine the text only in relation to the preestablished lines of inquiry. In both cases the power of engaging one indirect discourse with another practical world would be lost because the texts were not allowed to generate their own dialogue and aspects of comparison and similarity. The distinction is between making comparisons on theoretical terms generated by the text and making comparisons about the issues and clearings created in contrasting practical lived worlds. The aim of interpretive phenomenology is to use indirect discourse to uncover naturally occurring concerns and meanings. Three narrative strategies provide the basis for entering practical worlds and understanding socially embedded knowledge: (a) paradigm cases, (b) thematic analysis, and (c) exemplars.

Paradigm Cases

Paradigm cases are the most usual point of entering the dialogue with the text. Paradigm cases are strong instances of concerns or ways of being in the world, doing a practice, or taking up a project. To identify a paradigm case does not require the researcher to identify in advance what he or she is "looking for." Nor does it require determining what the contrast cases might be prior to collecting them. Researchers may choose to begin the interpretive analysis with a paradigm case that they think they understand well or may choose to do a case that they find puzzling or unsettling. This is a discovery process that allows the everyday skills of perception and understanding to guide the selection of the paradigm case. Usually one has some notions about the paradigm case. For example, when beginning to develop a paradigm case about a carpenter who "hated his work," I later discovered that this man was as much or more lost and depressed than anyone when he was out of work. So I had to revise my initial understanding of alienation and disengagement from work. It turned out that he had an engaged, adversarial form of connection to his work. Though he did "hate his work," he also drew structure, challenge and a large measure of his sense of self from meeting his adversary daily, and became depressed, falling into a "drink nap" routine, when not working (Benner, 1984b). This open descriptive approach to the initial identification of paradigm cases allows the researcher to understand the case in its own terms. Though it helps to clarify why the researcher thinks she or he is choosing the paradigm case, this is only an assumption that must be challenged once the interpreter begins to read the case.

First, the whole interview text is read for a global understanding of the story. Then topics, issues, concerns, or events are selected for a more detailed interpretation. Often it is helpful to look at the way the speaker moves from one topic to another or, in a small group interview, to look at what similar and dissimilar stories are created by hearing a particular story. The interpreter seeks to identify the everyday reasoning and associations made by the participants. A systematic moving from the parts back to the whole text allows the interpreter check for incongruities, puzzles, and unifying repeated concerns. The interpreter does not assume that the text will be "rational" or that there will be a match between ideology and practice. Nor is the assumption made that the interpreter will exhaust the meaning of the text. The goal is to present the text as fully as possible, identifying puzzles, incongruities, and mysteries. This is a phenomenological corrective to the hermeneutics of faith or suspicion. In a hermeneutics of faith, one looks for the concerns and notions of good that the participants are living out. In a hermeneutics of suspicion, one is trying to identify through theoretical terms, such as "power relationships" or "independence and dependency," or larger theoretical systems, such as psychoanalysis, ego psychology, or a Marxist theory of culture, what is going on in the text. In contrast, the interpretive researcher seeks an insider's account. Understandings of the researcher are confirmed or negated by the participant where possible, or else consensual validation is sought from people who have a similar experience or culture.

The interpretive phenomenologist seeks to understand the language used by the participants. Typically this interpretation will be "clearer" than the experience itself, and in that sense the interpretation focuses the lived experience. By using whole paradigm cases, the interpreter offers the reader an opportunity to engage in the practical world of the participant and come closer to the lived experience, the understanding of the transition as it unfolds, or a particular way of being in the world (Heidegger, 1927/1962). Often this practical engagement with everyday understandings of the world will challenge existing theoretical perspectives (see Chapters 8, 9, 10, and 15). The sources of commonality within the text are not assumed to be generated by a particular form of logic or rationality (see p. 102). Nor does one seek to reduce the text by the use of one single-factor or multifactorial theory. The text is assumed to be meaningful if only in being an account of poorly understood events (Rubin, 1984). The text is meaningful in that it participates in and flows from multiple traditions, particular language, a socially organized set of practices, and a variety of experiences, all of which form a community and a culture. The interpreter seeks to articulate those multiple aspects of the text, identifying the naturally occurring questions and dialogue within the text, and to articulate the understandings created by the process of reading the text (Taylor, 1991, 1992).

Once one paradigm case is developed, a second case is examined in its own terms and in light of the first paradigm case. After completing the paradigm case as fully as possible, the researcher asks questions such as: "How would Paradigm Case A (the "case" can be a group, person, community, or event) act or respond, or how would the event unfold in this situation?" "What would happen if the context were different?" "Would the same issues and concerns show up for the two cases?" "What events, concerns, and issues show up in Paradigm Case A that do not show up in Paradigm Case B?" The practical world of one paradigm case creates a basis for comparison of similarities and differences with other paradigm cases. This is similar to Kierkegaard's use of indirect discourse, in which dialogue is created through letters (narratives about spheres of existence or world) between different people in different worlds (Rubin, 1984). The aesthete corresponds and engages in dialogue with Judge William, who is firmly grounded in the ethical world. Through their different concerns and eyes we more fully see the practical world of both. One naturally occurring practical world sheds light on another.

This is similar to cross-cultural comparisons, in which cultural meanings and patterns are examined in their own terms but are sharpened and clarified by cross-cultural differences and similarities. A phenomenological account has advantages over moving too quickly to a theoretical level of discourse because it allows practical meanings and concerns to show up in their own terms. This follows the interpretive phenomenological assumption that practices and concerns are a way of being and knowing in their own right. One does not imagine that there is a greater "truth" behind the text (Dreyfus, 1991a).

Paradigm cases are used as a strategy of perceptual recognition and understanding early in the research process, but they are also used as a presentation strategy. By the time they are used in the writing-up process, it should be clear to the researcher why the particular paradigm cases are chosen and what contrasts and similarities are being made between the cases, and the reader should be given enough textual evidence to challenge the researcher's practical reasoning.

Thematic Analysis

A thematic analysis may also be done across cases to clarify distinctions and similarities. The analysis is called thematic because meaningful patterns, stances, or concerns are considered rather than more elemental units such as words or phrases (see Chesla, Chapter 9). The interpreter moves back and forth between portions of the text and portions of the analysis (from themes and situations, and from thematic analyses to paradigm cases). This shifting between texts and between parts and wholes of the text allows the interpreter to confront and develop new interpretive questions. Inconsistencies and even incoherent aspects of the text may be encountered. The interpreter struggles to understand the text, but this struggle must not end in making the practical world more rational, coherent, or consistent than it really is. People live with great incongruities between different spheres of their lives (Leonard, 1993). Also there can be great gaps between stated ideologies and beliefs and actual practices (MacIntyre, 1993). This is where the researcher confronts all the ways in which real lives and actual practices are not like a literary text, which has internal consistency and perspective and whose destination and conclusion are already known (Wrubel, 1985). Lives are projected into an ambiguous future, and the past and present are experienced in qualitatively different ways (Merleau-Ponty, 1962). One can have an account of inconsistencies and incongruities that may or may not be recognized by participants. Because

there are sources of commonalities between embodied human beings constituted by similar cultures, we do have access to dialogue and understanding.
Though we do not all experience or live in the same worlds, these worlds can
be described, talked about, and discovered. Even bias, often considered only
negatively, is an essential aspect of everyday understanding and perceptual
grasp (Gadamer, 1975; Merleau-Ponty, 1962). We always come to a situation
with expectations, sets, and a preunderstanding (Benner & Wrubel, 1989),
and depending on our ability to be open and listen, these biases and preunderstandings can be challenged and changed. Dialogue cannot occur without
our own personal knowledge (Polanyi, 1958) being challenged. This process
requires that the interpretive researcher develop coping skills and personal
knowledge. For example, students who enter research as a way of gaining
distance and control that they could not achieve in their clinical practice may
find interpretive phenomenology in conflict with their intellectual and personal goals. Likewise the clinician who is comfortable with action, even
inarticulate action, may have difficulty learning the skills of description and
uncovering the "obvious" (the taken for granted). As noticed earlier, the
action-oriented clinician may feel impatient with the level and demands of
reflection required by interpretive research.

Just as the interpretive researcher moves back and forth between the parts
and the whole of the text, the stance of the interpreter must shift from
understanding and imaginatively dwelling in the world of the participant to
distancing and questioning the participant's world as other. The interpretive
researcher engages in cycles of understanding, interpretation, and critique.
It is a common experience during the initial phase of identifying and understanding to idealize the situation and participant. This can serve as a positive
bias as long as it is later held up for scrutiny and corrected. It is difficult to
understand the world of another if his or her world is objectified or rejected.
An interpretive maxim is that the other person's world is livable. Total
rejection or excessive idealization means that the interpreter has not yet
grasped the lived world of the participant or situation. When the researcher
experiences total rejection or acceptance of a situation or participant, this is
usually a sign that the complexity, particularity, and otherness of the situation
or participant have not been adequately understood, and it is at this point that
an interpretive colleague should be brought in to provide an alternative
interpretation and perspective.

Exemplars

Paradigm cases can be augmented by exemplars and thematic analyses.
Once the interpretive researcher has identified a pattern of meaning, common

situation, or embodied experience, exemplars may be extracted from the text to demonstrate the similarity or contrast. Exemplars convey aspects of a paradigm case or a thematic analysis. Exemplars substitute for "operational" definitions in interpretive research because they allow the researcher to demonstrate intents and concerns within contexts and situations in which the "objective" attributes of the situation might be quite different. For example, multiple exemplars of the healing relationship (Benner, 1984a) may transcend traditional clinical boundaries, and each exemplar may add nuances and qualitative distinctions that were unavailable in previous exemplars. A range of exemplars allows one to establish a cultural field of relationships and distinctions. In developing clinical promotion programs for nurses, exemplars are used to illustrate characteristic performance of different caring practices and diagnostic and monitoring skills of nurses (Benner, 1984a; Benner & Benner, in progress). The continued collection of exemplars can capture a growing, living tradition.

In developing a research report, the goal is to develop a range of exemplars that allows the reader to recognize the distinctions the interpretive researcher is making in practice. This is evident in the exemplars that Chesla (Chapter 9) uses to illustrate different parental care patterns. The pattern of "engaged care" is not a set of techniques, procedures, or behaviors, but rather a way of being a parent. It is the working out of a particular tradition of being a parent. With the use of exemplars, Chesla is able to illustrate the large pattern of engaged care so that a clinician could recognize the pattern, without presenting a narrow, objectified, formulaic account of this mode of engagement. Theoretically, the collection of exemplars is open-ended because it is not possible to completely explicate or freeze a particular cultural meaning, concern, or habitus (Benner, 1984a; Bourdieu, 1990). In doing interpretation, keeping track of exemplars selected as illustrative of a pattern allows the researcher to follow his or her own train of thought. The collection and aggregation of exemplars is central to the interpretive task. The researcher is developing his or her practical reasoning and understanding in the exemplars and usually can see an evolution in his or her understanding of qualitative distinctions. For example, in *From Novice to Expert* (Benner, 1984a) I had not initially delineated distinctions between the coaching function of "making culturally avoided aspects of an illness approachable and understandable" and the healing function of "creating a climate for and establishing a commitment to healing" (pp. 49-94). Indeed, "finding an acceptable interpretation or understanding of the illness, pain, fear, anxiety, or other stressful emotion," an aspect of coaching, was also an aspect of the healing relationship, but the coaching role had more to do with social negotiation and working with the patient's understanding of illness, treatment and recovery. It was only through many distinct exemplars that these nuances were established. In the interpretive process, these exemplars were all grouped together, and it was only through further refinement of the grouping of similarities and dissimilarities of the exemplars that the two practical intents and distinctions were clarified. The goal is to make qualitative distinctions having to do with intents and meanings. These qualitative distinctions are not the same as establishing mutually exclusive categories with no shared attributes. For example, in nursing practice coaching involved a narrower set of practices with a different intent than the healing relationship, though sometimes coaching is integral to a healing relationship (Benner, 1984a). By identifying both intents and practices in their contexts, each became clearer. This is an articulation strategy that allows practical distinctions to be identified. The exemplars form a family resemblance to one another (Kuhn, 1970).

Exemplars can become teaching and curriculum documents that give the clinician (nurse, physician, teacher, social worker, lawyer) concrete examples of distinctions made in practice. This is different from the traditional approach used in casuistry, in which quandary or puzzle cases are presented to teach principles or illustrate exceptions to rules (Jonsen & Toulmin, 1988) because the exemplars may or may not be breakdown or puzzle cases. Indeed, puzzle or breakdown exemplars are used only to illustrate contrasts to strong instances of the pattern, concern or meaning (Benner, Tanner, & Chesla, in press).

Sources of Text

It is beyond the scope of this chapter to discuss in detail the methodological issues and skills required to interpret different types of text, but multiple sources of text are always preferable. The interpretive studies in Part 2 of this book have a range of textual sources. The sources of text are selected depending on the lines of inquiry and with an eye toward context and studying typical and nontypical situated actions, breakdown, and smooth engaged action. Multiple data sources and contexts are preferred in order to create a more naturalistic account and to prevent an overly narrow perspective on the situation. Participant observation and interviewing in the situation are almost always required because taken-for-granted actions, skills, and habits will be too much a part of the participant's world to be discussed in interviews. The study of nonreflective aspects of the person's life requires observation and dialogue.

Narrative accounts are essential to gain access to the participants' ways of understanding and structuring the situation. Stories may be told for the first time or may be repeated, having been told many times before. This is an important distinction, since presumably a story told for the first time is more immediate and less structured by prior experience. However, a repeated story may be a rich source of uncovering qualitative distinctions and moral concerns because the emphases in the story may be more carefully constructed by the participant. The oft-told story is closer to shared memories, ideology, and beliefs than the unrehearsed first telling. For example, family lore is constructed through often-told stories, and these stories take on a life of their own, conveying the moral lessons and distinctions important to the family. That they have been told before and are subject to layers of social constructions does not make them less informative, but it is important for the interpretive researcher to make the distinction between a first-told story, which will be more immediate and closer to the lived experience, and a frequently told story. Direct first-person narrative accounts give a closer view of everyday lived understandings than generalizations about what one believes or what one usually does. The interpretive researcher may be interested in ideology, generalizations, and beliefs and how these relate to stories told and practices observed, but the distinctions and types of inferences that can be drawn are different between generalizations and narrative accounts or observations.

Videotapes of live, real-time events are particularly useful for studying craft and skills. Though it is expensive and time-consuming, a video camera can record continuous action and events and sequencing, noise sources, and responses to the environment that would be missed or altered by a person present in the room at intervals. Videotaping a therapy session or a nursing encounter and having the therapist or nurse talk about the video is yet another strategy for getting the participant's perspective. Videotape and photography have the advantage of disclosing aspects of the situation that may be overlooked or unattended by the participant observer intent on certain lines of inquiry. Televised documentaries and news clips (for example, news coverage of disaster studies) can also provide visual and textual data sources.

Photographs may also serve as visual textual sources (Savedra & Highley, 1988; Stainton, 1985). Because photography is a common cultural practice, having participants do their own photographic essays of their experience can give an access to their concerns and feelings that may not show up in conversation (Savedra & Highley, 1988). Photography gives another access to perception that may not be available to the participants. Photographs are valuable for demonstrating embodied skilled social practices. Postures, facial expressions, and responses can be captured by multiple photographs in varying situations.

Films, novels, biographies, or, in health and illness, first-person accounts of illness experiences can be rich sources of texts on everyday practical understanding. Specific illnesses have their own narratives based upon bodily and cultural commonalities (Frank, 1991; Kleinman, 1988). First-person experiential accounts reveal cultural meanings and moral dimensions of illness.

Naturally occurring social events, such as patient support groups, clinic visits, and encounters in waiting rooms, can be rich sources of everyday encounters and practices. Documents, patient records, and other unobtrusive measures can augment the textual sources created by the interviewer. These unobtrusive measures (Webb, Campbell, Schwartz, & Sechrest, 1966) offer a social record of communication patterns and actions. For example, Chesla (Benner, Tanner, & Chesla, in press) discovered that new graduate nurses typically structure their day by the various reports and documentation they are required to do. However, documentation is not typically constructed with this intent in mind. Uncovering the relationship required participant observation and a discussion of the documentation. The phenomena of interest must determine the design of the data collection and the selection of textual sources. The use of interpretive phenomenology for interpreting visual sources of data is not yet well developed, but visual data are central to many lines of inquiry amenable to interpretive phenomenology, particularly social practices, embodied skills, and the study of lived experience. Cultural anthropologists have long used visual data in their interpretive studies, and that body of literature can enrich written and verbal textual sources.

The Clearing, Body, and World

For Heidegger, the understanding of being is lodged in language, cultural conventions, social practices, and historical understandings, all of which create *the clearing* that allows us to encounter anything at all (see Plager, Chapter 4). Merleau-Ponty (1962) extended Heidegger's thought by discussing how the body is sentient and responds to meaningful situations. One's ways of being in the world are characterized by certain postures, gestures, habits, and skills. The social and lived body reveals long-term habits, meaning, and comportment that allow us to be in the world and be shaped by it. As Merleau-Ponty (1962, pp. 136-137) says:

> The life of consciousness—cognitive life, the life of desire or perceptual life—is subtended by an "intentional arc" which projects round about us our past, our future, our human setting, our physical, ideological and moral situation, or rather which results in our being situated in all these respects. It is this intentional arc which brings about the unity of the senses, of intelligence, of sensibility and motility. And it is this which "goes limp" in illness. . . .

It is in the same way theoretically understandable that mental illness may, in its turn, be linked with some bodily accident; consciousness projects itself into a physical world and has a body, as it projects itself into a cultural world and has its habits: because it cannot be consciousness without playing upon significances given either in the absolute past of nature or in its own personal past, and because any form of lived experience tends towards a certain generality whether that of our habits or that of our "bodily functions." These elucidations enable us clearly to understand motility as basic intentionality. Consciousness is in the first place not a matter of "I think that" but of "I can." [This term "I can" is the usual one used in Husserl's unpublished writings. Note by Merleau-Ponty]

Here the body is understood as irrevocably connected to the world. The body is set to action and is sentient, reflecting the understandings of the situation, so that by the time the nurse is at a competent level of performance she or he is already able to evaluate a situation by whether she or he feels confident, wary, unsure, or clear about what is going on and needs to be done (Benner, Tanner, & Chesla, 1992). Doolittle's research (See Chapter 11) on persons recovering from stroke captures their frustration when the once-familiar world no longer contains the same bodily meanings as the graspable rail or the climbable stairs. Kesselring (1990) captures the cancer patient's experience of living in the world of "I cannot" instead of the world of "I can." The body reflects the world where embodied social practices, postures, and gestures allow one to skillfully perceive, communicate, trade, negotiate, make love, work, and so forth. Likewise the world solicits the body engaging and training responses (see Schilder, 1986). McKeever's (1988) study of menopause illustrated the difficulty of standing outside oneself and describing physical changes. Menopause was experienced as vague, ambiguous, and associated with physical sensations, contextual events, and aging. Even so, common bodily and culturally imposed meanings could be described. Furthermore, describing the physical and emotional sides of the passage could help women to understand the transition and develop practical strategies to manage the symptoms and socially negotiate the transition (McKeever, 1988).

Clinical Ethnography

The term *clinical ethnography* represents the use of interpretive phenomenology in the study of illness experience (see Doolittle, Chapter 11). It follows in the ethnographic tradition of Geertz (1973, 1983). If meanings and self-understandings constitute the self and the situation, and one holds to the phenomenological paradox that the self both creates and is created by the situation, then clinical ethnography is a method well suited for studying meanings, distinctions of worth, associated emotions, practical knowledge, and physical signs and symptoms. A phenomenological approach to studying illness holds that cultural and social contexts create the conditions of possibility for the illness experience, coping, treatment, cure, and care. Areas of interest and sources of commonality in clinical ethnographies are:

1. Practical knowledge in terms of symptom perception, treatments, and resources
2. Skilled know-how evident in patterns of behavior, skilled actions, and self-care
3. Embodied knowledge and ways of being in relation to the illness, including bodily sensations, perceptions, emotional responses and feelings related to the illness, and social negotiation of the illness experience
4. A careful description of the lived experience and understanding of the illness
5. Informal models of causation
6. Self-care practices related to preventing and treating the illness
7. Help-seeking patterns, both professional and informal

Clinical ethnographies uncover practical experiential knowledge gained by patients in recovery or in management of a chronic illness. New therapies and practical knowledge about the actual skills associated with self-care in the context of daily living may be uncovered. Instead of looking for "compliance" or "noncompliance," the clinical ethnographer seeks to understand the illness, self-care, skilled know-how, illness meanings, and coping patterns of the person in the situation. This approach can help the clinician better understand the issues of caring for an illness. The focus is on understanding rather than explanation because explaining the disease without understanding the illness and care issues does not enable the clinician or patient to learn and care for the illness in his or her own context (Benner, 1985b, 1994; Doolittle, 1990; see also Benner et al., Chapter 12 of this book). One may explain all the pathophysiology without ever addressing the practical issues of how to manage symptoms, adjust medications, or prevent complications in the context of one's daily life.

The word *clinical,* as it is used here, denotes attention to recording a natural history of bodily events, bodily experiences, coping, and self-care practices. The purpose of the clinical ethnography is to understand the relationship between the lived experience of an illness (the bodily experience and know-how) and the illness as domesticated and understood theoretically and "scientifically" by medicine. Of course, there is no "uninterpreted disease" from a phenomenological perspective. Once a disease is named and domesticated by medical technology and medical interpretations, the experience and even the capacities for recovery may be drastically influenced by the naming and technological interventions and rituals. *Clinical* as intended here implies a naturalistic study, a precise recording of actual events, and a quest for understanding a lived experience. In the everyday world of health care, *clinical* is understood as a form of practical knowledge. A clinical understanding is gained directly from studying the patient and the patient's symptoms, the focus is on understanding, and it is this understanding of "clinical" and "clinical way of knowing" that is intended by the term *clinical ethnography*. The word *clinical* is not intended to refer to a medical perspective or the "clinical gaze" in Foucault's terms (Foucault, 1975). Breaking things down into elements and assuming a mechanical interpretation-free causation—a Cartesian or medical view of the illness—is a position held up for scrutiny rather than taken up as a background assumption. A clinical ethnography has an informal counterpart in nursing practice in the nursing history and represents a nursing access to understanding illness.

Developing Implications for Public Policy, Therapies, and Community Development

Interpretive phenomenology provides a critique of instrumental reasoning and objectification. The goal is to respectfully understand the lifeworld, critically evaluating what is oppressive, ignorant, or troublesome from the perspective of the participants and identifying sources of innovation and liberation within everyday practices. Therefore the philosophical stance of interpretive phenomenology is not one of social engineering, where that is understood as an enlightened objective view of the lifeworld that needs to be rationalized and better controlled by public policy (Bellah, 1982). However, interpretive phenomenology does have a major role to play in public policy by its power to make the concerns, voice, habits, and practices of people visible and in recommending public policy that is attentive to differences and cultural concerns. Of course, there are no guarantees that interpretive phenomenology will not be used in manipulative, unethical ways. No research method can transcend the character and ethics of the researcher and the community of researchers and readers who evaluate the research. Because interpretive research focuses on understanding and the possibility of uncovering concerns and notions of the good life, it offers a needed corrective (not a replacement) to public policy designed to adjudicate rights and privileges because it allows us to consider how our construal of particular rights and privileges supports or impinges on the constituents' notions of the good life. Understanding makes it possible to consider the notions of good and ethical concerns that we hold in common and in distinction. When developed wisely, interpretive phenomenology can be a powerful recognition practice that allows other voices to be heard, offering an alternative to an ever-increasing economic, exchange-oriented view of a society made up of isolated individuals with rights (Sandel, 1982). Interpretive studies can uncover and extend notions of the good life, common goods, and how to go about treating one another with increased powers of understanding without diminishing others through diagnosing deficits and normalizing each other (see SmithBattle, Chapter 8, and Stuhlmiller, Chapter 15). Interpretive phenomenology holds promise for making practical knowledge visible, making the knack, tact, craft, and clinical knowledge inherent in expert human practices more accessible. A strong exemplar, paradigm case, or effective thematic analysis offers not only understanding but a powerful way to increase perceptual acuity, recognition ability, and moral imagination. The method cannot transcend the talent or the moral character of the interpreter, but when the canons of textual evidence and consensual validation and dialogue are followed, a citizenry of critical readers and practitioners can discern better and worse interpretive accounts and better and worse ways of articulating common everyday taken-for-granted understandings. Practice will have gained a way to influence and shape theory more directly and effectively.

References

Aristotle. (1985). *Nicomachean ethics* (T. Irwin, Trans.). Indianapolis: Hackett.

Bellah, R. (1982). Social science as practical reason. *Hastings Center Report, 12*(5), 32-39.

Benner, P. (1984a). *From novice to expert: Excellence and power in clinical nursing practice.* Reading, MA: Addison-Wesley.

Benner, P. (1984b). *Stress and satisfaction on the job: Work meanings and coping of mid-career men.* New York: Praeger.

Benner, P. (1985a). Quality of life: A phenomenological perspective on explanation, prediction, and understanding in nursing science. *Advances in Nursing Science, 8,* 1-14.

Benner, P. (1985b). The oncology clinical nursing specialist: An expert coach. *Oncology Nursing Forum, 12,* 40.

Benner, P. (1991). The role of experience, narrative, and community in skilled ethical comportment. *Advances in Nursing Science, 14*(2), 1-21.

Benner, P. (in press). The role of articulation in understanding practice and experience as sources of knowledge. In J. Tully & D. M. Weinstock (Eds.), *Philosophy in a time of pluralism: Perspectives on the philosophy of Charles Taylor.* Cambridge, UK: Cambridge University Press.

Benner, P. (1994). Discovering challenges ethical theory in experience-based narratives of nurses' everyday ethical comportment. In J. F. Monagle and D. C. Thomasma (Eds.), *Health care ethics: Critical issues.* Gaithersburg, MD: Aspen.

Benner, P., & Benner, R. (in progress). *The use of narrative in developing clinical promotion programs based on clinical expertise.*

Benner, P., Wrubel, J., & Phillips, S.(in progress). *Critical caring: The knowledge, skill and ethics of helping.* (Book-length manuscript)

Benner, P., Tanner, C., & Chesla, C. (1992). From beginner to expert: Gaining a differentiated world in critical care nursing. *Advances in Nursing Science, 14*(3), 13-28.

Benner, P., Tanner, C., & Chesla, C. (in press). *Expertise in nursing practice: Clinical knowing, clinical judgment, and skillful ethical comportment.* New York: Springer.

Benner, P., & Wrubel, J. (1982). Skilled clinical knowledge: The value of perceptual awareness. *Nurse Educator, 7*(3), 11-17.

Benner, P., & Wrubel, J. (1989). *The primacy of caring: Stress and coping in health and illness.* Reading, MA: Addison-Wesley.

Borgmann, A. (1984). *Technology and the character of contemporary life.* Chicago: University of Chicago Press.

Bourdieu, P. (1990). *The logic of practice* (R. Nice, Trans.). Stanford, CA: Stanford University Press. (Original work published 1980)

Corbin, J. M., & Strauss, A. L. (1990, Spring). Grounded theory research: Procedures, canons and evaluative criteria. *Qualitative Sociology, 13,* 3-22.

Doolittle, N. D. (1990). *Life after stroke: Survivors' bodily and practical knowledge of coping during recovery.* Unpublished doctoral dissertation, University of California, San Francisco.

Dreyfus, H. L. (1979). *What computers can't do: The limits of artificial intelligence* (rev. ed.). New York: Harper & Row.

Dreyfus, H. L. (1991a). *Being-in-the-world: A commentary on Heidegger's "Being and time,"* Division I. Cambridge: MIT Press.

Dreyfus, H. L. (1991b). Heidegger's hermeneutic realism. In D. R. Hiley, J. F. Bohman, & R. Shusterman (Eds.), *The interpretive turn* (pp. 25-41). Ithaca, NY: Cornell University Press.

Dreyfus, H. L., & Dreyfus, S. E., with Athanasiou, T. (1986). *Mind over machine: The power of human intuition and expertise in the era of the computer.* New York: Free Press.

Foucault, M. (1975). *The birth of the clinic* (A. Sheridan, Trans.). New York: Vintage.

Fox-Keller, E. (1985). *Reflections on gender and science.* New Haven: Yale University Press.

Frank, A. W. (1991). *At the will of the body: Reflecting on illness.* Boston: Houghton Mifflin.

Gadamer, H. (1975). *Truth and method* (G. Barden & J. Cumming, Trans.). New York: Seabury. (Original work published 1960)

Geertz, C. (1973). *The interpretation of cultures.* New York: Basic Books.

Geertz, C. (1983). *Local knowledge.* New York: Basic Books.

Glaser, B. G., & Strauss, A. (1967). *The discovery of grounded theory: Strategies for qualitative research.* Chicago: Aldine.

Gordon, S. (1991). *Prisoners of men's dreams.* Boston: Little, Brown.

Guignon, C. B. (1983). *Heidegger and the problem of knowledge.* Indianapolis: Hackett.

Hacking, I. (1983). *Representing and intervening: Introductory topics in the philosophy of natural science.* Cambridge, UK: Cambridge University Press.

Hauerwas, S. (1990). *Naming the silences: God, medicine and the problem of suffering.* Grand Rapids, MI: Eerdmans.

Heidegger, M. (1962). *Being and time.* (J. Macquarrie & E. Robinson, Trans.). New York: Harper & Row. (Original work published 1927)

Heidegger, M. (1975). *The basic problems of phenomenology* (A. Hofstadter, Trans.). Bloomington: University of Indiana Press.

Husserl, E. (1964). *The idea of phenomenology* (W. Alston & G. Nakhikan, Trans.). The Hague: Nijhoff.

Jonsen, A. R., & Toulmin, S. (1988). *The abuse of casuistry: A history of reasoning.* Berkeley: University of California Press.

Keller, C. (1986). *From a broken web: Separation, sexism and self.* Boston: Beacon.

Kesselring, A. (1990). *The experienced body: When taken-for-grantedness fails.* Unpublished doctoral dissertation, University of California, San Francisco.

Kleinman, A. (1988). *The illness narrative: Suffering, healing, and the human condition.* New York: Basic Books.

Kuhn, T. (1970). *The structure of scientific revolutions* (2nd. ed.). Chicago: University of Chicago Press.

Kuhn, T. (1991). The natural and the human sciences. In D. R. Hiley, J. F. Bohman, & R. Shusterman (Eds.), *The interpretive turn: Philosophy, science, culture* (pp. 17-24). Ithaca, NY: Cornell University Press.

Lazarus, R. S., & Folkman, S. (1984). *Stress, appraisal, and coping.* New York: Springer.

Leonard, V. W. (1993). *Stress and coping in the transition to parenthood of first-time mothers with career commitments: An interpretive study.* Unpublished doctoral dissertation, University of California, San Francisco.

MacIntyre, A. (1981). *After virtue.* Notre Dame, IN: University of Notre Dame Press.

MacIntyre, R. (1993). *Sex, power, death and symbolic meanings of T-cell counts in HIV+ gay men.* Unpublished doctoral dissertation, University of California, San Francisco.

McKeever, L. (1988). *Menopause: An uncertain passage.* Unpublished doctoral dissertation, University of California, San Francisco.

Merleau-Ponty, M. (1962). *Phenomenology of perception* (C. Smith, Trans.). London: Routledge & Kegan Paul.

Packer, M. J. (1985). *The structure of moral action: A hermeneutic study of moral conflict.* Basel: Karger.

Polanyi, M. (1958). *Personal knowledge.* Chicago: University of Chicago Press.

Rubin, J. (1984). *Too much of nothing: Modern culture, the self and salvation in Kierkegaard's thought.* Unpublished doctoral dissertation, University of California, Berkeley.

Rubin, J. (in press). Impediments to the development of clinical knowledge and ethical judgement. In P. Benner, C. Tanner, & C. Chesla, *Expertise in nursing practice: Clinical knowing, clinical judgment, and skillful ethical comportment.* New York: Springer.

Ruddick, S. (1989). *Maternal thinking: Toward a politics of peace.* Boston: Beacon.

Sandel, M. (1982). *Liberalism and the limits of justice.* London: Oxford University Press.

Savedra, M. C., & Highley, B. L. (1988). Photography: Is it useful in learning how adolescents view hospitalization? *Journal of Adolescent Health Care, 9*(3), 218-224.

Schaefer, C. (1983). *The role of stress and coping in the occurrence of serious illness.* Unpublished doctoral dissertation, University of California, Berkeley.

Schilder, E. J. (1986). *The use of physical restraints in an acute care medical ward.* Unpublished doctoral dissertation, University of California, San Francisco.

Stainton, C. (1985). *Culture and cue sensitivity: A phenomenological study of mothering.* Unpublished doctoral dissertation, University of California at San Francisco.

Suchman, L. A. (1987). *Plans and situated actions: The problem of human machine interaction.* Cambridge, UK: Cambridge University Press.

Tanner, C., Benner, P., Chesla, C., & Gordon, D. (1993). The phenomenology of knowing a patient. *Image: The Journal of Nursing Scholarship, 25*(4), 273-280.

Taylor, C. (1964). *The explanation of behaviour.* London: Routledge & Kegan Paul.

Taylor, C. (1985a). *Philosophical papers* (2 vols.). Cambridge, UK: University of Cambridge Press.

Taylor, C. (1985b). Interpretation and the sciences of man. In C. Taylor, *Philosophical papers* (Vol. 2, pp. 15-57). Cambridge, UK: University of Cambridge Press.

Taylor, C. (1985c). Social theory as practice. In C. Taylor, *Philosophical papers* (Vol. 1, pp. 42-57). Cambridge, UK: University of Cambridge Press.

Taylor, C. (1989). *Sources of the self.* Cambridge, MA: Harvard University Press.

Taylor, C. (1991). *The ethics of authenticity.* Cambridge, MA: Harvard University Press.

Taylor, C. (1992). *Recognition practices and the politics of multiculturalism.* Cambridge, UK: Cambridge University Press.

Taylor, C. (1993). Explanation and practical reason. In M. C. Nussbaum & A. Sen (Eds.), *The quality of life* (pp. 208-241). Oxford, UK: Clarendon.

Tronto, J. C. (1993). *Moral boundaries: A political argument for an ethic of care.* New York: Routledge.

Webb, E. J., Campbell, D. T., Schwartz, R. D., & Sechrest, L. (1966). *Unobtrusive measures: Nonreactive research in the social sciences.* Chicago: Rand McNally.

Wrubel, J. W. (1985). *Personal meanings and coping processes: A hermeneutical study of personal background meanings and interpersonal concerns and their relation to stress appraisals and coping.* Unpublished doctoral dissertation, University of California, San Francisco.

7

✤

MARTIN, a Computer Software Program

On Listening to What the Text Says

NANCY L. DIEKELMANN

ROBERT SCHUSTER

SUI-LUN LAM

There is an apprehension among interpretive textual researchers that, in addition to its other potential negative effects (Apple, 1988; Streibel, 1988), technology has a reductive effect on the interpretation of complex phenomena. At the same time, researchers face a troubling but real dilemma: how can voluminous textual materials be studied, shared, stored, and retrieved efficiently without benefit of technology? Regardless of the validity of their apprehension, it can be argued that not utilizing technological tools can have as great an impact on research as using them by limiting studies to those that are smaller, less complex, and more realizable.

The mental and physical tasks of interpretive work are daunting, and this dilemma has pushed the computerization of textual research. Software designed to speed searches, to promote retrieval, and to facilitate analysis and the preparation of research manuscripts has been available for some time and is becoming increasingly common. One consequence is that computerization has begun engendering serious debate about the nature of interpretive methodologies themselves. In that debate, there is hope that if by embracing computerization there is a risk that research may lose its way, there is also the potential that the reflective development and use of computer software will generate methodological insight (Richards & Richards, 1991; Seidel & Clark, 1984; Walker, 1993).

Through an instructional grant from IBM's Project Trochos, the authors were given the opportunity to explore the nature of Heideggerian hermeneutic research and its methodologies by developing software to foster learning among graduate-level nursing students (Diekelmann, Lam, & Schuster, 1990, 1991). Difficulties in teaching and learning hermeneutics are that it is time-consuming because its materials are written, that hermeneutic methods and thinking can be demonstrated but not described, and that hermeneutic research often involves teamwork in which the thinking of the individual is difficult to distinguish. Experience at the University of Wisconsin-Madison School of Nursing indicated that the most meaningful learning is accomplished through experience rather than written or structured instruction. What we wanted was to allow students to follow the thinking of real researchers interacting with real texts. We wanted students to experience the discovery that happens when researchers are open to the possibility for anything to emerge. We also wanted to create a tool to help research teams come together. It was our hope, therefore, to add a playback mode to existing software and thus to make it possible for novices to learn by following the analytic turnings of expert hermeneutic researchers, and to enhance consensual validity by allowing experienced members of the research team to see how themes emerged from the text for other members of the team.

To that end, we began with a review of software already in use by other qualitative methodologies. Because software based on artificial intelligence techniques was still in its formative stages and not conducive to learning through demonstration, we disregarded it. Instead, we examined examples of software designed to assist the experienced researcher as a tool in the analytic process. Among these software tools were programs designed to search source materials, to catalog and retrieve passages extracted from source materials, and to probe relationships among passages.

Search Software

Search software focuses on the task of locating textual passages significant to the researcher. Most search strategies utilize the capability of the computer to find sequences of characters, strings, matching a specified search string. Even the least capable of computers can search for all occurrences of a given word or phrase with greater speed and accuracy than can the researcher. Combined with database-like counting functions to summarize the results of searches, such software has been in use for decades for stylistic studies of literature. With the addition of concordance or thesaurus strategies utilizing word or phrase sets, search programs have increased the potential for the location of passages meaningful to the researcher. The development of software that permits the use of Boolean logic in the construction of search terms has further increased the effectiveness of text searches. It is possible now to target passages that match one or more search sets, that include one and exclude another, or that satisfy some more complex formula.

The utility of this family of software for hermeneutic studies is limited. Though statistical summaries of language patterns or vocabulary are of use in textual studies such as content analysis, in hermeneutics, where the focus is on the context in which meaning resides and not vocabulary, the richness of human expression seemingly ensures that searches cannot locate all or even the most relevant passages. A simple example is a search set that includes the words fear, trepidation, anxiety, dread, foreboding, misgiving, uneasiness, and all of their variants. Whether the goal is to find passages matching all members of the set or to differentiate between members, the search would not find a passage like the following, in which the sense of fear is expressed implicitly but not stated explicitly:

A: I didn't want to.
B: Why didn't you want to?
A: (Laughing) I knew the needle would be this big (holding hands far apart).

For hermeneutic readings, the utility of such a search is primarily to relocate a passage or phrase whose language remains prominent in memory but whose location in the text has been lost during the course of reading.

Retrieval Software

Retrieval software in contrast focuses on the task of systematically reviewing textual passages that have already been found and in some fashion catalogued. The programming model for retrieval software is similar to that used to create electronic card catalogs, mailing lists, and bibliographies. Fundamentally, these are all traditional database applications. To make retrieval possible in textual research, each passage noted during the course of analysis becomes a new record in the analyst's database, either intact as text or by reference to its source document and its location in that document. In addition, each record must be identified by a label that is part of an objective and systematic labeling scheme. Without labeling, passages in the database exist only in reference to their source and the chronology of their creation. Through the addition of a label (whether it consists of one or more words or phrases), passages assume relationships to other passages. Many software packages allow for multiple labels.

This second family of software has more utility for hermeneutic studies than the first, because sense or meaning can be identified and coded systematically by the researcher through the use of labels related to theme, pattern, or practical knowledge. Whereas search software could not locate the sample passage illustrated earlier, the researcher using a retrieval package has the opportunity to label the passage, once noted, as an example of the meaning of fear, apprehension, or uneasiness, or perhaps all three. It could also be categorized as an example of the preservation of personhood or the reduction of pain in patients undergoing invasive procedures. Subsequently it can be linked to other passages of similar significance.

The third software type the authors examined builds on the traditional database structure of retrieval software but adds a dedicated logic to the retrieval process to facilitate further analysis. For some interpretive methodologies—grounded theory, for example—it is necessary to recall passages in correspondence to the branching points in a thematic hierarchy. If fear is the most generic of themes in an analysis, foreboding and uneasiness may be distinct thematic branches. Analytic software designed to support these relationships as well as relationships to other potential sub-branches must allow not only passage labeling; it must also allow the researcher to specify the position of the label in the hierarchy. The software then is able to retrieve passages at their appropriate points and to allow for refinement of subdivisions as analysis progresses. At its most basic, this requires the ability to create and manage a second database, dedicated to labeling, in addition to the first, dedicated to the passages themselves. In hermeneutics, where the importance is on both where one has arrived and how, this structured retrieval is reframed.

Each of the three software genres we examined is best begun with a preconceived structure of key words, labels, or thematic categories. Unless the researcher is willing merely to poke around for words or phrases that may show up in a stack of source materials, search software is most rewarding when it is used to scan for well-constructed sets of words and phrases. Although label fields in retrieval and analytic software databases can conceivably be left blank, relationships between passages cannot be established within the software until the blanks are filled in. In practice, filling in the blanks or refining a labeling scheme after it has been applied is laborious at best.

In contrast, Heideggerian hermeneutics requires that the researcher approach each text with openness and as much awareness of preconceptions as possible so that these can be challenged by the text. The researcher both influences and is influenced by the readings. A consequence of this respectful approach to interpretive work is that as understanding evolves the researcher may not immediately be able to see and identify themes as they are encountered. Nevertheless, particular passages stand out for the researcher. Within the Heideggerian context, ideas that may seem ungrounded when they occur can later point to new understanding. They can also be central to an understanding of the evolution of ideas.

We concluded that we needed to develop a new approach to software and to software development that was more reflective of the experience between the hermeneutic researcher and the text, one that would allow the researcher to dwell more closely and respectfully with the text and to move toward capturing fluid and evolving understandings. Yet we wanted to utilize the advantages the computer brings not only in not having to retype but in effortlessly bringing passages together in a way that evokes new thinking and understanding. To develop this new approach, we began by observing and discussing the experiences of a Heideggerian hermeneutical researcher working through texts from initial readings to a final research report. The technique used was to have the researcher think aloud while doing an analysis. All moves through the text were observed, recorded, and discussed.

During the early encounters with paradigm texts, we noted that frequently there is a lengthy period during which the researcher must read and reread, abandon and come back to the text as it begins to speak. As the text begins to resonate for the reader, what it says and means often remains obscure, as if spoken in a language not yet learned but felt and understood. Passages may be noted, but their meanings may not fully be understood. Nevertheless, the researcher continues to accumulate them and eventually to hear them with greater clarity and insight.

Thinking and the conditions out of which thinking emerges are of issue to the researcher. For the hermeneutic researcher, the opacity of these early hearings evokes thinking, but only when there is an openness to hearing. For Heidegger, "We never come to thoughts. They come to us." (Heidegger, 1971, p. 6). We were interested in the lived experience of thinking and in exploring how understanding begins to emerge. As a team, we sought to reveal more of thinking-as-comportment.

We observed numerous movements through, with, and across texts in these early stages. Many of these were individualized even to the point of apparent eccentricity, and there was a temptation to disregard them. At best, we thought, many moves were too inefficient to justify codifying them in software designed to accompany research. On further reflection, however, we concluded that even the most eccentric among these moves represented thinking comportment toward understanding and must therefore be respected and a place created for them. *If the computer is to accompany and not redefine interpretive methodology, the software must attend to all stages in which the text says and understanding emerges.*

Taking a cue from the flexibility inherent in the traditional cut-and-paste and index card techniques, we began to look for a computer environment that metaphorically, at least, could reproduce the researcher's desktop. The graphical user interface (GUI) then being popularized by Microsoft Windows made available the concept of self-contained screen objects known as windows. Using the windows concept, we designed a window to serve as the equivalent of a printed source document. Not only could the text be scrolled for reading, but multiple texts could be displayed simultanously, each in its own window.

Among the most common of the early moves we noted was that jottings are often made in the margins of a text reflecting the first tentative steps toward insight. Sometimes these are a personal reminder of something to look up later, perhaps a comparison, such as: "Sounds like interview 027, search for teacher-as-learner?" Sometimes they were ideas or insights. Those ideas or "flashes of insight" are respected and written down even when the meanings to the text are not obvious or apparent. These marginal notes are utilized during initial readings before any particular passage emerges, and later, as passages begin to stand out.

To create the possibility for adding notes to the text, we designed a second window type for entry of researcher notations. Each note window generated by the researcher inserted a marker in the text that could be detached at any time, moved, or discarded. There was utility in this note window as well for the other comments that come to mind during an analysis and are written in the margins, such as: "This statement is a good example of maxims embedded in texts—could be used in the interpretive nursing research course." In addition, note windows served to contain small ideas such as: "Is it the teacher as learner or the teacher learning that matters here? Seems like focusing on learner is like focusing on evaluation instead of testing. Not sure."

We also noted that researchers often utilize sets of mental markers before meaningful patterns emerge from the data. These nonverbal notations, which may include colors and symbols, are used as temporary markers or reminders. They may say merely that here is a word or phrase that must be attended to again later. Or they may represent an initial sense that here is a passage that represents something other than that last passage. What is important is that they support emerging thoughts at a stage that is too early for verbalization.

Finally, we noted that researchers often develop a relationship to the text that is spatial in nature. Having read through a text, for example, the researcher may recollect that there was something back there of importance that was near the top of the page and over near the right margin. As with the marker techniques identified above, these spatial relationships appear very early in thinking and precede verbalization. This spatial aspect is also evident among researchers who use index card and cut-and-paste techniques in their analyses. Stacks of cards or cuttings develop spatially on the desktop without any apparent, overt logic. This card needs to go in that stack over there by the phone; it doesn't go next to the coffee cup. Again, such examples appear to represent thinking at a preverbal stage, but they also endure beyond the beginning of verbalization and may simply represent thinking that does not require verbalization.

As a parallel to these early moves, we designed another window type to generate the equivalent of an index card that could be moved around the screen and stacked with other thematically similar cards. These card windows were designed to display a copy of the selected text passage, equating with cut-and-paste techniques. As text was pasted into the window, there was also provision for adding a lengthy descriptive label. Because the significance of the passage was related to its placement on the screen, the label was optional and not functional except for its utility to the researcher. Supplementing the label descriptor, each card was also given a notes window designed to provide the researcher a way to attach comments as well as lengthy analysis to the passage. At this point, we also realized that note windows could be left blank, their mark in the text serving as a correlative to preverbal mental markers for later attention.

We added one more window type extending the card window idea to support the researcher's recognition of textual themes and patterns. Theme windows were designed to hold cards as a way of formalizing the informal groupings of cards on the desktop, while pattern windows were designed to formalize groupings of theme and other pattern windows. As with the card windows, both were given a labeling option and a notes window. We felt these last windows were essential because as we followed the researcher beyond the initial readings and into stages of more complex understanding, we found that the need to support thinking before it could be verbalized remained important. Even at the point at which particular passages would be underlined in traditional paper and pencil readings or identified by line number and added to a retrieval database in existing computer software packages, this need continued to be evident. As with the unlabeled stack of index cards next to the telephone, the researcher early on sees and hears what the text says. The researcher knows that passages A and D belong together but may not yet know how to refer to them or what they represent. The collective windows offer a way of keeping a grouping of cards together and represent the first steps toward an understanding of textual patterns even before they can be named.

As the software program was developed and tested, the HOW of thinking and the nature of the relationship between the software and the researcher emerged. Eventually, we felt that we had created a tool that could accompany the interpretive process in real time. To test that compatibility, we distributed copies of the software to qualitative researchers utilizing a variety of qualitative methodologies at 13 sites around the country and internationally. Their feedback both confirmed our sense of the effectiveness of the program and stimulated the creation of additional features.

Of three major suggestions, two stood out as having roots in existing textual analysis software. Several sites requested that a search feature be added to the text windows. It was of interest to us that the rationale for its addition was not to support initial scans of paradigm texts but to find passages that had been noted during initial readings and that were recollected as specific words or phrases. Uniformly, the search feature was perceived to be a time-saving utility and not a substitute for an expert reading.

Complementing the perceived need for a textual search function was a recommendation that a key word labeling feature be added to the card windows to facilitate retrieval of passages with thematic relationships as perceived by the researcher. Although we had viewed that as duplicative of the theme and pattern windows, reviewers viewed it as adding flexibility and economy to the process of rethinking interpretations.

Finally, many reviewers expressed discomfort with the labels we had assigned to the various windows in the software: paradigm, notion, theme, and pattern. On one level, we expected that researchers utilizing methodologies other than Heideggerian hermeneutics would necessarily prefer their own labels and regarded these suggested changes as cosmetic. As we considered the suggestions, however, we perceived that they paralleled the individualized moves utilized early in the process of interpreting texts. There is something significant in naming, as there is in being able to use personal symbols, that goes beyond mere habit. Naming becomes a gateway or a pathway to understanding. We accommodated that need by changing our naming to match the real objects found on the desktop, cards and folders, and by adding a feature by which users could change menu and window names to match their own conventions.

Having developed a computerized research tool that appeared to complement a variety of qualitative methodologies, and having modified it to meet numerous suggestions, we returned to the question of how MARTIN could be used by research teams. Windows is equipped with a utility that records every keystroke, menu selection, and mouse movement. Having the researcher turn on the recorder at the beginning of an analysis proved to be an effective way to preserve even the subtle and nonlinear processes of textual analysis. In addition, the notes feature can be used to build in the asides of the researcher as teacher to the student or comments between and among research team members. Rather than being dependent on a lecture format of one teacher to many students, we had a tool in which one student could have many teachers. That is, the student could repeat and compare the movements of several studies and so gain a breadth of understanding including that of personal style in the interpretative process. It is not uncommon in graduate education that students and teachers study difficult texts together in reading courses. MARTIN can be used by teachers to show annotated interpretations to students in advance of class. Students can then add to or comment on previous comments, and the interpretations can be saved. In this way, it is also possible to read across text.

The Future

Technology shapes thinking. Computer software formalizes methodological pathways. Software that becomes the standard of a community of users itself contributes to the language and the understandings of its community. Furthermore, increasing reliance on it in order to remain productive also encourages increasing dependence.

Use of and changes in software, then, must always be approached thoughtfully. How is the technology appropriating users, and how is it opening up new possibilities it has itself helped to reveal?

In the light of those questions, we have found it meaningful to note the suggestions for changes and additions that have grown out of the experiences of MARTIN users in working with our software. Many of these lived experiences have revealed ways to increase the speed of the interaction between the researcher and the text: the need to cut keystrokes in moving a card from one folder to another, to streamline the procedures for bringing text into MARTIN from the word processor, to simplify the revision of folder and group organization. Researchers also describe the importance of continuing to enhance the ability of the computer to follow their movements during an interpretation. In observing that transferring cards between folders is cumbersome, researchers speak of how distracting this is to thinking. That is, to the degree that the mechanics of reading draw concentration away from interpretation, there is a barrier to immediacy within the text.

Understanding thinking comportment and the lived experiences of interpreting texts has revealed a new approach to developing software. What is missing in software is the hearing and seeing. The possibility of interpreting not only written paradigms but, in the form of audio and video recordings, the embodied experience of speaking is a possibility primarily only through the computer and is being explored.

We hope to respond to the continuing experiences emerging from practicing interpretive researchers and students we also hope to continue development of software that accompanies interpretive research and that respectfully allows meanings, insights, and understandings to emerge through the thinking comportment of the researcher. To that end, we have learned the importance of dialogue about our experiences in using software as an integral part of interpretive research. In this way, we both shape and are shaped by the tools we use as a community of interpretive researchers as we move toward hearing what our texts say.

References

Apple, M. (1988). Teaching and technology: The hidden effects of computers on teachers and students. In L. E. Beyer & M. W. Apple (Eds.), *The curriculum: Problems, politics, and possibilities* (pp. 289-311). New York: State University of New York Press.

Diekelmann, N., Lam, S., & Schuster, R. (1990). *MARTIN* [Computer program and user guide]. Madison, WI: University of Wisconsin-Madison School of Nursing (K6/152 Simonds Center, School of Nursing, 600 Highland Ave., Madison, WI 53792-2455).

Diekelmann, N., Lam, S., & Schuster, R. (1991). *MARTIN* [Computer program and user guide] (rev. ed.). Madison, WI: University of Wisconsin-Madison School of Nursing (K6/152 Simonds Center, School of Nursing, 600 Highland Ave., Madison, WI 53792-2455).

Heidegger, M. (1971). *Poetry, language, thought* (A. Hofstadter, Trans.) (p. 6). New York: Harper & Row.

Richards, L., & Richards, T. (1991). The transformation of qualitative method: Computational paradigms and research processes. In N. G. Fielding & R. M. Lee (Eds.), *Using computers in qualitative research.* (pp. 38-63). Newbury Park, CA: Sage.

Seidel, J., & Clark, J. (1984). The ethnograph: A computer program for the analysis of qualitative data. *Qualitative Sociology, 7*(1/2), 110-125.

Streibel, M. (1988). A critical analysis of three approaches to the use of computers in education. In L. E. Beyer & M. W. Apple (Eds.), *The curriculum: Problems, politics, and possibilities* (pp. 259-288). New York: State University of New York Press.

Walker, B. (1993). Computer analysis of qualitative data: A comparison of three packages. *Qualitative Health Research, 3*(1), 99-111.

Part II

Interpretive Phenomenological Studies

8

❖

Beyond Normalizing

The Role of Narrative
in Understanding Teenage Mothers'
Transition to Mothering

LEE SMITHBATTLE

Our modern understanding of parenting in general, and teenage mother-ing in particular, is increasingly shaped by abstract formal knowledge that virtually excludes narrative accounts and practical understanding of everyday experience. After briefly describing how scientific-technical normalizing practices have become the privileged form of explaining young mothers' lives, skills, and competence, I argue for narratives as a source for recovering the experiential terms by which young mothers and their families understand their lives. Tammy's story is told to demonstrate the role that narratives play in showing lives to be situated and organized by practical, rather than disengaged, rationality.

AUTHOR'S NOTE: This study was made possible by the financial support from several sources. I gratefully acknowledge the Fahs-Beck Fund for Research and Experimentation; the Century Club, UCSF School of Nursing; the Graduate Division of the University of California, San Francisco; the Alpha Eta Chapter of Sigma Theta Tau; and the National Center for Nursing Research for a National Research Service Award (NR1F31NR06266). Names and identifying information have been changed to maintain confidentiality.

Tammy's narrative is highlighted for a second reason. In the course of a phenomenological-interpretive study, her story raised questions about the struggles, constraints, and possibilities for becoming a responsive self in the context of an unresponsive community (SmithBattle, 1992). Her story introduced new ways of "hearing" teenagers' stories that recommended a search in the complete text for similarities, contrasts, and changes in young mothers' self-understanding along with the turning points, obstacles, conflicts, and resources for becoming the mother one wanted to be. Her moral tale called attention to the formative possibilities of mothering and how these possibilties are revealed and potentially extended in the very process of storytelling. As such, her story is consonant with a narrative conception of development (Freeman, 1984, 1991) and a research process predicated on dialogue and understanding.

Deficit-Filling and Finding Approaches

Since the 1960s, the academic discourse on teenage pregnancy and parenting has undergone a rather remarkable shift from the consideration of teen pregnancy as a moral problem of "promiscuous" girls to be condemned and shunned to a scientific-technical approach that commends remediation and treatment. Informed by the scholarship of Foucault, Arney and Bergen (1984) describe how this shift was in part created by a scientific discourse bent on discovering the "facts" of teenage pregnancy. In asking the question, "How did teenage pregnancy as a moral problem become redefined as a scientific-technical one?" they examine how normalizing science creates the "truth" it claims to have discovered. They summarize their cogent argument below:

> In broad strokes our claim is that pregnant adolescents used to be a moral problem. Now they are a technical problem. They have not lost their problematical character, but a moral problem invokes a different kind of solution than does a technical problem. Moral problems create oppositions to the natural order of things and invite punishment and practices of exclusion. Technical problems are deviations from a natural order. They are not excluded or punished for their lack of conformity. They are, instead, subjected to technologies of correction and normalization designed to get them to conform to their true nature, the truth of which is known by experts. (p. 11)

In describing the earlier moral system of blame and shame, they cite popular and public health literature of the 1940s and 1950s in which high rates of premarital pregnancy met with moral condemnation (potentially avoided through marriage) and *did not* require a scientific explanation and a search for causes. Beginning in the 1960s, however, this moral understanding began to give way to a scientific-technical order; no longer objects of moral condemnation, pregnant teens were becoming simultaneously visible in popular magazines and available to the scientific gaze. Through scientific practices of unitizing and generalizing (Guignon, 1983), social scientists isolated the teens' behaviors, thoughts, feelings, attitudes, and features of their social context from the complex interrelationships in which they were embedded and then reconfigured these "brute" facts, via statistical techniques, into a model that explained or predicted some aspect of teen pregnancy or parenting. In this way, young mothers' competence, knowledge, and development were mapped out and evaluated for how they conformed or deviated from an ideal, normative grid of parenting and the life course.

Scientific criterial norms abound in the empirical-rational research on teenage parenting and lead to the study of maternal behaviors and knowledge in isolation from personal history, meanings, relationships, family practices, and sociocultural contexts. Mothering is thereby misconstrued as individually derived rather than historically and socially embedded. As scientific experts purport to discover the objective "truth" or structure of the problem along with its variations and deviations from the norm, a scientific-technical language of problems to be solved by technical means is advanced.

Erikson's (1963) theory of psychosocial development, wherein development is achieved by progressing through formal stages, is often cited to highlight how mothering during adolescence jeopardizes identity formation (Holt & Johnson, 1991; Poole, 1987; Sadler & Catrone, 1983; Young, 1988). In this conception, the formal tasks of adolescence and motherhood are antithetical, not because of the teen's social disadvantage and vulnerability in current social arrangements that make parenting a private affair, but because of the teen's failure to first achieve autonomy and become a differentiated self.

Adherents to formal notions of development and the life course disregard how the timing of adolescence and pathways to adulthood vary for different groups of teenagers, reflecting local and societal conditions related to the educational system and entry into the labor force. For example, in circumstances in which opportunities for education and employment are bleak, varied configurations in the life course are limited so that mothering is often accepted as an inevitable and important rite of passage to adulthood (Burton, 1990; Gabriel & McAnarney, 1983; Ladner, 1971; Stack, 1974).

In presuming a normative, formal path to adulthood, current research portrays teenage mothering as an aberration of the normal life-course trajectory, one that "risks the future" of mother and child (Hayes, 1987). The modern "sin" that parenting teenagers commit lies in their failure to rationally choose among alternatives to become a productive, successful adult. This extremely individualistic notion of the self, where choosing one's self and the direction of one's life is viewed as an ultimate value, overlooks how goals and purposes are not strictly chosen on the basis of rational calculation but are given on the basis of one's participation and membership in the activities of one's family and defining community. The methodological individualism of scientific practices, by denying the role of personal and family meanings and concerns in local and cultural contexts in shaping pathways to becoming an adult, ends up treating teenage mothering as a "syndrome":

> This syndrome includes failure to fulfill the functions of adolescence, failure to remain in school, failure to limit family size, to establish a vocation and to be self-supporting, failure to have healthy infants, and failure to have children who reach their full potential. (Klein, 1978, p. 1151)

Syndromes compel diagnosis and treatment of individuals. Programs serving teenage mothers, to the extent that they embrace criterial norms of mothering and the life course, emphasize "training" and "rehabilitation" to lessen the negative effects of a first pregnancy, to delay a second pregnancy, and to improve the mother's long-term economic self-sufficiency. Although these are worthy goals, barriers to their success are often located in the young mother's personal characteristics (lack of self-esteem or personal control, etc.) rather than in social sources of disadvantage. For example, in addition to providing educational, job training, and health services, programs often include training in self-esteem, motivation, and personal control along with a heavy emphasis on formal knowledge of childrearing. The unfortunate result is that teenagers are further blamed when short-term interventions based on these models fail to demonstrate positive long-lasting results (see Fine, 1988).

The scientific-technological paradigm, focused on filling norm-based deficits and failures, correlates with an idiom of control rather than understanding and supports a rather narrow set of scientific-technical solutions aimed at having individuals come to certain beliefs or adopt behavior that will presumably ensure health and development, but where health and development are considered in a vacuum, divorced from personal meanings, relations, and context. In the end, emphasizing conformity to behavioral norms as a solution to young mothers' difficulties can become an even greater source of oppression, stigma, and exclusion and fails to bring into public debate discussions of the common good that might transform our understanding and response to teenage parenting.

In summary, normalizing science presumes that the "truth" of teenage pregnancy exists independent of sociohistorical contexts and prior to scientific practices. The specialized knowledge and practices of scientists are privileged over the everyday experience and self-understandings of the people studied. These limitations warrant an alternative approach that moves beyond studying objectified behaviors and formal tasks of mothering and identity to understand young mothers' meanings, purposes, and concerns as organized, promoted, and/or imperiled by family and social contexts. A narrative conception of development and the life course is one approach concerned less with how one event predicts another, and deviates or conforms to prespecified, ideal ends, than with the temporal unfolding of varied "ends" through a retrospective narrative accounting that attends to the role of meanings, concerns, and the situation in shaping what is understood to be a good and meaningful life (Benner & Wrubel, 1989; Freeman, 1984, 1991; Packer, 1991; Polkinghorne, 1988; Tappan, 1991).

Recovering Narrative Understanding

The technological paradigm of control privileges formal, abstract knowledge and disengaged reasoning over the understanding of lived experience and practical rationality. Stories are accordingly dismissed as prescientific and considered unwieldy compared to the stringent methods of social scientific survey research; they are therefore suppressed in interviews and disregarded as a methodological tool (Mishler, 1986). Yet stories remain an indispensable source for understanding ourselves and others and for understanding human action as situated and temporal (Benner & Wrubel, 1989; Packer, 1991) and lives as storied (Bruner, 1987; Polkinghorne, 1988; Rosenwald, 1992).

Consider the ways that reading or listening to a story opens up the world of the narrator, replete with the concerns, possibilities, intentions, options, contradictions, and impossibilities given in that person's world. The first-person rendering of a story provides an inside-out perspective essential to understanding the terms in which the narrator understands his or her life. Narratives therefore recover what formal theories necessarily overlook, how we are inherently social and historical beings. By revealing the context within which narrators act, stories demonstrate that meanings are lived out on the background of shared understandings that develop within a sociocultural tradition. Mair (cited in Howard, 1991) grasps the significance of how our stories (and our actions) are always socially embedded in traditions that precede us:

> Stories are habitations. We live in and through stories. They conjure worlds. We do not know the world other than as story world. Stories inform life. We inhabit the great stories of our culture. We live through stories. We are *lived* by the stories of our race and place. It is this enveloping and constituting function

of stories that is especially important to sense more fully. We are, each of us, locations where the stories of our place and time become partially tellable. (p. 195)

Stories capture the "practical rationality" that informs and organizes people's activities, where one does what it makes sense to do in similar situations based on the meanings, concerns, and purposes that are constituted by one's membership and participation in a family, community, and culture (Benner & Wrubel, 1989; Dreyfus, 1991). Within the interpretive tradition, much of what people do does not require explicit decision making or rational calculation but reflects the prereflective and embodied grasp of situations that we have on the basis of being socialized into shared understandings of living in the world; even explicit decisions that come up regarding personal reproductive behavior reflect much that is already taken for granted about a shared world. Children become teenagers with a familiarity of the possibilities for completing school, for becoming employed, or for going on to college that fit with the social organization of schooling and employment of a particular locale that in turn shape fertility patterns. The understanding of human action associated with interpretive phenomenology further assumes that activities are meaningful and situated, are open to mystery and contingency, and do not follow lawlike necessity (Benner, 1985; Dreyfus, 1991; Leonard, 1989; Packer, 1985; Taylor, 1989; Williams, 1987).

Tammy's Story: "Growing Up Together"

Tammy told her story as a participant in an interpretive-phenomenological study that examined teenagers' transition to mothering as shaped by personal meanings and concerns, the family's caregiving practices, and the mother's participation in a defining community (SmithBattle, 1992). Participants were encouraged to give narrative accounts of their experience of mothering so that meaning in context could be captured (Mishler, 1979). This was fostered by granting the young mother the position of acknowledged expert by virtue of her experience and by an active style of listening that encouraged a detailed account of what she actually did, thought, and felt in specific situations. No effort was made during interviews or later during analysis to abstract experience and life events from their contextual and narrative dependence.

Thin in appearance and steely in temperament, Tammy was easily drawn into telling her story as she kept a watchful eye or deftly attended to blonde and curly-headed Joy, her year-old daughter. From our initial meeting, Tammy struck me as a tenacious, impetuous, sometimes hot-tempered 17-

year-old. Her scrappy nature and brash language fit her self-described stubbornness.

Tammy's 49-year-old mother also participated in the study but never divulged her longstanding alcoholism during our two interviews. I learned of her drinking from Tammy, who spared few contemptuous words for her mother's frank neglect, occasional abuse, and numerous liaisons with men after divorcing Tammy's father. Episodes in which Tammy was physically abused remain indelibly imprinted in her memory in stark detail; more common was the trauma of bearing her mother's verbal abuse and drunkenness, mitigated only by an older sister's attempts to care for Tammy or by weekends spent with her father.

Given her mother's different liaisons, Tammy was "uncertain of exactly where my father fit in," but he certainly represents a more nurturant and positive example of parenting in contrast to Tammy's tumultuous home life.

> **T:** I guess just because he was always there when we needed him. You know, we'd be at my mom's house and we'd wake up in the middle of the night and nobody would be there, and we'd call my dad and he'd come and get us.

Tammy described her father as reliable, someone who "didn't take his own troubles out on his kids." He helped Tammy with homework without yelling at her as her mother did and "he let us know it was time to be okay and to behave and listen to what he had to say, and we respected him for that." When Tammy began running away at age 10 to escape her mother's drinking, her father's home became a safe refuge. Tammy attributes her resilience to her father's example, "who laid it all out to people but without violence, which I like, but my mother is a woosh, she doesn't stand up for anything." Her resilience, she claims, was honed once and for all the night her father died of cancer:

> **T:** My attitude changed the night he died. Because my mom woke me up at 3 a.m. and told me, and I said, "Don't lie to me." And she said, "No, he's really dead, he's gone." And I said, "Well, I want to go to see him," and she said no.

In storming out of the house and finding her way to the hospital (at age 12), she claims:

> **T:** I was stronger because I went to see him in the hospital and went to his grave and my sister never did. My sister couldn't handle it, so she didn't get all the anger and the frustration and stress out yet. But I did.

> I got it out right there cause I didn't want to all my life dwell on it.
> Because it's not worth it. He's gone.

Tammy's teenage sister became involved in drugs and in turn introduced them to Tammy at age 7, which Tammy concedes was a way to escape her tumultuous home life. It should be no surprise that she did not do well in school and that she eventually got in trouble with the juvenile system for frequently running away. At age 15, she ran away to Los Angeles for 4 months where she did "a lot of bad things" and conceived her first pregnancy. Because it was unplanned and unwanted, she had no hesitation about aborting:

> T: When I had the abortion, I didn't care. I didn't want the baby—I didn't
>   want that thing inside of me and I felt gross. . . . I had been doing a lot
>   of drugs. And I knew that would affect the baby. I wasn't ready for it
>   because I still wanted to party and I still wanted to do drugs, and I still
>   wanted to go out. And um, so I kept it up, I kept partying, I kept doing
>   drugs.

About a year later, she deliberately planned a second pregnancy with her boyfriend and conceived after 3 months of being drug-free "so that I knew that everything was out of my system." When the pregnancy was confirmed at 2 months gestation, she also abstained from smoking cigarettes for the duration of the pregnancy. Here are her reasons for getting pregnant:

> T: . . . and then I figured, you know, that I have to be responsible and that
>   I want somebody to love. You know, I wanted someone to care about
>   and to take care of, and um, me and [my boyfriend] discussed and we
>   figured that we could have a baby and that's how it all started.
> I: Was it hard to quit [drugs]?
> T: No, because the drugs weren't hard because I knew that that wasn't
>   important to me. And I knew that the baby was important to me cause
>   of the love that I had for her father. And I saw how he wanted a baby,
>   and how I wanted a baby. And we were going to work together on this.
> I: Why was it important to get pregnant?
> T: Because I wanted a baby. I don't know how to tell you. I don't know.
>   I guess, I'm guessing, I don't even know. Maybe I was afraid that he'd
>   leave someday and I didn't want him to go. . . . And plus, I just wanted
>   to settle down and have a baby.

Amidst family turmoil and drug addiction, Tammy imagines that caring for a baby might help her abstain from drugs and reorient her life. An apparently mutual decision proved less significant to her boyfriend. Although he also, by his own report, quit drugs initially, their relationship eventually soured. When he urged Tammy to relinquish the baby for adoption, she refused and resolved to raise the baby on her own.

At the time of Joy's birth, Tammy was living at home with her mother, but when her mother resumed drinking 3 months later, Tammy was desperate to move out and did so into an equally deplorable living situation:

> **T:** It was difficult, and everybody's self-esteem down there was like really low. Nobody worked and they had to beg their parents for the rent money. Me too. I had to ask my mom for money. Um, they'd sit around and get high all day, and of course I'm in the room so it's a contact high for me. And Joy was in the room, and I'd have to take her upstairs and go in the room, and just everything there, everyone, the whole environment, the neighborhood, everything got me down. And so I was depressed and feeling bad, which made Joy fussy. And I'd be stressed out and I'd yell at her and I'd felt so bad afterwards I'd just lay in bed and cry. And that's what I did usually the whole time I was there. And then my mom always made sure that Joy had food when I was living there. That was about it. I didn't eat. . . . I didn't have any money to take the bus so it was really hard, and it was stressful on me because. . . . And then I'd go downstairs and there'd be like 20 people in the house. [And I'd say,] "You guys have to leave." "Well, Ron said we could stay." "Well, I'm living here. My kid's upstairs sleeping. Get out!" And then they'd go get Ron. And then Ron would say, "We'll be quiet, we'll be quiet." At about 3:00 in the morning, I wake up with Joy screaming and people are downstairs yelling and stumbling everywhere, drinking beer. It was just really hard on me cause you know I couldn't handle them plus the baby plus my own feelings plus not eating didn't make me too happy. . . . Without Jim telling me I could live here, it would have been worse. And probably I would have had Joy taken away.

Fortuitously, upon learning of Tammy's circumstances, an older divorced friend invited her to live in his home. Tammy hesitated at first, not wanting to be "pitied," but she agreed and moved into his household. This proved to be a much more stable situation for Tammy and Joy: no drugs are allowed and there is no raucous late-night partying. Compared to the previous living situation, Tammy's daily routine is now fairly predictable. Her housemates will sometimes feed breakfast to Joy, giving her more time to sleep, but once they leave for work, she mostly plays with Joy and visits with friends who stop by. While Joy takes her afternoon nap, Tammy cooks dinner for the household. After dinner together, the housemates clean the kitchen and Joy becomes the evening center of attraction as friends visit. Joy has a regular bedtime, sleeping in her own crib in her mother's room.

Throughout her interviews, Tammy describes the power and directedness that issue from being a mother. Here is how Tammy describes her transformed world:

> **T:** I think that having Joy made me more mature, made me wake up and realize that life isn't just a piece of cake and you don't have to just get up in the morning and go out and party and come home and go to sleep. That's not what life is about. Plus, I was, you know, I never had to pay for anything and now I do and now I feel a lot more responsible. You know, cause, and now I have someone to take care of so I have to take care of her and I like feeling that way. I like having that sense of responsibility.
>
> **I:** And how has being a mother changed who you are as a person?
>
> **T:** My personality, my attitude.
>
> **I:** Oh, it has?
>
> **T:** Yeah.
>
> **I:** In what ways has it changed?
>
> **T:** I'm not, I'm not such a smartass, and my goals aren't just to go out and think of me.
>
> **I:** What are your goals now?
>
> **T:** My goals are just to live my life with my daughter and raise her the best way that I can.
>
> **I:** So how is it to make that switch?
>
> **T:** How does it feel?
>
> **I:** Yeah.
>
> **T:** It feels better. Cause she's a part of me.

How might we understand Tammy's story—as romantic self-delusion or as a credible possibility issuing from her experience? If we assume, as others do (Musick, 1990), that mothers reorganize themselves as they adapt to their new role by acquiring knowledge from an increasingly detached perspective, then we might agree that teenagers are unlikely to have the capacities *within themselves* to carry out such redefinition. But this stance assumes that mothers are fully self-contained and neutral selves who stand outside the situation, unmoved by their experience and the way the baby matters. When mothering is understood as a practice that pulls and guides the mother to perceive, feel, think, and behave in ways that accord with the particularity of the mother-child relationship within an already meaningful social and practical context, then Tammy's selfappraisal and living out of a "corrective narrative" (Benner, 1991) seem plausible. The world of mothering works a moral change in Tammy's life, giving birth to a relational self, a self born out of emerging skills, meanings, and habits of caring for and responsiveness to a specific child.

> T: I always wanted to go out and I always wanted to party and I always wanted to be where everybody was. I had to be the center of attraction too and now I don't. . . . We'd always go out and get drunk or stoned or whatever—anything. We'd always go to concerts and, um, I was always the center of attraction; I was always the one that made everybody laugh out of the bunch. And I still do that, but I'm sober and now I'm more smart. You know, I realize how stupid I was. I was stupid.

Tammy's new concerns as Joy's mother provide a new ethical framework and directedness that reorganizes her activities. She is moved to act in new ways because of her connection to Joy—"she's a part of me"—that overturns her previous self-absorption and meaninglessness. The new concerns that arise in being Joy's mother strengthen her resolve to become "a better person" and a good example to her child. Even though she sometimes falls short of her aspirations and hopes, these aspirations and hopes only show up for her as Joy's mother. When I ask her, "What is a good mother like?" she replies:

> T: There is no just one good mother. You're just the best person you can be. Everything you think about, everything you do, if you think about how it would affect your kid, that's the best mother you could be. Because everything that goes through my mind, I think about what would come out of it for Joy.

She elaborates by recounting a friend's motorcycle accident in which she could also have been hurt if she had agreed to go with him. In thinking of the possible repercussions for Joy, she continues:

> T: Everything I'm gonna do is going to affect her in some way—the kind of people I'm around, things I consider doing.
>
> I: Is that a constraint?
>
> T: I don't feel like it's a burden. I like that feeling because then I'm watching out for myself too. You know, if I do something wrong. I think it helps me. Cause if I went out on every single urge I had, I'd be in jail right now. Being in the wrong place at the wrong time.

Here Tammy points to how doing better for herself is intertwined with doing better for her child in ways that create a privileged space *for the mother*; the experience of loving and being loved by a child offers a corrective experience that contrasts with her own painful and troubled past. Tammy fondly remembers the early months of feeding Joy at night when she would "just stare at her, I just couldn't believe she was mine." She recalls with deep emotion the recent time that Joy first said, "Mommy, I love you." These emotional experiences are corrective for Tammy and create a new moral horizon, a possibility described by Swidler (1987):

> In loving and being loved, people give themselves over, at least for brief periods, to intensely moving experiences through which they achieve new awareness of self and others. Love can make possible periods of crystallization or reformulation of the self and the self's responsibility to the world. (p. 108)

Loving and caring for Joy reorganizes Tammy's world, pulling her to be the kind of mother she wants to be for Joy. Below, she describes how important it is for her to create practices that contrast with her mother's abuse in order to create that "bond that nobody can break because I never had that with my own mom":

> **T:** But I don't want [friends] to put forth help when I'm here because she's mine. Like I don't let people change her diaper for me. Well, I do sometimes and it's nice, but usually I can do it myself. Because I don't want to get too dependent on them doing it. Because I'm afraid I would slack off on being a mother to her—that's always been a concern—because my mom did it to me. I'm afraid if they kept doing it, I'd be—oh, okay, I can go do this or that, and I don't want to be that way because that's the way my mom was to me. From one minute to the next I didn't know who I was going to be with. And that's not right and that's not fair at all.
>
> I'm not trying to cut her off from the world. Everybody's involved with her—my family and friends. It's ok if my sister takes her for a day or so, but when I'm there, I'm the one who does everything for her so she knows that I'm the one that's her mother.

This passage and others show Tammy's heightened sense of responsibility that arises in having to create a world in opposition to her mother's example. Because she cannot rely on a worked-out, stable set of caring practices in raising Joy, she is vigilant, guarding herself from becoming like her mother. Because of the meaning of being left in the care of others, Tammy feels compelled to do everything for Joy. Help offered to her cannot be accepted or refused based on the immediate situation but is read for how much she is like or unlike her mother. Tammy's "hyper-responsibility" (see Benner, Tanner, & Chesla, 1992, for a similar response in learning to be a nurse) reflects a deliberative style of mothering in which one is obliged to invent a set of practices out of whole cloth without the stable significance provided by being fluent or at home in a working tradition. In the absence of working family traditions, lacking stories and practices that cultivate notions of the good and rituals of responsiveness and love, the usually prereflective know-how of mothering that gets passed on implicitly through habits and routines must now be learned more deliberately and built up by way of contrast and imagination. Although this is probably the case for many modern parents to some extent because of rapid demographic and sociocultural changes impacting family life and the peculiarly modern striving to become "perfect" parents (Walkover, 1992), it is especially true for those with abusive histories in which caring practices from their past provide a thin and shabby guide for developing practices of responsiveness to a particular child. Where sources of good mothering are limited, mothers must rely on their will and imagination to build up corrective habits and routines, an alternative mood and style of mothering that is animated, in part, by protestation over an abusive past.

But Tammy's story also depicts, in however fragile terms, an emerging moral framework in the sense described by Taylor (1989), which is not a belief system but an orientation to the good incumbent in loving and caring for a child. Her experience is directed not only by her protestation against her past but by skills, meanings, and notions of the good lived out in being Joy's mother. The moral distinctions she adopts as a mother provide a ground from which to evaluate her behavior, lead her to live a drug-free life, and direct her to take a strong stand regarding what her friends can and cannot do in Joy's presence. For example, when Tammy is contemplating moving in with her boyfriend and two other couples, she calls a meeting with prospective housemates:

> T: . . . that if I live here, things all have to be for the benefit of my daughter. There can be drinking but not like a party and not all the time. But I just told them I don't want parties there, and if there were going to be parties there, then to let me know a week ahead of time because I don't want to inconvenience you, because it's your home, but it's going to be my home too. And I have to set down some rules. If I'm going to live here, you're going to have to understand. I got everyone down and everyone gave their opinions on it because I can't fool around. I don't have time for someone to say something and not to stick by it. I have my life to live.

Tammy also informs them that if she moves in, smoking pot in the house is not acceptable because of the example it would set for Joy. Although she admits to having smoked pot a couple of times since Joy's birth, she says, "I don't like the feeling because I'd end up worrying about her, thinking about something and getting paranoid, and that's not fun to me." It is also of utmost importance to Tammy that her friends show an attentiveness to the baby. Unlike several other teens who participated in this study, Tammy is not jealous of the attention Joy receives from family and friends. She experiences the attention bestowed on her child as self-affirming:

> **I:** So tell me about a recent memorable situation.
>
> **T:** Well, me and Joy went over to my girlfriend's school and we saw our friends, and everybody just like went crazy over Joy, they loved her. And they wanted to hold her and they wanted to play with her and she was being really cute. She was being really cute. And she'd like play and she'd talk, and they'd say "pretty baby" and she'd say it back, and it was really cute. It made me feel good that people cared about my baby and not just me. You know, they weren't just friends with me but they cared about Joy too.

Tammy admits that she is more "cautious" now, taking fewer risks in potentially dangerous situations. For example, on New Year's Eve, she opts not to go out with friends who will be drinking but stays at home with Joy:

> **T:** [New Year's Eve] was fun. You know, cause I like being alone with her. For a lot of people think it's boring, but I don't think it's boring; cause if you don't make it boring, if you love the person, it shouldn't be a problem.

Other aspects of her life also come in for review. For example, she no longer wears tight-fitting, immodest clothing:

> **T:** . . . the clothes that I wore—like I'd wear spandex and stuff like that, and it's just—I can't get into wearing things like that anymore, cause I don't want her wearing things like that.

The world of mothering—with its perspective, demands, and relational capacities—introduces a deep desire to do the right thing that fits with the shared background practices available in the culture. This is not primarily a matter of willing, desiring, and highly deliberative thinking but of adopting and being led by the possibilities that show up in a specific mother-child relationship as shaped by the webs of one's history. Although in Tammy's case, her mother's negative example compels her to be conscious of acting differently—"to make damn sure that I'm not that way to Joy"—her conscious deliberation is first conditioned by the background significance of Joy mattering to her. The fact that she has had counseling that "helped her to get her life organized" and to come to terms with her deprived past has no doubt opened up possibilities available in mothering:

T: Well, it made me understand what I was going through throughout my pregnancy, and it made me understand how my mother is, and how my family is and how they're not going to change.

Below, Tammy offers a dramatic example of her mother's self-absorption when I ask if her mother was a good mother to her:

T: I think she thought she was, but she really wasn't. I mean, it was like—she was the kind of person, she was the kind of mother that was there for you, to give you the loving feeling when it was right timing for her, you know. And whenever it was the right time for her. I mean, we'd go to hug her and kiss her goodbye when she goes on a date, and she'd actually yell at us and slap us for touching her fucking hair. Okay? Her hair! All right? I mean, stupid whore went out all the time, you know. It's just. And for touching her hair! Okay, I mean, that's pretty stupid. That's how stuck on herself she was.

Tammy's attentiveness to Joy is revealed throughout her interviews and in the following excerpt in which she allows time "to relax with the baby" when dropping Joy off at her mother's before going to work:

T: She doesn't like me just to leave her and go. Just to drop her off and go.
I: Okay. So it's a way of settling her and—how did you learn that?
T: Because it's just, when you just say, "Okay, bye," and you just leave, they start crying, they feel really bad.
I: So 20 minutes sort of allows her to . . .
T: Yeah, to get her mind off of it, and then I go talk to her and I always tell her that I'm going to come back.
I: And what's it like when you come back, is she still up?
T: Oh, yeah. She's—oh, my God, she gets so excited. She goes, "OOH." And she walks around the house going, "oh, oh, oh." It's so funny. She does that all the time now. She'll walk around going, "Oh, oh, mommy." And she'll run up to me and she'll hug me and I'm going, Joy, you are weird. It looks so cute and it makes me feel so good that she cares like that.

Other examples give credence to Tammy's assessment of her more engaged involvement compared to her mother's vacillating moods and unpredictable behavior:

I: How would you say your mothering style is different or similar to your own mother's style?

T: I think it's different because I'm more aware of Joy and I'm thinking more of Joy and not of myself. Everything revolved around [my mother].

The excerpt below shows how Tammy's responsiveness to Joy develops from knowing her baby, where knowing depends upon working out the notions of the good in a particular mother-child relationship:

I: And how does a parent know what a child needs?

T: If you're really close to them, you just feel it, just by their actions.

I: Can you give me a for instance?

T: Like when Joy's walking around the house, around the house moaning, going "ooh, ooh," like that and she'll just kind of cry but she'll just keep walking around the house—she wants her bottle, or she's hungry.

I: Oh. How do you think you get to understand that?

T: Just by being around her and by studying, you know, the way she is. And, you know, like her actions towards me.

At my last visit when Joy was 15 months old and exhibiting the temperament of a curious and sometimes willful toddler, Tammy did not become embroiled with her daughter's growing independence. Tammy readily acknowledges in the coping episode below that her child's fussiness is sometimes taxing, annoying, and perplexing:

T: Uh, I guess when she's—she's really, um, tired it makes it really hard.

I: What's hard about it?

T: Oh, she gets really mean like her father.

I: Like what does she do?

T: She scratches you in the face, she hits you in the face. She throws tantrums when you put her down. Um, then she screams at the top of her lungs in bed when she's fighting sleep.

I: So, can you remember a recent situation like that?

T: Um, yeah. A week ago she just threw a temper tantrum; I don't know what was wrong with her. She didn't want to eat, she didn't want her bottle, she wasn't wet, she didn't want me to put her down, she didn't want me to pick her up, and then on Christmas, that was worse. I've never seen her have a tantrum as bad as she did. She started screaming and crying, and all these people were here, and she'd just, like, she freaked out, and I took her in the other room and she would scream at the top of her lungs; her face was beet red and I did not know what was wrong with this kid and so I just put her in her bed, I mean I rocked her a little bit and me and my sister were in my mom's room talking to her and stuff, but she just—and then she finally calmed down and I put her down.

> **I:** How did you feel during it?
>
> **T:** I was pissed cause I didn't know what was wrong, and then I was scared because I'd never seen her react that way before. You know, I thought something was wrong. But nothing was wrong; she just threw a fit. I guess it's because maybe she was so excited because there was so many people here, that was the only thing I could think of.

Because of Tammy's abusive childhood and her own impetuousness, one wonders how she copes with sudden uncontrollable anger. She volunteered an early episode within 3 months of giving birth when Joy's continuous crying almost unhinged her. Rather than striking out at Joy, she put Joy in her crib and left the room until she could calm herself. In telling the story, she credited a teacher's words for what to do in potentially abusive situations—"Put the child in a safe place, leave the room, calm yourself before going back to the baby." Learning that she *could* control herself in such a situation has been an important lesson. She denies that she has ever come that close in the year following this episode.

Although Tammy is affectionate and comforting with Joy, her typical style of being with others is much less yielding and more tough and at times downright defiant. As she says, "I don't let people get over on me." With so little comfort and safety in her past, she learned to protect herself by being separate and defiant. Her interactional style of overcoming others to protect herself, brought forward from her precarious and abusive past, leads her to be combative and reckless at times. Without a doubt, she remains impetuous and too quick to fight with peers, but her fighting now shows up as an issue for her. She notices when she falls short of her intention not to fight:

> **T:** Like the other day I almost got into a fight. But I don't fight anymore. I'm trying not to fight cause I'm supposed to be responsible, and I am. . . . Most people who do fight, it's like they're hurting inside and that makes them get angry, and then they fight. And that's the way I used to be. Cause little things like my boyfriend or just little things, would set me off and I'd fight. And, um, I'm not sad about anything or depressed about anything. So I just kind of, you know, I have a big mouth but I talk more than I fight. But if it came down to it, I wouldn't care, I'd still fight. But I try not to because what if, like we were in, in that store or whatever, and a cop came by. I can't get arrested. I will not have anyone take me away from my kid cause then I'd end up hurting the cop. I'm serious. Nobody would take me away from my kid. So I got to watch what I do. And that's the only thing that would get me in trouble. Fighting.

Tammy intimidates friends and strangers whose comments or inattention to the baby offend and provoke her. One episode in which Joy fell off the bed while being watched by a friend angered Tammy so that a fight almost ensued. In another situation with a fellow employee, she describes the mood and embodied responses developed during childhood that overtake her intent not to fight:

> **T:** I was in the mood to fight, but I'm not like that anymore, but it just kind of popped up. I mean, I am but I'm trying not to because it doesn't show that I have responsibility. I mean I know that I do, but to other people looking back on me and my child, it makes them think, "Well what kind of standards does she have?"

In wanting to set a good example for her daughter, Tammy claims she never fights in her daughter's presence. But she worries that her daughter might eventually learn about her fighting from "war stories":

> **T:** . . . because it's not right and it doesn't make you look cool. I want her to know self-defense so she can protect herself, but I don't want her to fight like I did because it didn't get me anywhere. I've gotten my ass beat three times and I've fought since I was 11. I want her to stick up for herself, but I don't want her to antagonize people.
>
> **I:** How do you want your daughter to handle problems with people?
>
> **T:** I want her to talk them out, but if somebody's hitting her, then I want her to beat their ass. And if she doesn't, to go back for more. And if she's really scared of the person, then I'm going to go with her.

Tammy has a harder time imagining behavior and a future for her daughter that differ from her own ways of being in the world. It is perhaps easier for her to create practices that differ from her mother's than her own embodied responses to growing up in an abusive household.

Tammy's aspirations for the near future pivot on being Joy's mother. Being a homemaker and mother takes precedence over a "career" while Joy is young:

> **T:** Because I wanna eventually be a housewife when I find the right person.
>
> **I:** Oh?
>
> **T:** I mean, I wanna have a career but not yet, not until Joy's like 10 years old.
>
> **I:** Really? Describe why that's important to you.
>
> **T:** So, so, I can, I can grow up with her. So we can grow up together. I think that's why it's good for you to have a kid when you're fairly young because then you're growing together.

Tammy's future may diverge considerably from her present hopes. There may be little opportunity for her to have a "career" or to be a full-time housewife because the first is dependent on a good education (she is not a high school graduate) and the second is dependent on marrying a stable provider. It is perhaps more feasible to imagine her struggling to support herself as a single mother who becomes dependent on welfare or low-paying service or clerical jobs. Tammy, in fact, begins a poorly paying part-time telemarketing job during the study period that may be a portent of things to come, particularly when she loses her Supplemental Security Income (SSI) benefits at age 18. She dislikes the job because it is "boring" and because she is away from Joy during that time. But the added money helps her savings account grow and sets an example of work and self-discipline for Joy that she never had growing up. Early in the job, she begins to experience the competing demands of work and mothering:

> **T:** I hate going to work. Not because, not because I don't enjoy it, just because I don't like being away from her.
> **I:** So how do you cope with it?
> **T:** I just forget about it, or get on the phone and call. I do that a lot.
> **I:** So tell me what's the most frequent number of times you've called home?
> **T:** Five. Within a 4-hour period. Only a 4-hour period and they talk to you on the phone, and the only thing she says is "hi," but I can talk to her for the longest time. The most she's ever said is "Hi, baby." And I say, "Hi, how you doing, Joy? I love you." And she goes, "Hi, baby, hi, baby, hi, baby." That's all she says. And I can talk to her forever.

By the end of the study, Joy sometimes accompanies Tammy to her job with her supervisor's approval. Her supervisor permits Joy to be in the office even though he could be fired for doing so because "he's a good friend and knows I have responsibilities." Joy is welcomed by staff, who are amused by her as she plays with a play telephone in the area set up by staff.

This scene has little in common with Tammy's prepregnancy account of a drug-filled, self-destructive existence. Joy has created existentially a "place" for Tammy that allows more responsiveness, restraint, and affection than Tammy ever experienced in her own childhood. Tammy has not remade herself as much as mothering has remade her by giving her corrective experiences and a set of practices that introduce significance, meaning, identity, and a future within the possibilities and constraints of her immediate situation and the wider social understandings of what it is to be a woman and a mother. In her instance, the formative possibilities of mothering have most likely been fostered by counseling that helped her to understand and face the story of her impoverished past.

Commentary

". . . nothing living resembles a straight line . . ."
(Marge Piercy, cited in Howell, 1975, p. 25)

Tammy's story offers a dramatic example of the self's remarkable capacity to adopt new meanings and concerns and the vulnerability of doing so in the absence of a positive maternal legacy and responsive community. With moral sources of care lacking in her past, Tammy must depend upon her own experience and imagination for weaving a new web. She is guided by the moral claim of the baby to create a new narrative of comfort and care in opposition to family norms and peer relations. She must create a new world for her child and herself in relative isolation and separation, spinning a web of her own without the backup or invisible safety net of care and responsiveness to sustain her vision of the good, building new skills and routines that contrast with her painful and bitter childhood memories. To create a world for herself and her child is a remarkable human possibility captured in Adrienne Rich's poem "Integrity":

> Anger and tenderness: the spider's genius
> to spin and weave in the same action
> from her own body, anywhere—
> even from a broken web.

[The lines from "Integrity" are reprinted from A WILD PATIENCE HAS TAKEN ME THIS FAR, poems 1978-1981, by Adrienne Rich, by permission of the author and W. W. Norton & Company, Inc. Copyright © 1981 by Adrienne Rich.]

In the midst of a frayed and threadbare community, pulled forward by her desire to overcome her past and to meet her baby's needs for care, Tammy scrapes together an altered future. The shape and direction of that future remains open-ended; understanding its course will remain forever inexplicable to the cool, dispassionate language of normalizing science, which, in overlooking context, meanings, and notions of the good, blunts distinctions and treats human being as a raw resource to be controlled and disciplined in line with a moral order based on technical rationality (Borgman, 1984; Foucault, 1979; O'Neill, 1985; Rose, 1989; Schwartz, 1986). Understanding the unevenness of a human life and the situated possibilities that emerge (that fully escape the technological paradigm) is captured, if at all, in a story, as George Eliot (cited in Coles, 1989) so eloquently reminds us:

> Every limit is a beginning as well as an ending. Who can quit young lives after being in long company with them, and not desire to know what befell them in their after-years? For the fragment of a life, however typical, is not the sample of an even web: promises may not be kept, and an ardent outset may be

followed by declension; latent powers may find their long-waited opportunity; a past error may urge a grand retrieval. (p. 809)

The Power of Narrative

Tammy's story demonstrates the power and validity of narrative accounts for moving beyond deficit-finding and filling approaches wherein formal evaluative criteria are privileged over the concerns, possibilities, limitations, shortcomings, obstacles, and notions of the good that are worked out in a specific mother-child relationship. Whereas young mothers' stories are curtailed and their voices silenced in scientific-rational discourse, stories of everyday experience provide an opportunity to engage a young mother in a dialogue that reveals her situated understanding and notions of the good that are fused with and organized by the family and social worlds she inhabits.

That a young mother may find possibilities for becoming a responsive self ultimately depends on the extent to which her vision of the good is sustained and nurtured by others. For many participants in this study, an interviewing style that presupposed their narrative competence and actively solicited ordinary accounts of mothering sometimes helped them to find and respond to their own voices, legitimated their concerns, and clarified their dilemmas and difficulties, with the result that their practical understanding of their situation was sometimes deepened (Mishler, 1986; Rosenwald, 1992; Tappan, 1991; White & Epston, 1990). For Tammy, the opportunity to talk to an attentive, engaged listener about what mattered to her and how she should live validated and confirmed the very possibilities she was trying to articulate. As Gilligan (1987) points out, giving teenagers the chance to describe their experience supports the teenager's emerging moral voice:

> Such questioning may reveal to teenagers that they have a moral perspective, something of value at stake, and thus that they have grounds for action in situations where they may have felt stuck or confused or unable to choose between alternative paths. The efficacy of the intervention may depend on the responsiveness of the research relationship, on whether the researcher engages with the teenager's thinking rather than simply mirroring or assessing it. For the adolescent, the realization that he, and perhaps especially she, has a moral perspective that an adult finds interesting, or a moral voice that someone will respond to, shifts the framework for action away from a choice between submission and rebellion (action defined in others' terms) and provides a context for discovering one's own terms. (p. 89)

The formative possibilities of storytelling became apparent to me once I realized how carving out a future and reorganizing her life around mothering had been *the* focus of Tammy's interviews. I was abruptly reminded of this 2 years later when I revisited Tammy. Upon greeting me at the door, she volunteered in unequivocal terms, "I don't fight anymore." These few words immediately reoriented me to the drama and force of her struggle to become the mother she wanted to be. As an empathetic witness who had helped to "midwife" her "corrective narrative" (Benner, 1991), she, without hesitation, launched into resuming her story where she had left off 2 years earlier. In the 9 months preceding my visit, Tammy's mother had stopped drinking, at least in part because Tammy delivered an ultimatum that she would no longer see her grandchild until she maintained sobriety. She was also excited to tell me about her engagement to a 21-year-old after a year-long relationship. They were in the process of saving their money from his full-time job as an assistant manager in a retail firm for a wedding in a year. She described this young man as more reliable and responsive than previous boyfriends, and she had no reservations about the kind of father he would be to Joy. As I was drawn again to consider the shape and direction of Tammy's ongoing story, I felt there were grounds for hoping that the redirection of her life was repairing old habits and making fewer demands that she remain so fiercely independent and that she might, given more responsive relationships, experience the comfort and care that was so tenuous in her childhood.

Other evidence for the formative possibilities inherent in storytelling comes from a study that investigated a short-term educational intervention with black teenage mothers in the first postpartum week (Greenberg, 1988). To control for the Hawthorne effect of time spent with the researcher, a contrast group of young mothers *did not* receive instruction in recognizing and responding to infant cues for interaction; rather, they were encouraged to talk about their experiences during pregnancy, labor, delivery, and early mothering. One month later, the mothers who received this "nonintervention" expressed more confidence as parents (as measured by a Parenting Sense of Competency Scale) than mothers in either experimental or control groups, and during a time of feedback with the researcher described how talking about their experience "helped them to think things through and sort out some of their feelings" (p. 70). This serendipitous finding led the researcher to recommend that active listening be added to educational programs. I, of course, agree and add that the tact of listening furthers a responsively engaged relationship and dialogue with the new mother that sets up the very possibility for tailoring an educational program to her experience, skills, concerns, and struggles, thereby curbing the modern impetus to impose interventions that may be irrelevant to the young mother's understanding and situated possibilities (see Smith, 1991, and Field, Widmayer, Stringer, & Ignatoff, 1980).

Tammy's story served as a paradigm case (Benner, 1985) that brought a fresh perspective to understanding young mother's lives. Although dramatic and deliberative, her story captures the struggles, conflicts, and constraints as well as the potential learning and moral development that comes from "growing with a child." Like others with an impoverished and shabby maternal legacy, Tammy must create practices in isolation without the example and support of trusted others. But her story also reveals her learning to set limits on the most dangerous and unreliable aspects of her community as the baby's needs for care led her to adopt and learn new responsive and responsible habits. Her narrative not only shows how the teenager's problems, conflicts, difficulties, shortcomings, and possibilities for growth and development are not strictly matters located in the self to be endlessly manipulated and controlled, but also articulates the possibilities and impossibilities of the family and social worlds one inhabits.

Conclusion

We can spin only what we hear, because we hear, and as well as we hear.
(Daly, 1978, p. 424)

Despite the two-decades-old social policy debate and the extensive literature and research on teenage pregnancy and parenting, we have given scant attention to the stories of young mothers and family members. Through the presentation of one entire case, I have argued that narratives, in recovering young mothers' voices, shift attention from a singular, narrow interest in identifying norm-based deficits and failures of teen mothers and capture instead, the difficulties, conflicts, notions of the good, and the possibilities for development experienced by young mothers. Tammy's story, in particular, highlights the working out of possibilities against the background of a fragile and unworkable maternal legacy, the burdens arising from hyper-responsiveness, and previously unnoticed sources of good, hope, and possibility.

My hope is that the stories of young mothers will move us away from the language, distance, and stigma of normalizing disciplinary practices to a dialogue that hears and heeds their words. Here I am referring not only to the numerous exchanges between young mothers, family members, and professionals who serve them but also to the many other "conversations" that foster or imperil young mothers' vision of the good and growth toward responsiveness. The reader is encouraged to consider how the stories of young mothers might shape the practices of educators, social workers, and health care providers in ways respectful of the meanings, obstacles, contradictions, options, and possibilities that their stories disclose, and how their words may challenge us as citizens to join the many "conversations" to create the neighborhoods, schools, health care institutions, and social welfare and corporate policies that preserve and extend responsiveness, care, comfort, safety, hope, and opportunity for all children.

References

Arney, W. R., & Bergen, B. J. (1984). Power and visibility: The invention of teenage pregnancy. *Social Science and Medicine, 18,* 11-19.

Benner, P. (1985). Quality of life: A phenomenological perspective on explanation, prediction and understanding in nursing science. *Advances in Nursing Science, 8,* 1-14.

Benner, P. (1991). The primacy of caring: The role of experience, narrative and community in skilled ethical comportment. *Advances in Nursing Science, 14,* 1-21.

Benner, P., Tanner, C., & Chesla, C. (1992). From beginner to expert: Gaining a differentiated clinical world in critical care nursing. *Advances in Nursing Science, 14*(3), 13-28.

Benner, P., & Wrubel, J. (1989). *The primacy of caring: Stress and coping in health and illness.* Reading, MA: Addison-Wesley.

Borgman, A. (1984). *Technology and the character of contemporary life.* Chicago: University of Chicago Press.

Bruner, J. (1987). Life as narrative. *Social Research, 54,* 11-32.

Burton, L. M. (1990). Teenage childbearing as an alternative life-course strategy in multigeneration black families. *Human Nature, 1,* 123-143.

Coles, R. (1989). *The call of stories: Teaching and the moral imagination.* Boston: Houghton Mifflin.

Daly, M. (1978). *Gyn/Ecology.* Boston: Beacon.

Dreyfus, H. L. (1991). *Being-in-the-world: A commentary on Heidegger's "Being and time," Division I.* Cambridge: MIT Press.

Erikson, E. M. (1963). *Childhood and society* (2nd ed.). New York: Norton.

Field, T. M., Widmayer, S. M., Stringer, S., & Ignatoff, E. (1980). Teenage, lower-class, black mothers and their preterm infants: An intervention and developmental follow-up. *Child Development, 51,* 426-436.

Fine, M. (1988). Sexuality, schooling, and adolescent females: The missing discourse of desire. *Harvard Educational Review, 58,* 29-53.

Foucault, M. (1979). *Discipline and punish: The birth of the prison (A. Sheridan, Trans.).* New York: Vintage.

Freeman, M. (1984). History, narrative, and life-span developmental knowledge. *Human Development, 27,* 1-19.

Freeman, M. (1991). Rewriting the self: Development as moral practice. *New Directions for Child Development, 54,* 83-102.

Gabriel, A., & McAnarney, E. R. (1983). Parenthood in two sub-cultures: White, middle-class couples and black, low-income adolescents in Rochester, N.Y. *Adolescence, 18,* 595-608.

Gilligan, C. (1987). Adolescent development reconsidered. *New Directions for Child Development, 37,* 63-91.

Greenberg, R. (1988). *The effects of a short term perinatal intervention on stress and parenting attitudes, perceptions, and behaviors of black adolescent mothers.* Unpublished doctoral dissertation, University of Michigan.

Guignon, C. (1983). *Heidegger and the problem of knowledge.* Indianapolis: Hackett.

Hayes, C. D. (1987). *Risking the future: Adolescent sexuality, pregnancy, and childbearing* (Vol. 1). Washington, DC: National Academy Press.

Holt, J. L., & Johnson, S. D. (l991). Developmental tasks: A key to reducing teenage pregnancy. *Journal of Pediatric Nursing, 6,* 191-196.

Howard, G. S. (l991). Culture tales: A narrative approach to thinking, cross-cultural psychology, and psychotherapy. *American Psychologist, 46,* 187-197.

Howell, M. D. (l975). *Helping ourselves: Families and the human network.* Boston: Beacon.

Klein, L. (1978). Antecedents of teenage pregnancy. *Clinical Obstetrics and Gynecology, 21,* 1151-1159.

Ladner, J. (l971). *Tomorrow's tomorrow.* New York: Doubleday.

Leonard, V. W. (l989). A Heideggerian phenomenologic perspective on the concept of the person. *Advances in Nursing Science, 11*(4), 40-55.

Mishler, E. G. (l979). Meaning in context: Is there any other kind? *Harvard Educational Review, 49,* 1-19.

Mishler, E. (1986). *Research interviewing: Context and narrative.* Cambridge: Harvard University Press.

Musick, J. S. (l990). Adolescents as mothers: The being and the doing. *Zero to Three, 11*(2), 7-8, 23-28.

O'Neill, J. (1985). *Five bodies: The human shape of modern society.* Ithaca, NY: Cornell University Press.

Packer, M. J. (l985). Hermeneutic inquiry in the study of human conduct. *American Psychologist, 40,* 1081-1093.

Packer, M. J. (1991). Interpreting stories, interpreting lives: Narrative and action in moral development research. *New Directions for Child Development, 54,* 63-82.

Polkinghorne, D. E. (1988). *Narrative knowing and the human sciences.* Albany: State University of New York Press.

Poole, C. (1987). Adolescent pregnancy and unfinished developmental tasks of childhood. *Journal of School Health, 57,* 271-273.

Rich, A. 1981. *A wild patience has taken me this far: Poems 1978-1981.* New York: Norton.

Rose, N. (1989). Individualizing psychology. In J. Shotter & K. J. Gergen (Eds.), *Texts of identity* (pp. 119-132). Newbury Park, CA: Sage.

Rosenwald, G. C. (1992). Conclusion: Reflections on narrative self-understanding. In G. C. Rosenwalk & R. L. Ochberg (Eds.), *Storied lives: The cultural politics of self-understanding* (pp. 265-289). New Haven: Yale University Press.

Sadler, L. S., & Catrone, C. (l983). The adolescent parent: A dual developmental crisis. *Journal of Adolescent Health Care, 4,* 100-105.

Schwartz, B. (l986). *The battle for human nature: Science, morality and modern life.* New York: Norton.

Smith, L. (1991). Critique [of family-focused tertiary prevention with the adolescent mother and her child.] In S. S. Humenick, N. Wilkerson, & N. Paul (Eds.), *Adolescent pregnancy: Nursing perspectives on prevention* (pp. 155-168). Birth Defects: Original Article Series, Vol. 27, No. 1. White Plains, NY: March of Dimes Birth Defects Foundation.

SmithBattle, L. (1992). *Caring for teenage mothers and their children: Narratives of self and ethics of intergenerational caregiving.* Unpublished doctoral dissertation, University of California, San Francisco.

Stack, C. G. (l974). *All our kin: Strategies for survival in a black community.* New York: Harper & Row.

Swidler, A. (1987). Love and adulthood in American culture. In R. N. Bellah, R. Madsen, W. M. Sullivan, A. Swidler, & S. M. Tipton. (Eds.), *Individualism and commitment in American life* (pp. 107-125). New York: Harper & Row.

Tappan, M. B. (1991). Narrative, authorship, and the development of moral authority. *New Directions for Child Development, 54,* 5-25.

Taylor, C. (1989). *Sources of the self: The making of the modern identity.* Cambridge, MA: Harvard University Press.

Walkover, B. C. (1992). The family as an overwrought object of desire. In G. C. Rosenwald & R. L. Ochberg (Eds.), *Storied lives: The cultural politics of self-understanding* (pp. 178-191). New Haven: Yale University Press.

Williams, R. N. (1987). Can cognitive psychology offer a meaningful account of meaningful human action? *Journal of Mind and Behavior, 8,* 209-221.

White, M., & Epston, D. (1990). *Narrative means to therapeutic ends.* New York: Norton.

Young, M. (1988). Parenting during mid-adolescence: A review of developmental theories and parenting behavior. *Maternal-Child Nursing Journal, 17,* 1-12.

9

✚

Parents' Caring Practices With Schizophrenic Offspring

CATHERINE A. CHESLA

We have many fictional and historical depictions of the family as a context in which members are cared for with solicitude, affection, and skill. Lasch (1977) suggests that the family remains a unique and important repository for these romantic illusions. Present-day families, however, live in a culture in which rationality prevails, science holds tremendous power, and technological advancements encroach on or replace many traditional cultural practices (Borgman, 1984). Although it seems reasonable to assume that family care has been shaped by this modern culture, the practical ways that families take up the care of their ill or vulnerable members have not been well examined.

In this investigation, family care was examined through parents who cared for offspring with schizophrenia. Although many aspects of the caring practices that were discovered would be particular to schizophrenia, the ways that parents undertook this care might have commonalities with family care of other chronic mental illnesses (Rolland, 1984). Discovering these potential commonalities begins with a detailed description of the experience of

NOTE: This project was funded by National Research Service Award #1F32 NRO6214 from the National Center for Nursing Research. The helpful comments of Dr. Patricia Benner are gratefully acknowledged.

167

caring for a schizophrenic son or daughter, using the parents' own stories and terms.

Problems arising from schizophrenia for both the individual and the family have been well documented (Bernheim, Lewine, & Beale, 1982; Chesla, 1988; Seymour & Dawson, 1986). Schizophrenics fit poorly into a society that values achievement because the illness drains the individual of motivation to accomplish valued goals. The negative symptoms of the illness (Andreason, 1984) read like a list of vices in our culture: apathy, social withdrawal, anhedonia, amotivation. Matters are worsened by the fact that these symptoms are present in physically healthy adults, who appear to be able to work. The positive symptoms of the illness, particularly hallucinations and delusions, set schizophrenics apart, making it difficult for them to share common understandings of everyday life. Families have identified the demands of living with schizophrenic offspring as (a) breakdowns in meanings shared by schizophrenic and parent, (b) changes in the schizophrenic's person, (c) lack of clarity in the boundaries of the illness, and (d) regression in the schizophrenic's abilities to manage life responsibilities (Chesla, 1988).

The aim of this project was to provide an interpretive account of parents' caring practices that evolved in response to the demands of living with schizophrenic offspring. The study focused on parents' ongoing practical activity directed to care for their ill family member. Their ongoing involvement in their child's care was studied directly through observation and indirectly through narrative accounts. The study's overarching goal was to discover what care meant to these parents and to understand their concerns and practices as they provided that care.

Background

In studies of family care of the chronically mentally ill, traditional scientific methods have predominated and have emphasized the rational and technical aspects of care. In a recent review, the foci of these studies have been identified as: (a) impact of family environments on illness course; (b) the impact of care on the family/caregiver, or family "burden" research; and (c) families' perceptions of their resource needs (Chesla, 1989a). In these investigations care has been consistently conceptualized as tasks or burdens that place the family at risk (Pai & Kapur, 1981; Runions & Prudo, 1983; Thompson & Doll, 1982). Alternatively, the affective quality of the care has been conceptualized as a risk for the ill member (Kanter, Lamb, & Loeper, 1987; Koenigsberg & Handley, 1986). Within these dominant conceptualizations, empirical studies have identified families and schizophrenic members at risk for negative outcomes in physical or mental health. However, by focusing on the risk factors, these investigations have ignored what the experience means to the family, as well as the myriad of ways that they have undertaken the care (Bowers, 1987; Gubrium & Lynott, 1987).

Interpretive studies of the experience of caring for mentally ill or vulnerable family members have served as an important adjunct to empirical work. Nurses have discovered variations in family caring practices, emotional adjustments, and resolutions that went well beyond the understandings captured in the prevailing theoretical accounts (Bowers, 1987; Davis, 1980). In addition, nurses have identified new meaning constructs that captured aspects of the care previously unnamed; for example, mutuality and coping with negative choices (Hirschfeld, 1983; Wilson, 1989). A brief review of these works highlights how the interpretive accounts extend prevailing empirical studies.

Bowers (1987) found that adult caregivers were not primarily concerned with caregiving tasks, the central focus of much caregiving research, as they cared for their elderly disabled parents. She identified five categories of care: anticipatory, preventive, supervisory, instrumental, and protective. Only instrumental care encompassed the tasks of hands-on care, while the four remaining categories focused on emotional and interpersonal responsibilities and concerns. Family caregivers themselves identified protective care as the most central and demanding type of care, because it flowed from a concern to protect the elder's personhood and esteem and to maintain the relationship between the caregiver and elder even if it required withholding the most efficacious physical or medical care. This work highlighted a "hidden" aspect of care, that of protecting the elder, which exerted a powerful influence on caregiving decisions, yet was not acknowledged in prior conceptualizations of family care.

While exploring the family care of members with three types of disabilities—mental retardation, chronic mental illness, and disabilities of aging—Davis (1980) found that family adaptive responses to care responsibilities were evident across disabilities. She noted four distinct resolutions of the family's emotional adaptation to care demands: (a) positive action, (b) commitment to duty, (c) accommodation or growing accustomed, and (d) conflicted resolution that alternated between acceptance, rejection, and resentment. These adaptive patterns extended conceptions of family care by specifying a family-level response and by examining the adaptation to the demands of caring, rather than examining only the negative impacts.

Wilson (1989) identified a central demand in the care of a family member with Alzheimer's dementia as coping with negative choices and typified the family's coping process as one of surviving on the brink. In her sample of 20 community-based caregivers, she highlighted the variability in the family's coping over time; she identified distinct stages of coping with the crisis, chronic, and terminal phases of the disease and identified the coping strategies unique to each phase. Prior investigations of family coping have conceptualized coping as a static process; thus Wilson's work highlights the need to examine changes over time.

Finally, Hirschfeld (1983) found variability in the degree to which caregivers experienced mutuality with their elder family member with dementia. From the caregiver's perspective, mutuality was the ability to find gratification and meaning in the care relationship and to perceive reciprocal emotion from the impaired person. Four different levels of mutuality were statistically related to caregivers' morale, tension, attitude toward institutionalization, and the ability to manage.

In summary, interpretive nursing investigations have demonstrated the complexity and variability of care relations and caring practices for the chronically mentally ill. Each study described meaningful dimensions of family care that had not been previously noted in more empirical, abstract, risk and burden research on family care. Although these insights must be examined and extended in further investigations of family care, they evidence the importance of interpretive work in correcting and extending theoretical constructions about care.

Caring Practices

In this chapter caring practices are interpreted from a naturalistic study of families' care of their schizophrenic members. Background for understanding caring practices was derived from the work of Heidegger (1962) and Kierkegaard (1843/1985) as explicated by Dreyfus (1991) and Rubin (in press). Benner and Wrubel (1989) have pointed to the relevance of these philosophical orientations for nursing knowledge development and practice; caring practices are defined as "organized, specific practices related to caring for and about others" (Benner & Wrubel, 1989, p. 408). These practices are particular, historical, and contextually and situationally elicited and delimited. Practices grow from a tradition, in this case the tradition of family care and parenting practices, that is enriched by an ethic or notion of what is good and practical knowledge.

Such a phenomenological orientation to caring practices offers an alternative to a normative or pathological view of care. Care is not viewed as strictly attitudinal, but rather as a set of concrete practices that arise from caregivers' unique backgrounds, ways of being, skills, and understandings. The important interpretive task is to understand how certain aspects of the person and the situation open up possibilities and close down others in parents' care.

Benner (1984) has demonstrated that caring practices can be understood through narratives about real life experience in meaningful contexts. In contrast to abstract detached discussions about what care is or what it should be, which yield explanations of care, narratives move closer to the actual experience. They reveal caregivers' concerns, aspects of the situation that were salient, and the skills and practices that came into play when care was discussed. Caring practices are best described in exemplary stories of care that demonstrate the complex relations between the situational constraints and demands, and caregiver concerns and actions. The caring practices described in this paper are drawn from full narratives of parents' care experiences presented elsewhere (Chesla, 1988).

Method

The study was designed within the interpretive tradition of hermeneutics (Packer, 1985; Packer & Addison, 1989). The philosophic underpinnings and assumptions of the method have been detailed (Benner & Wrubel, 1989; Dreyfus, 1991; Leonard, 1989; Taylor, 1985) and exemplified in the work of Benner (1984) and others (Brykczynski 1989; Chesla, 1989b).

Twenty-one parents from 14 families who cared for a schizophrenic member in the community were recruited from family support groups and were followed for 3 months. Families were selected if the schizophrenic had been diagnosed for at least 1 year, was 20 to 35 years old, and lived with or had at least weekly contact with the parents. Consent to participate in individual and family interviews and observations was obtained from each participating family member, including the schizophrenic member.

Parents who participated were predominantly middle-aged, married couples. Thirteen parents were married (one father refused to participate), six were divorced, and two were widowed. Their mean age was 56 (range 50-77). Participants belonged to middle or upper middle class families. Most fathers held undergraduate or graduate degrees. Approximately half of the women had completed high school or some college, and the other half had under-graduate or graduate degrees. All of the men, even those who had retired from one career, were employed full time in professions such as teaching, law, engineering, middle management, or skilled labor. Five women were house-wives, and four women each were employed on a full-time or part-time basis in predominantly secretarial or clerical positions.

Their schizophrenic offspring had a mean age of 29 years (range 24-35) and had been ill for an average of 8.5 years (range 1-22). All but two of the schizophrenics in this sample were males. To protect the anonymity of the small number of families with daughters, all are referred to as males. Most of the schizophrenics had completed high school (seven) or some college (six), but only one had a college degree. Most were involved in some activity outside of the home. Six worked part time in clerical or labor jobs, two participated in day treatment, and one attended school on a part-time basis.

All members of each participating family, typically the father, mother, and schizophrenic, were individually interviewed by this author once a month using the Berkeley Stress and Coping interpretive interview (Benner, 1984; Lazarus & Folkman, 1984; Wrubel, 1985). Parents were asked to name positive and negative episodes of care and elaborate on their context, what they considered troublesome, the ways that they coped, the alternative courses of action they considered, their emotions, and the outcome of each episode. Each of the 21 parental caregivers described six to nine care episodes over the 3-month period. The author also observed 25 hours of care in the home of each family over an average of eight visits with half the sample. Extensive observation notes were made by hand during observational periods and transcribed into a family file immediately after the observation ended. Finally, the author attended family support groups in two separate counties for 12 months to learn about the generalizability of the episodes reported by study families. Interviews of parents from the same family were interpreted separately; thus the caring practices are described from their individual perspectives. Family-level interpretations and the schizophrenics' perspectives will be the subjects of other papers.

Hermeneutical interpretation is made up of three interwoven processes: thematic analyses, interpretation of exemplars, and interpretation of paradigm cases (Benner, 1985). The thematic interpretation of the interviews and observations proceeded through the following steps:

1. The complete notes from five families were reviewed for patterns of difficulties and care.
2. An interpretive outline was formed, which addressed lines of inquiry from both the original research questions and the categories of interest that arose consistently in the data.
3. Each case was then examined in detail, and the portions of text that were relevant to each portion of the interpretive outline were transferred to the outline, thus creating a new "coded" case file.
4. Across-case comparisons continued throughout the interpretive process but intensified after most cases had been coded.

5. Findings were validated (a) by repeatedly reading and testing texts against proposed interpretations, and (b) by presenting findings to the families' support groups for validation.

In addition to the general themes, "coping episodes," specific examples of stressful or difficult events that were cited by participants, were culled from the Stress and Coping Interviews. All relevant aspects of each coping episode were coded together, including (a) the caregiver's recollection of what preceded the episode, (b) how the episode unfolded, (c) the caregiver's emotions at the commencement and throughout the episode, (d) the actions considered and taken, (e) the direct and indirect clues to what was at stake for the caregiver, and (f) the caregiver's retrospective reworking of the situation; for example, would he or she change the action taken? In their complete form, these coping episodes served as exemplars of particular patterns of action that included a rich description of the situation and responses that evidenced the caregiver's intentions, concerns, and practices.

A paradigm case is a strong concrete instance of a pattern of things that go together in a particular way. Often, the patterns evident in a concrete paradigm can be identified consistently but cannot be reduced to a set of elements or rules that describe what the paradigm is and is not. In this project, paradigm cases of caring practices were identified by noting similar whole patterns of care that were evident in different families.

Caring Practices With Schizophrenic Offspring

Four qualitatively distinct forms of caring practices were evident in this sample of families and are the overarching ways in which parents undertook care: Engaged Care, Conflicted Care, Managed Care, and Distanced Care. They represent the parents' orientation to their children and how they worked out their concerns. The forms of caring were not pure; nor were they mutually exclusive. However, each parent did demonstrate one predominant form of caring over all others. This study did not permit the systematic investigation of how different forms of care evolved over time; thus there is no suggestion of how one form of care developed into another.

Engaged Care

Parents who provided Engaged Care were solicited by the child's difficulties and undertook care in a way that gave their lives content and direction; they characterized their care as an extension of their parental responsibilities.

Their interviews lacked an emphasis on personal suffering and focused instead on the satisfactions they derived from the care and the care's significance. Instead of attempting to balance giving and receiving, these parents were personally drawn to and fulfilled by the care.

> I think [caregiving] is like motherhood you know? You just do these things without even thinking about them. I always have watched my children. And I think I know them quite well, even though sometimes they think I don't. [laughs] I think it's because we have been so interested in the kids. They've been the *most important things in our life.* And anything else really was secondary.

Parents are expected to devote themselves to the care of their child during infancy and childhood. But it becomes suspect to continue this form of care into the child's adulthood. Some theories label such parents as overinvolved or dysfunctional (Beavers, 1982). Although these parents suffered stigma because they chose to support their adult schizophrenic children financially, socially, and practically, they did not waiver in that support. Rather, they characterized their care as something they were called to do and, in the words of one mother, they found it "honorable, difficult, and *for* me."

Parents involved in Engaged Care exhibited a level of acceptance with the situation as it stood. They found possibilities for living within the bounds and limits that the schizophrenia placed on their lives. One father noted, "I've missed a lot with him that I would like to have had with a son. But you learn to realize that he's sick and you live within the parameters of the sickness." Parents did not achieve a "state" of acceptance that was fixed once and for all, but participated in a continual process of accepting what the disease turned out to be. What was fixed was their engagement in the process.

Engaged Care parents tried to understand the ill family member's thoughts, actions, and worries. They sought access to the child's world and worked to engage him in the real world.

> I poured a concrete wall for a walkway in the yard. He comes down and sits and talks to me. It's good [to be] in an association like that, we can talk and relate a little bit, and that always helps. Then whenever I can, I ask his opinion on things. I like to have him come to me and have him try to help me. Otherwise I'm shutting him out. To me, it would be devastating to shut him out. He gets enough of that all day long, people shutting him out. He's difficult to talk to.

Other parents also sought ways to access the child's world and to engage them in their real world as much as possible. One mother purposefully searched the television channels for programs on animals, knowing that her son loved these programs and that they could watch them together. Another

mother demonstrated exquisite skill in selectively attending to the schizophrenic's chatter. While visiting in the home, I could not make sense of his
statements, but his mother knew the consistent themes and knew, by his tone
or manner of speaking, when there was a new theme or a greater level of
anxiety.

Engaged Care parents demonstrated that they were most interested in
fostering the schizophrenic's self-esteem and that they were only secondarily
concerned about improving his functioning. One father demonstrated this
priority.

> We have one of these instant hot water taps in the kitchen. The darn thing
> sticks. My wife says, "He is fixing the hot water faucet." [laughs] Like it's go-
> ing to be a disaster. We had a feeling he was going to really screw this up. He
> didn't fix it. But rather than telling him "leave it alone," to me it is worth
> even buying a new hot water faucet than to discourage him.

These parents maintained a supportive stance by lowering their expectations
and by accepting their child's limits.

Finally, the parents who gave Engaged Care demonstrated a capacity for
joy, satisfaction, or "high notes" with their schizophrenic children. One
father told me:

> He bought me a nice Father's Day card. And that's a high note, when he does
> little things like that. That was a high moment. [Pause] Doesn't take much of
> a good thing to be called a high moment, with our son.

This bittersweet statement reflects the father's sad acceptance of what was
possible for his son given the bounds of schizophrenia.

These parents had difficulty setting limits and asking the ill member to
change noxious behaviors. Consequently, their lives were disrupted by the
symptoms to a greater extent than other families. For example, one schizophrenic son collected garbage and stored it in large visible piles around the
parents' home. Although the parents were distressed by this practice and
embarrassed with the neighbors, they could not limit their son's collecting
because they feared that they would upset him and cause him to be self-
destructive.

Conflicted Care

Conflicted Care parents were always dissatisfied, disgruntled, and angry
at their situation. The anger arose from the thwarted hopes for themselves
and their child. The child solicited them and enlisted their efforts but at the

same time created conflicts in terms of their concern for their own well-being. The conflicts that held them were so intense and pervasive that their care was a struggle, which was evident in their descriptions of care as "a pain in the ass" or "annoying as hell." They admitted they felt "cheated" and "resentful" about their responsibilities.

One father's discussion of his son's dogs demonstrated the conflicting concerns. He supported the dogs because they provided companionship and a source of personal responsibility, yet he detested the dogs' messes.

> He likes the dogs; the dogs like him. And I think that people with many forms of mental illness can benefit from having dogs. And these are exceptionally nice dogs. And sometimes I think it would be nice if maybe they got run over. On the other hand, I love 'em. [Laughs]

Parents tried to cope by not letting care disrupt their lives too much. They tried to find a "middle road" or a balance between their own concerns and their concerns for the schizophrenic. Striking this balance was seldom successful and the parents remained dissatisfied. For example, the father quoted above was disgruntled because his dream of traveling the world after his early retirement had been disrupted by having to monitor his son for psychosis. Yet love and concern for his son's safety would not allow him to leave his son unattended. This father comforted himself by buying an expensive sports car, but it was clear from his interviews that the car never healed the disappointment of the loss of an easy retirement.

Amidst their conflicting concerns, these parents resisted learning the schizophrenic's idiosyncratic thoughts and meanings. For example, one father ignored his son's delusional discussions or told the young man that he didn't want to talk about it. Other parents tried to argue the schizophrenic out of his delusions. In contrast to the parents who were engaged in care, these parents were not interested in understanding the schizophrenic's world from the inside.

Only Conflicted Care parents interpreted the schizophrenic behavior as manipulation. They suspected that irritability, repetitive requests, or sleep disturbances might be manipulation rather than "true" schizophrenia. One father believed his son was "freeloading," and a mother described her son as "very manipulative, mind-wise."

A form of coping that was not available to parents who gave Conflicted Care was to let things run their own course. They could not tolerate inaction with the child's illness. Even in incidents when they coached themselves not to interfere, they seethed emotionally with every action by the schizophrenic that contradicted their hopes or expectations. As a group, these parents were the most emotionally distressed and dissatisfied, both with the schizophrenic and with themselves.

Managed Care

In the third form of caring practices parents demonstrated objectivity, clear plans for their interventions, and relatively unambiguous end goals for care. They considered themselves as managers, with specialized knowledge about how to help their children function at a higher level or achieve a better biochemical balance. They remained objective, even when the schizophrenic was seriously ill or distressed, because they believed that care was best administered with an eye to long-term goals.

Parents who practiced Managed Care found possibilities for the child in external ideals or from the scientific literature, rather than from the ill member's demonstrated capabilities. They were not overly concerned about understanding the illness from the ill member's perspective because that perspective was tainted by the disease. Instead, they sought out and analyzed scientific and lay information on schizophrenia to plan their care. They were the most active of all parent groups in creating therapies to improve the child's functioning.

> So each year, I'd try to sort of [sic] set new priorities. The first year was just to kind of civilize him again so we could take him in public, get him to dress up, get him clean. The second year was just more of the same. More activity so he would know the weekend from the weekday. We sort of looked at it all in stages.

Those who practiced Managed Care characterized their efforts as treatment. They thought of themselves and at times represented themselves to others as the schizophrenic's psychologist, social worker, or therapist.

> If I hired a psychiatric nurse, the nurse would have to have a certain number of hours off, and since I really consider that the role I'm playing now is that of a psychiatric technician, I have to have a certain number of hours off to be able to have enough ability and strength to go back.

Contrast this self-identification with Engaged Care parents, who described care as an extension of parenting. Engaged Care was not bounded by time or role definition, but was all-encompassing and personally defining. Parents who managed care viewed caregiving as a role with specified responsibilities and boundaries.

Because of their diligent efforts and insistence on long-range goals, children under Managed Care experienced remarkable achievements, given their disabilities. One mother, for example, structured pet, music, cooking, and shopping therapies for her son over the years, and he improved to the point that he attended college.

> I began to try to figure out all the ways that I could maybe . . . work with him with all of those disabilities, which are rather enormous disabilities, and still do something that would be creative and that he wouldn't realize was therapy, and nobody else would realize was therapy, and would also help *me* to pass the time.

In Managed Care, parents leapt in and took over for the child. They tried to interpret the schizophrenic's world, overriding his internal impressions and at times objectifying the child. For example, when one schizophrenic who was attending college began to have some difficulty in a course, his mother decided to investigate. Without her son's knowledge, she wrote to the instructor and the school nurse explaining her son's history and asking them to complete a "behavioral checklist" so that she could "see what was happening." In her eagerness to assess and help her son, she disclosed his illness to significant people in his life and ignored his wish to pass as normal in public settings. Similar incidents arose repeatedly in Managed Care, because parents structured their care on external principles rather than on carefully reading and weighing the child's concerns and intentions.

Difficulties arose in Managed Care because parents felt that their care was work, but yet it lasted 24 hours a day. They yearned for time away from care, and devised strategies to obtain it such as a "do not disturb" sign or rules for when they couldn't be interrupted. One mother admitted she worked part time because it gave her a reason to leave the house regularly and be away from her son. Other parents hired tutors, miscellaneous caregivers, and "friends" to share the work. Parents continued to feel burdened by the care, which one mother described as a "20-ton weight" she had had to carry for 10 years. Another mother felt that she was a "prisoner of the disease," although she accepted it as her fate for life.

Distanced Care

The parents involved in care from a distance were fathers who relied on their wives to undertake the hands-on direct care of the ill member. These fathers were interested in the ill member's well-being and were concerned that his needs were met, yet they were not personally involved in discovering or meeting his needs. Distanced care required only occasional attention, and fathers accepted periodic reports from their wives. These fathers had a global rather than a specific awareness of problems and understood illness fluctuations in gross terms rather than in finely tuned distinctions.

These fathers were emotionally vulnerable because they were unable to track the ongoing changes in the ill member. They suffered over the child's losses but were not able to participate in the schizophrenic's daily advancements. They were less in tune with the child and therefore suffered more severe images of what might go wrong. For example, one father had a persistent fear that his son was self-destructive or suicidal. This fear arose from an event many years earlier when the young man had been suicidal. Whenever the son embarked on his daily walks, the father feared he intended to harm himself and couldn't eat or sleep until the boy returned, sometimes 1 hour later, sometimes 6 hours later. The mother, who practiced Engaged Care with the son, knew the son's changing status and felt she would have advance warning if he were to become selfdestructive. Her assurances didn't calm her husband, but her knowledge of her son allowed her to be at ease during his daily walks, secure that he would return unharmed.

Discussion

The four forms of caring practices outlined here were distinctly different scenarios of how care was worked out in this small sample of families. Each form included its own notion of good and skilled know-how. Conflicted Care parents were predominantly angry, disgruntled, and dissatisfied with themselves, their adult child, and the outcomes of their efforts. Engaged Care parents were much more satisfied because they had found ways to support and protect the ill member, yet not be drained or burned out. The care they gave fulfilled the child's needs and defined and fulfilled the parents as well. Managed Care was energetic, hopeful, and goal directed. These parents were challenged by the problems the illness presented and were enthused about their own creative responses. Although their care was important work, it lasted 24 hours a day, and they felt drained. Distanced Care was relatively unencumbered but not without its emotional risks. Fathers who delegated care were less attuned to their child and therefore lacked firsthand knowledge of current issues and threats in their child's life. They also missed the daily possibilities for joy or satisfaction that were evident in those who grappled with direct care.

These descriptions of caring practices are a window on the world of parents' struggles to cope with the demands of schizophrenic offspring. Certainly the descriptions were shaped in a particular way by the theoretical perspective on care that structured the investigation; however, every effort was made to provide

descriptions that captured the tone and essence of the parents' caring practices in their own terms. Subsequent presentations of these findings to groups
of families who participated in the project and to parents who share their
plight have verified the accurate representation of their care.

These interpretive findings provide an empirical and critical basis for
examining prevailing theories about families who care for schizophrenic
members. Recent research on this population has been shaped by conceptions
of the family as burdened by care, or of family affect as a potential risk factor
in the course of schizophrenia. The parents' caring practices that were noted
in this investigation could not be adequately understood through either
conception, which shows that clinical work with families who care for
schizophrenics can be only partially informed by the prevailing theoretical
formulations.

If the parents studied here were examined through the theoretical grid of
family burden, variable amounts of burden might well be found. However,
the distinct nature and meaning of the burdens to parents involved in different
forms of care would be lost. For example, parents who practiced Conflicted
Care and Managed Care would probably rate themselves as significantly
burdened on most subjective burden scales. However, the nature of the
burden in the two groups was quite distinct. In Conflicted Care, parents
searched for a satisfactory way of relating to the situational demands. They
had not accepted the disease and were disgruntled, wishing a way out and
finding none. In contrast, parents who practiced Managed Care were at home
with the care situation because they found a way to care through personally
constructed "therapies" and found a space for hope in science. Their burdens
arose only because the child's need for therapy was unending; therefore,
caring was a drain. Although both groups of parents would probably rate
themselves as burdened, the qualitative distinctions in how they were burdened would be ignored by the theoretical grid of family burden.

A more serious problem in conceptualizing care as a burden is that it
systematically overlooks most of the content of care. As Gubrium and Lynott
(1987) note, the "horizons of the caregiving experience" are much broader
than studies of burden allow them to be. For example, caring practices with
schizophrenic offspring were directed toward understanding the schizophrenic's private world, promoting his feelings of self-worth, promoting his
capacity for personal accomplishments, and easing his suffering. The content
of these practices was broader and more significant than could be encompassed by any list of tasks and their potential burden value.

Similarly, a hazard of family affect research (Kanter et al., 1987; Koenigsberg
& Handley, 1986) is that the emotional expressions that place the schizophrenic at risk—parental criticism, hostility, and emotional overinvolve-

ment—might be misinterpreted as the only aspects of family involvement that deserve scrutiny. This study demonstrated the diversity of ways in which parents were involved and undertook the care of a schizophrenic child. If these parents were examined by the yardstick of family affect, few might be judged to be critical or overinvolved, according to the criteria for making such designations (Kuipers, 1979). Although it is important to identify risk factors, theory used to guide clinical work with these families cannot be solely shaped by concern over risks. Instead, an attempt to understand the complexity and richness of parents' caring practices seems an important adjunct to ongoing efforts to specify their deficits.

The Significance of Parents' Caring Practices With Schizophrenic Offspring

The different forms of caring practices described in this study might be considered as an extension of the practices that comprise parenting in our culture. That these parents were able to extend and adapt their parenting practices to respond to the special needs of a schizophrenic son or daughter is remarkable. Their efforts deserve careful examination, for they may have much to teach us about care of an injured, chronically ill, or "normal" child. In coping with the extreme breakdowns in expectations for their children and themselves, these parents had to find new meanings and practices for continuing their parenting.

This is a radical interpretation. Parenting practices with schizophrenics have historically been presented as paragons of dysfunctional family processes (Beavers, 1982). New understandings of schizophrenia as a genetically based, environmentally sensitive, biochemical disorder have loosened the hold of schizophrenogenic family theories (Halweg & Goldstein, 1987), but a suggestion that these families illuminate basic parenting practices will undoubtedly meet with skepticism. However, several aspects of care that simply belong to parenting today were centrally important to the parents in this project. Like all parents, these parents tried to demonstrate to their children that they were valued and loved, they fostered their personal autonomy, and they helped their children develop some capacity for work or meaningful accomplishments (Kagan, 1980). Each form of caring practice that was described in this study highlighted certain parenting concerns and diminished others.

Engaged Care parents were centrally focused on making the child feel valued and loved. Through variable symptoms, these parents were concerned with supporting the child and easing his pain and did not focus on their personal discomforts or disruptions to their lives. Care was simply not experienced as being burdensome. Rather, it felt like a calling or a commitment that gave their lives content and meaning.

Sensitive to the cultural press for adult independence, parents who practiced Conflicted Care were troubled by the child's lack of autonomy and continued dependence on the family. These parents experienced care in terms of a balance sheet. Answering the child's needs diminished the parents' fund of well-being. Providing for the child's dependence left these parents feeling personally cheated.

Managed Care was unique in its reliance on parenting technologies and scientific prescriptions for helping the child to experience achievement in some aspect of his life. A concern with promoting the child's functional capacities was the basis for this care, but parents relied on scientific theories rather than on an in-depth understanding of their particular child. At times their care, although it was well intentioned, mismatched their particular child's capacities and concerns.

In Distanced Care there was a clear division of responsibilities, with the mother responsible for all parenting tasks and the father primarily concerned with his work outside the home. Care from a distance can best be understood as a remnant of a time when men's and women's work were divided into distinct public and private spheres. Care from a distance was thus possible for men, and it remains unclear whether such a possibility might arise for women as roles change and women participate actively in public spheres.

Limitations

These interpretations must be considered in relation to a larger, more diverse, sample of families. In addition, this study makes no claim to be complete. Additional forms of caring practices not evident in this sample of parents may be discovered in other studies of family care of schizophrenia and other chronic illnesses.

Notes

1. Three combinations of parental care patterns within families were identified: (a) identical, (b) complementary, and (c) contending. In some families, both parents held identical care concerns and practices, and therefore most of their explanations and actions were in concert. Couples with complementary care patterns managed care in distinct but coordinated ways. The most common complementary pattern was a mother who practiced Engaged Care and a father who provided care from a distance. Contending patterns were observed least frequently but had

great impact on family interactions, since much of the parental time was spent negotiating the differences in concerns and care. The most common contending pattern occurred when one parent provided Engaged Care and the other provided Conflicted Care.

2. Dr. Judith Wrubel (1985) discussed various interpersonal concerns demonstrated by healthy middle-aged men and women in relation to their families, friends, and work. Her insights, particularly regarding "engaged care," allowed me to identify similar and dissimilar concerns in the care provided by parents of schizophrenics.

References

Andreason, N. C. (1984). *The broken brain: The biological revolution in psychiatry.* New York: Harper & Row.

Beavers, W. R. (1982). Healthy, midrange and severely dysfunctional families. In F. Walsh (Ed.), *Normal family processes* (pp. 45-66). New York: Guilford.

Benner, P. E. (1984). *Stress and satisfaction on the job: Work meanings and coping of mid-career men.* New York: Praeger.

Benner, P. E. (1985). Quality of life: Explanation, prediction and understanding in nursing science. *Advances in Nursing Science, 8*, 1-14.

Benner, P. E., & Wrubel, J. (1989). *The primacy of caring: Stress and coping in health and illness.* Reading, MA: Addison-Wesley.

Bernheim, K. F., Lewine, R. J., & Beale, C. T. (1982). *The caring family: Living with mental illness.* New York: Random House.

Borgman, A. (1984). *Technology and the character of contemporary life.* Chicago: University of Chicago Press.

Bowers, B. J. (1987). Intergenerational caregiving: Adult caregivers and their aging parents. *Advances in Nursing Science, 9*(2), 20-31.

Brykczynski, K. A. (1989). An interpretive study describing the clinical judgement of nurse practitioners. *Scholarly Inquiry for Nursing Practice: An International Journal, 3*(2), 75-104.

Chesla, C. A. (1988). *Parents' caring practices and coping with schizophrenic offspring: An interpretive study.* Unpublished doctoral dissertation, University of California, San Francisco.

Chesla, C. A. (1989a). Mental illness and the family. In C. Gilliss, B. Highley, B. Roberts, & I. Martinson (Eds.), *Toward a science of family nursing* (pp. 374-393). Menlo Park, CA: Addison-Wesley.

Chesla, C. A. (1989b). Parents' explanatory models of schizophrenia. *Archives of Psychiatric Nursing, 3*, 218-225.

Davis, A. J. (1980). Disability, home care and the care-taking role in family life. *Journal of Advanced Nursing, 5*, 475-484.

Dreyfus, H. (1991). *A commentary on "Being and time," Division I.* Cambridge: MIT Press.

Gubrium, J. F., & Lynott, R. J. (1987). Measurement and the interpretation of burden in the Alzheimer's disease experience. *Journal of Aging Studies, 1*, 265-285.

Halweg, K., & Goldstein, M. J. (1987). Introduction. In K. Halweg & M. J. Goldstein (Eds.), *Understanding major mental disorder: The contribution of family interaction research.* New York: Family Process Press.

Heidegger, M. (1962). *Being and time* (K. Macquarrie & E. Robinson, Trans.) (pp. 1-7). New York: Harper & Row. (Original work published 1962)

Hirschfeld, M. (1983). Homecare versus institutionalization: Family caregiving and senile brain disease. *International Journal of Nursing Studies, 20*(1), 23-32.

Kagan, J. (1980). The psychological requirements for human development. In A. Skolnick & H. Skolnick (Eds.), *Family in transition* (3rd ed.) (pp. 427-438). Boston: Little, Brown.

Kanter, J., Lamb, R., & Loeper, C. (1987). Expressed emotion in families: A critical review. *Hospital & Community Psychiatry, 38*, 374-380.

Kierkegaard, S. (1985). *Fear and trembling* (A. Hannay, Trans.). Princeton, NJ: Princeton University Press. (Original work published 1843)

Koenigsberg, H. W., & Handley, R. (1986). Expressed emotion: From predictive index to clinical construct. *American Journal of Psychiatry, 143*, 1361-1373.

Kuipers, L. (1979). Expressed emotion: A review. *British Journal of Social and Clinical Psychology, 18*, 237-243.

Lasch, C. (1977). *Haven in a heartless world: The family besieged.* New York: Basic Books.

Lazarus, R., & Folkman, S. (1984). *Stress, appraisal and coping.* New York: Springer.

Leonard, V. W. (1989). A Heideggerian phenomenologic perspective on the concept of the person. *Advances in Nursing Science, 11*(4), 40-55.

Packer, M. J. (1985). Hermeneutic inquiry in the study of human conduct. *American Psychologist, 40*, 1081-1093.

Packer, M. J., & Addison, R. B. (1989). *Entering the circle: Hermeneutic investigation in psychology.* Albany: State University of New York Press.

Pai, S., & Kapur, R. L. (1981). Impact of treatment intervention on the relationships between dimensions of clinical psychopathology, social dysfunction and burden on the family of psychiatric patients. *Psychological Medicine, 12*, 651-658.

Rolland, J. S. (1984). Toward a psychosocial topology of chronic and life threatening illness. *Family Systems Medicine, 2*, 245-262.

Rubin, J. (in press). *Too much of nothing: Modern culture and the self in Kierkegaard's thought.* Cambridge, MA: Cambridge University Press.

Runions, J., & Prudo, R. (1983). Problem behaviors encountered by families living with a schizophrenic member. *Canadian Journal of Psychiatry, 28*, 382-386.

Seymour, R. J., & Dawson, N. J. (1986). The schizophrenic at home. *Journal of Psychosocial Nursing and Mental Health Services, 24*, 28-30.

Taylor, C. (1985). *Human agency and language: Philosophical papers 1.* Cambridge, MA: Cambridge University Press.

Thompson, E. H., & Doll, W. (1982). The burden of families coping with the mentally ill. An invisible crisis. *Family Relations, 31*, 379-388.

Wilson, H. S. (1989). Family caregiving for a relative with Alzheimer's dementia: Coping with negative choices. *Nursing Research, 38*, 94-98.

Wrubel, J. (1985). *Personal meanings and coping processes.* Unpublished doctoral dissertation, University of California, San Francisco.

10

❖

Parenting in Public

Parental Participation and Involvement in the Care of Their Hospitalized Child

PHILIP DARBYSHIRE

The desirability of encouraging parents to live in with their hospitalized child is widely accepted. In the latest U.K. government report, *Welfare of Children and Young People in Hospital* (U.K. Department of Health, 1991), it is stated that "A cardinal principle of hospital services for children is complete ease of access to the child by his parents, and to other members of the family. . . . This is not a luxury" (p. 16). This chapter examines the meaning of this "cardinal principle" for both live-in parents and pediatric nurses.

Hospitalization has long been recognized as a potentially stressful experience for both children and their parents. Since the publication of the Platt Report in the U.K. (Ministry of Health and Central Health Services Council, 1959), there have been various attempts to humanize pediatric hospitals by offering open visiting (Fagin & Nusbaum, 1978) and living-in facilities for parents (Hardgrove, 1980) and by encouraging parents to take a more active part in their child's care while in the hospital (Cleary, Gray, Hall, Rowландson, & Sainsbury, 1986; Sainsbury, Gray, Cleary, Davies, & Rowlandson, 1986).

However, there is evidence to suggest that although such changes may be desirable, their implementation has been more difficult than was first imagined (Consumers Association, 1980; Hall, 1978, 1987). Hospitals are complex environments, and phrases such as "encourage parents to live in with their child" and "encourage parents to participate in their child's care" gloss over the implications of this increased parental presence for both parents and pediatric nurses. Throughout the literature on pediatric hospitalization there is a lack of detailed description of how parents and nurses understand such rhetoric and how such principles of pediatric care are worked out in practice.

The Research Approach and Method

This research study explored the lived experiences of parents who decided to live in with their child during hospitalization. Lived experience was understood to be the ways in which people encounter situations in relation to their interests, purposes, personal concerns, and background understandings (Benner, 1985).

The wider study (Darbyshire, 1994) of which this is a part was carried out in a pediatric hospital in a large Scottish city. The research participants were 30 parents (26 mothers and 4 fathers) who either lived in with their child or spent most of the day with him or her. Twenty-seven qualified nurses also participated. Data were collected during a 9-month period of fieldwork in two wards of the hospital. One was a general medical ward where the "turnover" of resident parents was measured in days or 1 or 2 weeks. In contrast, the second study ward was a Burns Unit where parents were often living in for up to 2 to 3 months. The research participants engaged with me in informal discussions, individual and "couple" interviews, and focus group interviews that produced the essential data of 32 interviews. These were tape recorded and transcribed verbatim by the researcher for interpretive pheno-menological analysis (Allen, Benner, & Diekelmann, 1986; Benner, 1985; Van Manen, 1990).

These necessarily brief methodological details do not, however, tell the whole story of my struggles as a researcher within the qualitative and interpre-tive tradition. Accounts of published research tend to perpetuate the view that a particular method is selected at the outset and that this method is simply "used" unproblematically and unchanged throughout the study. My experience within this study was that as my understandings of phenomenological approaches and philosophy developed, my approaches to the interpretive analysis shifted in focus. For example, I began to see more fundamental differences between the grounded theory and phenomenological approaches that, at the outset of the study, I had imagined I could combine easily. I became concerned that I was using grounded theory's approach to coding and categorizing while recog-nizing that my interpretive insights were drawing increasingly on Heideg-gerian hermeneutic phenomenology.

This was a source of real frustration as I struggled fruitlessly to find a "Core Category" or "Basic Social Process" that would subsume all of the rest of the data. The only way in which all of my codes and categories would fit into an overarching core category would be if the category were so general as to be meaningless. It was not exactly a "research high," when I had spent months coding, memoing, and recoding, to come up with "something to do with relationships." Eventually, I began to sense that my grounded theory strategies were fragmentary and reductionist. My thinking was being forced into the construction of analytic laws and causal mechanisms that would "explain" the "reality" of the research setting. I needed instead to think in ways that helped me to dwell with the stories of the participants and enabled an interpretive uncovering of lived experience and practices that would preserve context. Such analytic thinking, in its search for closure, answers, and ultimate clarity, seemed to fail to acknowledge the circularity of understanding (Gadamer, 1960/1975). In contrast, "dwelling thinking" (Heidegger, 1959/1966) allowed for a keeping open, an essential incompleteness in the dialogue that left a space for the important presence of the reader.

A specific example of my growing dissonance with grounded theory was my initial attempt to keep both theoretical and observational notes, as suggested by Glaser and Strauss (1967) and Schatzman and Strauss (1973). This seemed a logical strategy initially, but I later questioned the philosophy underlying it. This approach seemed to assume that some data were interpreted and thus deemed to be theoretical whereas another class of "brute data" (Rabinow & Sullivan, 1979) were merely observational and thus presumably uninterpreted. Such an assumption seemed increasingly at odds with a central assumption of hermeneutic phenomenology, that there can be no interpretation-free "data" because we are all self-interpreting beings who are within our preunderstandings.

These comments are intended to enhance the reflective element of this study and to highlight that the philosophical and hence methodological basis of this study did not remain static over the 6 years of its undertaking. They are also intended to avoid the glossing over or ignoring of real methodological difficulties.

Parents, Nurses, and Participation

The initial focus is upon the parents' and nurses' respective expectations and understandings of what parent participation would and did entail, exploring similarities and discordances. This analysis is extended in a discussion of the creation, control, and determination of parent participation. I argue that interpretation of participants' accounts suggests that parent participation is more a set of unexpressed expectations than any form of mutual agreement between parents and nurses.

Parent participation as a concept and as a professional tenet begs the question of "Participation in what?" Here, the parents' accounts of how they perceived the nature of their participation were illuminating. I suggest that parental involvement, particularly in the early part of the child's stay, was limited to what parents themselves called "basic mothering work."

It was often assumed by nurses that parents could carry out these familiar tasks equally well within the different context of the ward. However, I found that nurses' and parents' understandings and expectations of parental participation changed during the parents' stay in the hospital in ways that called this assumption into question.

The demarcation of care into basic mothering work and the more technical work of nursing or medical procedures was more clearly delineated in the earlier part of a parent's stay, becoming less pronounced over the length of the child's hospitalization. The strategies used by parents and nurses to bring about participation and its development are also discussed.

Parents' Experiences of Participation

I use two terms in this chapter, *participation* and *involvement,* because I suggest that for the participants in this study, there was a subtle but important distinction between them. I take *participation* to refer to the more functional involvement of parents in their child's care—for example, in helping carry out everyday care. For the parents, *involvement* had a more holistic connotation, implying a deeper sense of being an integral and essential part of their child's hospital experience. It is parental involvement in this deeper sense that is addressed in this chapter. This section describes how parent participation was created, controlled, and experienced by both parents and nurses.

Though the parents had a general desire to help care for their child during their stay, they may have lacked sufficient or specific knowledge of the child's condition to allow them to do this confidently. Being a live-in parent was not a static "role," however. Changes in the child's condition, the length of the parents' stay, and parents' relationships with ward staff all influenced the nature of parents' participation. During the period of fieldwork, I met many parents whose levels and kinds of participation were different. Some were very happy to carry out only their child's basic mothering care and leave the more technical care to nurses, whereas others had learned some technical skills, such as nasogastric feeding, so that they could do this with their child.

There were also a small group of parents who had attained the status of what I will call "expert parents," whose autonomy and expertise regarding their child's care marked them out as being unique. This concept of the expert parent has important implications for the more general discussion of parental participation and will be discussed at the end of this chapter.

For the majority of parents, becoming increasingly involved in their child's care was an uncertain process. During the interviews and discussions with parents, I asked them about how they spent their day; this would usually elicit some information as to how the parents participated, if at all, in their child's care. I may also have asked how it came about that they began to do the particular things that they did for their child.

Determining Participation: Parents' Understandings

The parents who chose to live in with their child in the hospital seemed to have no clear idea as to what the nature or extent of their participation in their child's care might be. Some parents' ideas prior to living in reflected fairly outmoded concepts of pediatric care. For example, some expressed pleasant surprise at being "allowed" to do so much for their child. As one mother noted:

> I was surprised. . . . This is the first time I've been in hospital, and I was surprised that they let the mothers do so much, to tell you the truth . . . just because I didn't know what to expect, I mean, I thought a mother came to hospital and sat with her child all day and done nothing for her child, that they [the nurses] did everything . . . and I was quite pleasantly surprised to see that they allow you to do so much for them.

Parent participation did not appear to be an openly negotiated arrangement. Parents therefore had the task of steering an appropriate course through the uncertain and, as was often the case, uncharted area of participation in their child's care.

When I asked parents how they came to do the things that they did for their child in the hospital, they replied that this was an automatic or instinctive reaction. They tried to carry on as they would have done at home. As these parents explained:

> My wife just took it upon herself . . . typical mother like, she just got up and done it like with no asking.

> Just naturally . . . natural instinct.

I just did it automatically, he was my son, it was my responsibility.

These replies may seem to indicate that for parents there was a seamless continuation between their child care practices at home and in the hospital. However, this was often not the case and parents frequently found the process of participating in their child's care to be fraught with tensions. They were often uncertain and confused as to what exactly they were allowed and expected to do. Consequently, parents regularly remarked that they had learned the limits of their participation by the often chastening experience of trial and error—for example, experiences of being chastised for using the ward kitchen.

For the majority of parents in this study, parent participation was an unspoken agreement. As one mother noted:

> *No, no, no,* that [the mother's level of participation] was never discussed, never discussed, I just did everything. . . . No, it was never mentioned, Philip, I just took it as being the way.

Parents watched what other resident parents did for their child and took their cues from them. The nature of their participation was also determined by the severity of the child's illness or injury. Generally, the more seriously ill the child was, the less directly the parents would participate, even in basic mothering work. One mother's comments illustrated this clearly in relation to her baby son who was in an Intensive Care Unit:

> There was nothing we could do, he was on a ventilator, he was so sick. . . . He didn't need us at all, it's just that we were there cause we thought that every breath could be his last one . . . and we felt that we had to be with him. It's different now. [At this time the baby was in a close observation area within the main ward.] I can do things for him, I can change his nappy and I can give him his feeds down his NG tube, but that's still not really doing anything.

This mother's account was also illustrative of the ways in which the ethos of the ward tended to elevate the importance of the technical task or the physical procedure. Within such an ethos, parents' being present with their child, their bearing witness beside him when his hold on life was at its most fragile, was less valued and recognized. Their presence seemed synonymous with a useless passivity, a "doing nothing" for their baby who "didn't need" them.

Parents participated more when they were asked informally and unthreateningly by nurses whether they might like to help with a particular aspect of their child's care. This encouragement also extended to the performance of more technical tasks such as the giving of nasogastric feeds, although parents tended to be taught more formally how to carry out these procedures, rather than gently encouraged. Two mothers described this strategy:

> The nurse just said one day, "I'm going to wash Claire, do you want to help?" and I said "That's fine, am I allowed to?" and she said "Well, we quite encourage the mums to take part and do things with their kids."

> At first they always cleaned her and then they sort of said, "Do you want to do it?" and I sort of said "It doesn't bother me," and they said, "we're just sort of cleaning her," so I sort of took over.

The way in which nurses broached the subject of the parents' participating was important to parents. They were appreciative of nurses who allowed them to make their own choices as to whether and to what degree they wished to participate. It was particularly important in this respect that the parents were allowed to decide their own level of participation without feeling that they were being pressured. In this way they were able to vary their participation depending upon how they were feeling at any given time. These parents' accounts illustrate this point:

> You know, they didn't say, "Right, change his nappy," and if at any time I don't want to, I can just say, "No, I don't want to."

> They'll not say, "Right, you'll do it!" . . . They'll say, "Do you want to finish off or do you want me to carry on?" and I'll say yes. . . . It's a little bit of give and take.

It would have been almost unthinkable for parents to have taken it upon themselves to carry out aspects of their child's care that might have been thought the prerogative of nurses. These were not only the more traditional nursing tasks such as changing dressings and recording observations. Live-in parents quickly realized that what would previously have been considered basic mothering tasks, such as feeding, changing, and bathing the child, now required nurses' permission if they were to be done by parents. One way for parents to legitimize their participation was for them to portray their involvement not as interference in the working of the ward, but as a positive help to nurses. As this mother noted:

> I mean, you know that you're helping them, because one nurse maybe gets three bairns, but all she has to do with my one is take her temperature and pulse and she can

devote all her time to the other two, cause I'm in here the whole day, virtually seven o'clock in the morning till eight at night and on call if they want me.

It was important for parents to find a balance in the level of their participation. If this balance was upset they then felt expected to carry out too much of the child's care without adequate support. One mother described this feeling of being her child's sole caregiver while in the hospital:

> Well, I think I *have* been his care [laughs], I've been the one that's done it really . . . but I still think that there should be a back-up from the nursing staff. . . . Sometimes I wish that someone would come and give him a bath and you know, just get him changed.

As the nurses' accounts in a later section of this chapter suggest, the control and determination of the extent and level of parent participation lay principally with nursing staff. However, parents did carry out some of their child's care on their own initiative; for example, one mother told how she had decided to wash her child without seeking "permission":

> Jill was in here for about 3 days before I realized that nobody had washed her, I mean I'd washed her face when she'd been sick but nobody had come and washed her, and as soon as I had filled up the basin one of the nurses came up and helped, but I made the decision.

Another mother took this a stage further by initiating her own form of treatment for her comatose son, believing that in the absence of any other explicit treatment plan, she was obliged to do her best to devise something:

> Nobody has come up to me and said, "Look, we think this might be a good idea, if you talk about this or do this with John," there's nobody come over and suggested anything like that. . . . I've taken it upon my own back to take him out of his chair and walk him a couple of steps or put him in his bed for a little while.

Taking such participatory initiatives was not an easy option because it could render parents open to suggestions that they were overstepping the mark and encroaching into areas that were proper concerns of nursing and medical staff. Most parents were aware that they were performing a delicate social balancing act and thought it prudent to try to keep on the good side of nurses.

Having described how the phenomenon of parent participation came about, I now explore, from the parents' perspective, what such participation actually entailed.

Parents and Play: "Worse Than Working"

The importance of play for hospitalized children has been repeatedly emphasized in recent years (Betz & Poster, 1984; Jolly, 1981; U.K. Dept. of Health, 1991). Pediatric nurses have been encouraged to attend to the play and recreational needs of children as well as to their more physical needs. The introduction of Play Leaders in pediatric hospitals (Hall, 1977) has been another attempt to ensure that children's play needs are not neglected.

The literature on play has, however, largely ignored the active part that live-in parents play in keeping their child amused and occupied during their stay. Previous studies of play have also tended to characterize play solely as a diversionary activity for the child and have ignored the importance of the meanings that play has for parents. I suggest that these meanings were tightly bound to parents' understandings of their child's condition and prognosis and also to their own lived experience of being resident parents. In this section I therefore describe not only parents' involvement in play but, equally importantly, the ways in which parents' understandings of play could be altered by the nature of their child's condition.

Most parents will attest to the fact that keeping a young child amused, occupied, or entertained for a sustained length of time is not an easy task. For live-in parents this was made much more difficult by virtue of the child's illness and possibly restricted mobility and the physical restrictions of an unfamiliar environment. It was difficult for some parents to play with their child for long periods of time because this pattern of interaction was so different from what they usually experienced at home. A mother described this intensity of play involvement with her child:

> **INT.:** How did you find that you spent your day while you were here?
> **MOTHER:** By her bedside, as I say, half six in the morning till she went and slept at night, with the odd break in between, playing games with her.

The parents of comatose children in the medical ward who had sustained serious head injuries explained that there was no demarcation between verbal stimulation and play. Most of their efforts to amuse or play with their child centered on trying to elicit any type of response that could be favorably interpreted. Their major difficulty was in speaking to and stimulating their child, who before the accident had been active and talkative and who was now almost entirely unresponsive. These parents described painfully how the nature of everyday communication with their child had changed:

> [Play] . . . is worse than working. The hardest thing in there is sitting talking to Kim . . . because you know looking at her that she's lying sleeping, and it

makes you tired, you really feel exhausted, you know I just talk to her as much as I can and then I put her tapes on. . . . I think if she's lying there and she's listening to something it'll make her feel that there's no nobody sitting at all with her. . . . What do you say next? You've spoke about *every possible thing* you could say to her. . . . What do you do next?

The importance of the meaning of play within the context of the child's illness was memorably demonstrated during my interview with another mother of a head-injured child. She was almost in tears, partly sad and partly angry, as she told me how she had came into the ward one day to find her son, who was approximately 10 years old, holding, and in her view being expected to play with, a pillow, "Can you believe that, a pillow!" She repeated this phrase half-angrily, half-bewildered, several times as if she could scarcely comprehend the implications of what she had seen.

For this mother, play was not merely a diversion to amuse or entertain her child; it also had a normalizing function. She was adamant that her son should not have been given toys such as rattles or activity centers because, as she said, "he's not a baby." Although he was only just beginning to regain rudimentary purposive motor functions, his mother refused to see this as a second babyhood and insisted on age-appropriate toys for her son. Play for her was clearly not only a part of her child's therapy but an important part of the construction or, more properly, the reconstruction of her child's identity.

Play was also used by parents as a diversionary tactic to distract their child and to hopefully minimize the distress of painful or frightening procedures. Here, a parent described how she used play to lessen her daughter's fear of being anesthetized:

When we got into the anesthetic room she just screamed and burst into tears and there was no way. . . . We tried a little game, you know, blow up the bag on the thing, look it's a big balloon, try and blow it up for mummy, but no. . . .

Parents also used play as a way of monitoring changes in their child's condition. For example, one mother detected an improvement in her child when her daughter became less dependent upon her constant attention and began to show an interest in playing with some of the other children on the ward:

The first week or so she just wasn't interested in who was going past [the cubicle], she just wanted mummy and she just wanted someone to sit and read to her, play with her, a few games, but towards the end of the time she would watch people going past, and sort of, if one of the little ones came up to the glass and waved to her, she would wave frantically, and the girl round the corner was called Jill, and if she saw her it would be "Look, mummy, look, there's Jill!" . . . and she was obviously starting to feel better and want more contact.

Parents' stay in the hospital was temporary, and they anticipated the difficulties that might arise when they returned home with their child. A common parental concern here was that the child had become accustomed to having the virtually constant and compliant attention of his or her mother for several days or even weeks. The previous mother described how she tried to gradually withdraw her attention as the child's condition improved. In this way she hoped that the child would become less dependent upon her for play:

> I tried not to play with her constantly so that if she can amuse herself a bit, let her do it, cause I don't want her sort of, have her feeling that she was going to have me constantly there. . . . If she was playing with something, I would just sit and read or sit and knit, I would sort of push the chair back so that I wasn't totally with her, playing with her, so that she would play on her own for a bit.

If the phrase *parent participation* begs the question "Participation in what?" then the parents' accounts of their experiences and understandings of play provided a partial answer. Parents did not view play merely as something to keep their child occupied for the duration of their day. Play was viewed as integral to many other aspects of the child's condition, treatment, and recovery. In keeping with a central tenet of this study, play had unique, context-specific meanings for parents that could easily be overlooked if it was seen as a purely functional or instrumental part of parent participation.

Keeping Vigil

Parents who were carrying out their child's physical care or who were actively helping nurses with technical procedures were participating in highly visible ways. There were occasions, however, when parents felt themselves to be intensely involved with their child, yet may have seemed to be merely sitting beside the child's bed. Parents' accounts suggested that keeping vigil or being with the child was not simply a matter of being in close physical proximity to the child's bed but was more often an intense bearing witness with the child's plight.

Parents were often being with or presencing with their child in the existential sense (Benner, 1984; Benner & Wrubel, 1989; Reimen, 1986), whereby they were hyperattentive to their child and acutely sensitive to their needs, at times to the point where they seemed to exclude all other aspects of their environment. This was especially so when the child was seriously ill. One mother conveyed this well when she described a time when her baby's life was considered to be in real danger:

> **INT.:** While you were there [in the ICU], what did you actually do?
> **MOTHER:** Nothing [laughs nervously], just sort of sat and watched him . . . cried a lot . . . wandered about . . . just in total turmoil, we couldn't do anything, we could just sit. . . . We just sat and either watched him or sat and just thought. . . . Never said a word really, just sat and watched him. . . .

This powerful need to be with their child and to be there for him or her was expressed by several other parents. One father whose son had been badly scalded and who had been taken immediately from Casualty into the ward treatment room expressed the distress which he felt when he was unable to be with his son at a moment when he felt that his child most needed him:

> So we got to the hospital and they put us in a wee room at the side and the child was screaming and at this you were getting all tense and tense, *you want to go in, you want to go in.* . . .

This father also expressed a typical desire to be there for his child during the "tough times" when the child was most likely to be frightened, perhaps when undergoing a painful or distressing procedure.

For some parents, the desire to keep vigil with their child had a strong functional importance. They were very keen to work in some way with their child as well as to be available to respond to the child's other needs and wishes. One parent described an experience shared by many other parents when she described how the need to be beside her child was so strong that she could not detach herself enough, in any sense, to relax and enjoy a short coffee break. She explained that

> You think, "Oh, I'll just go for a drink," and then when you're in there you're thinking to yourself, "I shouldn't be sat here, I should be sat in there talking, or doing something."

Another mother explained how she tried to go home for a short break and to be with her other children for a while but found this impossible:

> I can't cook, Philip, I can't do it. I try to force myself . . . but if I'm in the house for any length of time I start breaking down about Kim and I've got to come right back in again.

An important aspect of keeping vigil was the length of time that parents spent in concentrated attention at their child's bedside. A father whose daughter was comatose spoke of sitting "for maybe 4 . . . 5 hours or whatever" when he visited the hospital. His wife also described how, when her daughter had developed a serious infection, she had "sat with her for 12 hours one day." She also brought out clearly in her account the unique meaning that the experience of keeping vigil had for her sense of being a parent:

> I've seen some mammies coming in with their babies and just walking out and leaving them crying. . . . Maybe they've got important things in the house to do, but I couldn't do that. I've got to sit with her, right up to 11 o'clock at night to make sure she's going to sleep, then I can go to sleep, but I can't come away till she's settled.

Parents also described how they simply had to be with their child at particularly significant moments, times that cannot be formalized within a framework of "functional reasons." For one mother this was on the anniversary of her father's death:

> I went in at one o'clock in the morning, and I sat with him till four o'clock, just sat and bubbled [cried] and cried cause it was 5 years ago on Saturday that my dad died . . . and it was the first year that I'd missed going to the crematorium cause I was through here with Ben. . . . I just sat and the way he was lying, I just held his hand. . . . I just sat there and bubbled and cried, I couldn't help myself.

This mother needed to be with her son at this particularly significant time in her life. Through this moment of vigil with her child she experienced a sense of connectedness that possibly helped her to cope with a particularly traumatic time. Nurses often expressed the hope that parents would "come to terms with" their child's illness or death. It is possible that this mother had found the act of keeping vigil and being with her son at this quiet and relatively private time to be a help as she tried to understand and "come to terms" with the circumstances surrounding his accident and injuries. It also seemed that being with her child was a source of comfort to her as she remembered her father and his death.

I propose here that keeping vigil was not the passive, uninvolved nonactivity that some previous studies have suggested (Meadow, 1969). Keeping vigil served several purposes for parents, although its meaning cannot be adequately captured in purely instrumental terms. It was a dwelling attentiveness and receptivity toward their child. It also helped the parents themselves to feel useful. By keeping vigil with their child parents felt that they were doing not only the right thing in the moral sense but the only thing that they could do. They were being of real help to their child at what were among the most traumatic moments of both of their lives.

Summary

The parents' descriptions of their participation suggested that this was not so much a deliberate nursing philosophy and strategy as an unspoken and haphazard arrangement. Their accounts also suggested that encouragement of participation seemed to be dependent upon the thoughtfulness of individual nurses who would try to enable and empower parents in ways that were comfortable and acceptable to them.

The participation of parents in their child's care seemed to exist mostly at the level of the parents' carrying out "basic mothering" work, which was viewed merely as a continuation of a mother's normal parenting practices at home. Some parents would become involved in more technical tasks such as suctioning their child or administering nasogastric feeds. I suggest, however, that the parents' participation could more meaningfully be called the parents' agreement to take over certain tasks from nurses.

Nurses and the Creation of Parent Participation

This discussion of parent participation has focused primarily on the parents. However, because a central proposition of this study is that social phenomena within the pediatric ward are cocreated by the respective participants, it is now appropriate to consider in more detail the perspectives and practices of the nurses.

Previous research literature has tended to focus exclusively upon nurses' attitudes toward the concept of parental involvement. It seems to have been largely accepted that parent participation was an occupational reality that nurses were either for or against.

Little consideration has been given to how pediatric nurses perceive the meaning of many of the phrases currently used to encapsulate this concept of parent participation. "Encourage parents to participate in their child's care" is but one of the expressions that has implications for pediatric nursing practice but that has remained unexplored.

In this section I draw predominantly on nurses' accounts to illustrate how the process of parent participation was created from the nurses' perspective. This involves examining more fully the nurses' influence in shaping the extent and nature of parent participation and also the nurses' understandings of the value of this arrangement.

I also explore further how the phenomenon of parent participation came about largely as an unspoken agreement, but now looking more from the nurses' perspective. In doing so I examine the strategies that nurses described when they encouraged parents to participate.

Parent Participation:
Nurses' Understandings and Practices

Nurses had particular expectations regarding live-in parents in relation to their cooperation, competence, and character. From the nurses' accounts and descriptions of parent participation, it seemed that a similar set of expectations were present regarding this particular aspect of living in. In addition to their first impressions, nurses described other influences on how they assessed a parent's "readiness" to participate in his or her child's care. They took readiness cues as indications upon which to base their assessments of parents' potential participation. This readiness included a consideration of parents' willingness, interest, timing, ability, and the nature of the task in which the parents may have been expected to become involved.

Nurses were sensitive to the importance of timing in their attempts to encourage parent participation. The nurses spoke of assessing parents' readiness to participate in care in ways that indicated that there was a temporal element to participation and that timing was important for parents if they were to be successfully helped to participate. For example, if a child had been admitted as an emergency to an intensive care unit, the severity of his illness or injury combined with the unfamiliarity of the surroundings would adversely affect the parents' readiness to help in their care. This did not suggest an unwillingness but illustrated that the parents' anxiety and dread would mean that the time would not be right for them to actively assist in care. The nurses' understandings of readiness suggested that parents needed time to adjust to each change in their child's condition and that they first had to accommodate such changes before moving on. One nurse described how she assessed and interpreted this lack of readiness in parents:

> Parents that run a mile when the doctors come to take blood, and immediately hand over their child at *any* procedure. I think they are the ones who take a bit longer to . . . you know . . . not that they're not capable but just that either they're frightened or they don't have the confidence.

This nurse brought out the temporal feature of this readiness by acknowledging that this was not synonymous with lack of capability and by understanding that parents could not call forth this participation until they felt ready within themselves.

A nurse from the Burns and Plastic Surgery unit described this temporal aspect of readiness in terms more resonant with a truly meaningful participation when she spoke of how she gauged parents' readiness by the extent of their acceptance or nonacceptance of the child's condition. For this nurse, it was important that parents and nurse shared a similar understanding of the nature and implications of the child's condition before any meaningful participation could be negotiated. This nurse felt that discrepant perspectives here would nullify any attempts that she might have made to involve or specifically teach the parent. She explained that

> Up the stairs [in the Burns and Plastic Surgery Unit] it's like, your initial . . . it's the way they react to the initial injury that makes you think, right, they've accepted this and this is how they go on from here. If they've got problems grasping, like what's happened and why it's happened you then have a problem that you can't . . . because they haven't understood what's happened, you can't teach them something to put an input into what you're trying to do.

Another nurse described the importance of this timing in ensuring that parents were not "forced" beyond their own sense of readiness:

> There are some parents you think, Oh well, maybe that is beyond them . . . so then you won't force that issue, as yet . . . perhaps in a little while, but not in the beginning, cause you don't honestly think that they're ready for it.

In assessing if and when parents were to be encouraged to participate, nurses set great store by their initial and intuitive judgments. For them, first impressions were important. When nurses replied to questions in this way, I asked them to try to think of any specific parental cues that might have influenced them as they made these initial assessments. The nurses looked for signs that parents were willing as well as ready to participate in their child's care. As this nurse noted:

> I think a lot depends on the parent, if they're willing, you know, you chat to them, and mention would you like to help do this? . . . and some are very apprehensive and just don't want to.

Parents showed such willingness by directly offering to help and by asking if they could carry out particular tasks. This was also shown more subtly by perhaps asking where the nappies were kept or whether they might have a clean bath towel. One nurse described this:

If they start asking, "Can I do that?" you obviously say certainly or "We'd rather we did it" or something like that. I think if they start saying something like "I feel a bit helpless, you know, Can I help? Can I do something?" Obviously you would let them do something.

The nurses also interpret parents' questioning as an indication of willingness to participate. As this nurse explained,

> I think it's the interest that they show when you're doing something, like if they're . . . say you're putting on a head bandage or something, and you're bandaging him up, if they're like having a good look and quizzing you about how you do it, you can then think, well . . . maybe they are capable of doing this, we'll let you try it.

The nurses spoke of how they also based their judgments of parents' ability to participate on their perceptions of the parents' competence. One nurse explained how she expected parents to be able to demonstrate their competence in a particular task:

> When they come in, if they're interested enough and want to know why you're doing things and are prepared to listen and prepared to give you an example of them doing that then you're quite happy, then I would go ahead and let them.

There were both general and particular aspects that nurses took to be indicative of parents' competence and consequently of their ability to participate in their child's care. Nurses noted the parents' general level and style of interaction with their child. As this nurse remarked, "just sort of maybe, how they generally handle the child." Another nurse gave a more detailed account of this:

> I think a lot of it is experience. . . . It seems a silly word to put on it at times, but I think a lot of it is, you seem to just know inside what parents can do more . . . what parents you can get to . . . what parents you can encourage and what others you're going to help a lot. I mean, I might not have known at first, a few years ago, but now you can more or less sense in the parents how much they want to do and also if they've been doing a lot, and when they're getting tired of doing everything then it's time for you to step in again.

It seemed from these accounts that assessing parents was largely intuitive and not part of a discourse in which nurses were comfortable in attempting to articulate their practice. This is a difficulty clearly recognized in the literature on intuition in nursing (Agan, 1987; Benner & Tanner, 1987).

The general aspects of the parents' approach to the child that were considered valuable indicators of their ability to participate were their expressed care and love for their child. Conversely, parents who seemed distant from their child, due to either less emotionally intense contact or a physical distancing such as "sitting away from the bed," were seen as being less likely ta be able to participate.

When asked if they could describe any specific parental factors that influenced their perceptions of parents' ability to participate, the nurses spoke of the importance of parents' giving the impression of understanding:

> The ones that understand what you're doing, you know, if you're trying to explain something and the parents don't seem to be taking it in, then there's no use asking them to do a certain procedure or wanting them to help because they'll just not know if they're doing wrong or what they're doing.
>
> If you've been explaining everything to them, how they've taken in the explanations, whether they're maybe too upset, if it's an emergency admission and they're too upset to listen properly, or just intelligence level . . . their understanding of the situation.

These accounts suggested that nurses assessed parents' ability to participate partly on how parents responded to the nurses' professional interpretation and explanation of the situation. How could parents show an understanding of the situation that would satisfy nurses that they were capable of participation?

Parent participation seemed to be shaped and determined by a dynamic process involving both parents and nurses. The nurses tended to make their assessments of parents' readiness, willingness, and ability to participate in their child's care on the basis of largely unarticulated intuitive responses to general cues and impressions given by parents. In this respect, nurses seemed to positively assess parents who showed obvious love and concern for their child as expressed through close physical contact and caring handling.

Nurses similarly assessed positively parents who showed keenness and interest in participating by either asking directly to do so or hovering interestedly beside the child while the nurse was carrying out some aspect of the child's care. If they did this, it was more likely that the nurse would then ask the parents if they would like to help. The influence of the child should not be overlooked, however, because his or her insistence that the parent was to stay with him or her and help with any particular care task also had an influence upon a parent's decision to participate.

The nurses described how they assessed which parents they thought most suitable to participate in care. Underlying this activity was the assumption that this participation had some value for the child, the parents, or the nurse herself, or indeed for all concerned with the hospitalization. I therefore asked the nurses about any benefits that they felt had accrued from having parents participating and also whether they felt that there were any disadvantages in this.

The nurses often claimed that it was valuable to have close contact with parents because they were the experts, the people who knew their child best. Similarly in their accounts of what they saw as advantages and disadvantages of parent participation, the nurses spoke of how they valued this expertise in terms of what the parents did for their child that might have been more difficult and time-consuming for the nurse. For example, nurses explained, parents could be helpful in monitoring their child's clinical condition:

> They tend to notice sooner if their child isn't the normal or if they're not acting normally or they're not taking their fluids as well as they normally do. . . . They know their normal a lot better, although we know a basic normal, they know their own child's normal.

This nurse described how parents' particular knowledge of their child was valued as a specific adjunct to the nurse's generic knowledge. But it seemed that such parental knowledge was valued, not only for its value to the child's care but for how it could benefit the nurses through reducing their workload.

Nurses and the Unspoken Arrangement

The nurses shared the parents' perception that participation was indeed an arrangement that was rarely discussed at the start of the hospitalization. Not only was this rarely discussed among nurses and parents, but some of the nurses commented that this seemed to them to be a strange question and one that they had "never really thought about before." What was largely an unspoken agreement for parents was similarly so for nurses.

The nurses were generally agreed that discussion with parents concerning participation did not take place at the outset of their stay, although some felt that this was something that should occur. As this nurse noted:

> We expect them to carry on their daily care, like their usual basic care, washing them, feeding them . . . and basically you expect them to do it, but it's never said to them.

The nurses seemed to view any developing parental participation as dependent on the developing relationship that the parents had with ward staff, rather than as the result of any clearly explicated guidelines or procedure. The individual nurse was therefore expected to anticipate and to be attuned to possibilities for participation. This was achieved by monitoring and interpreting parental cues that might signal the parents' desire or willingness to participate or to participate more fully. One nurse explained that

> It takes a very clever nurse to anticipate, does this mum want to be completely involved, partly involved, or hardly involved, say in the first instance when the child comes back from theater [operating room]. . . . It's really difficult.

Although the nurses' accounts seem to suggest that parent participation was simply something that happened in the absence of any negotiation, it would be wrong to imply that nurses took no part in the shaping of the participation process. Nurses described two principal approaches that they used in order to allow or encourage parents to participate. These approaches emphasized the common nursing perspective that participation was a gradual process whose pace was largely determined by parents themselves. This contrasts with the perspective of parents, who felt that their participation was more under the control of nursing staff.

The Inform-and-Leave Strategy. The nurses described an inform-and-leave strategy in which they gave parents what they felt to be sufficient information and encouragement to allow them to participate in part of their child's care if they so wished. Nurses described how this was done:

> It's very much, "There's the locker, the nappies [diapers] are in there and the towels in there and just get on with it."

> If the mums are there it's "Here's the bottle, here's the food, do you want to do it?" and you do it as the situation arises rather than beforehand.

The nurses appeared to presume that what they were doing was helping parents by allowing them to help, using minimum pressure. Implicit within this strategy was the sense that this allowed the parents the option of being able to help with the child's care if they wished to or felt ready to. However, as the earlier discussion of parents' experiences of participation showed, parents felt under pressure to participate in care and to establish their identity as good, useful, and willing workers.

There was a tension apparent in the accounts of the nurses as they described this seemingly laissez-faire approach to encouraging participation. For although they emphasized their wish to allow parents to participate at their own pace and as they wished, they were also clear that such participation was assuredly expected from parents. Such participation may even have been viewed as almost a condition of the parents' living in. As these nurses explained:

> If they're there for a large chunk of the day, resident-wise, we expect them to be there and you expect them to eventually, to take over from what you start to do.

> We seem to expect that they will, if they're going to stay, help with the care. . . . You expect from the fact that they're staying in that they will do some of the care, that they're not just going to sit there and be bystanders.

Parent participation was expected in basic mothering care. It seemed to be taken as a given by the nurses that this was work that parents could and should begin to undertake shortly after the child's admission or soon after the need for any form of intensive care or demanding medical treatment had passed.

One nurse explained that such participation in the child's basic care was indicative of normal parental responsiveness and that consequently its absence could be an indication of some pathological problem in the child-parent relationship. As this nurse observed:

> That's why they're there, I mean it's their child, even though they're in hospital. They would have to feed it at home. . . . I mean, you could have a 6-week-old baby, and if mum's sitting there and the nurse is feeding it you'd think there was something far wrong here.

The nurses seemed unaware that the tension between the inform-and-leave approach and their expectations regarding parents' participation could create problems for parents. As was revealed in the parents' accounts of participation, they often interpreted such a nursing approach as meaning that they had been simply left to their own devices. They saw their situation as being one in which they had to fend for themselves and learn what they could and could not do by trial and error, usually the latter. This strategy created a consequent problem for parents by placing them in the position whereby they were the ones expected to make approaches and requests to nursing staff. Nurses seemed to interpret this positively as being synonymous with parents' deciding upon their own extent and rate of participation. Parents, however, interpreted it more negatively. They described how having to regularly ask nurses for permission or assistance made them seem demanding or a nuisance.

The As-If-at-Home Analogy. Nurses also described how they tried to promote participation by encouraging parents to feel more at home. This was usually done by explaining to parents that they should feel free to do whatever they did for the child at home.

I interpret this approach in two ways. I believe that it was a well-meaning attempt by some nurses to try to minimize for parents the strangeness of their new situation. It also seemed to be an attempt to defuse or minimize any anxieties related to participating that parents might have had by likening their participation in the hospital to the everyday care with which they would be familiar at home. Another possible interpretation, however, is that this was a way in which nurses made more explicit to parents the notion that within the ward there was parental work and nurses' work. This would carry the hidden implication that by saying, "Just do whatever you would do at home," nurses were also implying, "Don't do any other things with your child because that is our work." This would also suggest that although parent participation was still largely an unspoken arrangement, some aspects of the demarcation of nurses' and parents' responsibilities were made explicit.

Several nurses described their use of the as-if-at-home approach:

> I expect them to take care of the nursing duties of the child, like, you know . . . the feeding, changing, bathing and things like that, obviously because that's what they would do at home.

> As far as the sort of condition is, I mean the normal things that they would do at home . . . the mothering type things, like washing and bathing, feeding. . . .

Nurses, however, seemed unaware of the difficulties that parents faced as they tried to sustain this as-if-at-home analogy within the different context of the ward. There were many aspects of their child's care that parents found it very difficult to simply "do as they would do at home." Discipline, for example, was described by parents as a very personal and private practice that was difficult to undertake within the ward, which was seen as the professional domain of child care experts. Another difficulty was noted in the case of certain burned children, whose parents could not simply wash and change them as they would have done at home because the nature and meaning of the child's injury had rendered this formerly straightforward care problematic.

A further difficulty that parents experienced in trying to participate in terms of both the as-if-at-home and the inform-and-leave approaches was revealed in their accounts of how they had tried to use ward kitchens. I had considered initially that the kitchen might have represented what Goffman (1959, pp. 114-115) termed "a back region or backstage," an area where there would be "no audience present" or, in this case, no parents. However, from my own pediatric nursing experience and from my observations and conversations during the period of fieldwork, I could find no evidence that the kitchen was used by nurses in this way.

Another interpretation of why parents' access to kitchens was restricted ties in with the ward kitchen being a metaphor for the home. This opens up the possibility that allowing parents unrestricted access to and use of the kitchen would be a logical but unacceptable conclusion of both the inform-and-leave and as-if-at-home approaches. If this is so, it may support the second interpretation of nurses' adoption of the as-if-at-home analogy. Nurses may have had unstated limitations in mind when they encouraged parents to "just carry on as normal" and to "do what you would do at home."

Parents described how this exclusionary practice confounded their attempts to participate in the ways suggested by the as-if-at-home analogy. For example, they may have been unable to simply go and fetch their child a drink if they were thirsty or make up their baby's feed or make their child a slice of toast for supper. In addition to contradicting the image of the ward as home that nurses tried to promote, this practice also placed parents in the uncomfortable position of having to risk the censure of nurses. This occurred if they were caught trying to enter the kitchen unnoticed to quickly get a drink or if they had to ask a nurse to do this for them and therefore undertake what the parents saw as a comparatively trivial and nuisance task.

The importance of these nursing approaches to encouraging parent participation lies in the unrecognized tension that existed between these articulated strategies and the unspoken expectations that the nurses held. This tension had a direct impact upon parents' lived experience of their participation. For although they received encouragement from nurses that they themselves should determine the nature and extent of their participation by carrying on in ways that were normal for them, there were clearly discernible nursing and institutional expectations and practices that contradicted this seemingly laissez-faire approach.

Conclusion

This research has examined nurses' and parents' accounts of their lived experiences related to parent participation within a pediatric ward. Interpretive analysis suggests that the concept of parent participation is very much a phenomenon cocreated by both nurses and parents. However, there seem to be significant tensions and incongruities within these respective understandings. For example, nurses had definite but often unexpressed expectations of parents, yet their strategies to encourage participation stressed that participation should be largely determined by parents themselves.

The term *parent participation* seemed to have a meaning for nurses and parents that implied an arrangement whereby one party, the parents, would be allowed by the other party, the nurses, to help with their child's care. This perception seemed to be underpinned by a view of the nurse-parent relationship that perceived the nurse as being the dominant power figure and the parent as being in a more secondary and compliant role. Within this perspective, it seemed more likely that the nurse would ultimately decide upon the critical aspects of participation and the parents would participate accordingly.

The impression gained from the study participants' accounts was of parents as helpers, functioning in a role akin to that of an unqualified member of the ward staff. The parents' efforts at participation were thus directed toward areas of care that were incidentally, if not primarily, useful for nurses to have done by others, for example, basic mothering.

What seemed to be largely missing from the nurses' and parents' accounts of participation was any real sense of involvement, reciprocity, and mutuality. By this I mean an involvement whereby parents felt that they had retained an acceptable control over both their own and their child's lives. This involvement would also be characterized by their feeling that aspects of both their child's care and their own role were truly negotiable and a proper subject for discussion and genuine dialogue, and their feeling that their participation in the child's care was of worth and value in terms other than those of helping out the nurses. In the absence of such involvement, I argue that the concept of parental participation was more akin to "parents who stayed for a long time and helped out the staff." On this point, one mother remarked ruefully:

FATHER: You do feel involved, the things that we do for the bairn . . .
MOTHER: Aye, but we're just visitors to them [the hospital staff].

Parental participation impacted upon the nurses' sense of professional identity. Nurses described a tension wherein they recognized the importance of allowing and encouraging parents to undertake more of their child's care, but also recognized that this could seem diminishing to their sense of self as nurses. For some nurses, sharing care with and involving parents was not a calling forth of greater connectedness with a whole family. Rather, it seemed that by "handing over" aspects of care that had traditionally been viewed as theirs, nurses then saw nothing of comparable value with which to replace them. There was a tension apparent here whereby some nurses felt that by encouraging parents to undertake more of their child's care, they as nurses were consequently diminished. This diminution was not only professional but also emotional and personal, in the sense that nurses spoke of no longer "being needed." For these nurses, it seemed as if encouraging parent participation was not a practice that was mutually empowering and satisfying but an alienating and exclusionary process that could deprive the nurse of contact not only with parents but, more importantly for them, with the child.

However, there were parents who described their experience of living-in in ways that showed that they had felt valued and useful and that other nurses had enabled them to be meaningfully involved in their child's care. These parents and nurses may well have agreed with Gadamer's insight that

> "Participation" is a strange word. Its dialectic consists of the fact that participation is not taking parts, but in a way taking the whole. Everybody who participates in something does not take something away, so that others cannot have it. The opposite is true; by sharing, by our participating in the things in which we are participating, we enrich them; they do not become smaller, but larger. (Gadamer, 1984, p. 64)

References

Agan, R. D. (1987). Intuitive knowing as a dimension of nursing. *Advances in Nursing Science, 10*(1), 63-70.

Allen, D., Benner, P., & Diekelmann, N. (1986). Three paradigms for nursing research. In P. Chinn (Ed.), *Nursing research: Methodology, issues and implementations* (pp. 23-38). Rockville, MD: Aspen.

Benner, P. (1984). *From novice to expert: Excellence and power in clinical nursing.* Menlo Park, CA: Addison-Wesley.

Benner, P. (1985). Quality of life: A phenomenological perspective on explanation, prediction and understanding in nursing science. *Advances in Nursing Science, 8*(1), 1-14.

Benner, P., & Tanner, C. (1987). How expert nurses use intuition. *American Journal of Nursing, 87*(1), 23-31.

Benner, P., & Wrubel, J. (1989). *The primacy of caring: Stress and coping in health and illness.* Menlo Park, CA: Addison-Wesley.

Betz, C. L., & Poster, E. C. (1984). Incorporating play into the care of hospitalised children. *Issues in Comprehensive Pediatric Nursing, 7,* 343-355.

Cleary, J., Gray, O. P., Hall, D. J., Rowlandson, P. H., & Sainsbury, C. P. Q. (1986). Parental involvement in the lives of children in hospital. *Archives of Disease in Childhood, 61,* 779-787.

Consumers Association. (1980). *Children in hospital: A Which? campaign report.* London: Consumers Association.

Darbyshire, P. (1994). *Parenting in public: A study of the experiences of parents who live-in with their hospitalised child, and of their relationships with pediatric nurses.* London: Chapman & Hall.

Fagin, C. M., & Nusbaum, J. G. (1978). Parental visiting privileges in pediatric units: A survey. *Journal of Nursing Administration, 8,* 24-27.

Gadamer, H-G. (1975). *Truth and method.* New York: Seabury. (Original work published 1960)

Gadamer, H-G. (1984). The hermeneutics of suspicion. In G. Shapiro & A. Sica (Eds.), *Hermeneutics: Questions and prospects* (pp. 54-65). Amherst: University of Massachusetts Press.

Glaser, B. G., & Strauss, A. L. (1967). *The discovery of grounded theory.* Chicago: Aldine.

Goffman, E. (1959). *The presentation of self in everyday life.* New York: Doubleday.

Hall, D. J. (1977). *Social relations and innovation: Changing the state of play in hospitals.* London: Routledge & Kegan Paul.

Hall, D. J. (1978). Bedside blues: The impact of social research on the hospital treatment of sick children. *Journal of Advanced Nursing, 3*(1), 25-37.

Hall, D. J. (1987). Social and psychological care before and during hospitalisation. *Social Science and Medicine, 25,* 721-732.

Hardgrove, C. (1980). Helping parents on the paediatric ward: A report on a survey of hospitals with "living-in" programs. *Pediatrician, 9,* 220-223.

Heidegger, M. (1966). *Discourse on thinking* (J. M. Anderson & E. H. Freund, Trans.). New York: Harper & Row. (Original work published 1959)

Jolly, J. (1981). *Communicating with children in hospital.* London: H.M. & M.

Meadow, S. R. (1969). The captive mother. *Archives of Diseases in Childhood, 44,* 362-367.

Rabinow, P., & Sullivan, W. M. (1979). *Interpretive social science: A reader.* Berkeley: University of California Press.

Reimen, D. J. (1986). The essential structure of a caring interaction: Doing phenomenology. In P. L. Munhall & C. J. Oiler (Eds.), *Nursing research: A qualitative perspective* (pp. 85-108). Norwalk, NJ: Appleton-Century-Crofts.

Sainsbury, C. P. Q., Gray, O. P., Cleary, J., Davies, M. M., & Rowlandson, P. H. (1986). Care by parents of their children in hospital. *Archives of Disease in Childhood, 61*(6), 612-615.

Schatzman, L., & Strauss, A. L. (1973). *Field research: Strategies for a natural sociology.* New Jersey: Prentice Hall.

U.K. Department of Health. (1991). *Welfare of children and young people in hospital.* London: HMSO.

U.K. Ministry of Health and Central Health Services Council. (1959). *The welfare of children in hospital* (Platt Report). London: HMSO.

Van Manen, M. (1990). *Researching lived experience: Human science for an action sensitive pedagogy.* Ontario: Althouse Press.

11

❖

A Clinical Ethnography of Stroke Recovery

NANCY D. DOOLITTLE

In the United States alone more than 2 million people are living with neurologic impairment secondary to stroke. However, the personal struggle of stroke survival and recovery is much more compelling than this dramatic number. Most biomedical research on stroke recovery has as its focus the return of physical functioning and independence in self-care. The perspective presented here is that living with lacunar stroke goes far beyond living with physical impairment, and that recovery involves much more than attaining functional independence. It is more than the return of limb movement and strength. Although clinicians mark recovery in terms of functional ability and movement, people who have had a stroke measure recovery in terms of how well and to what extent they can take up activities of concern. These activities are what matter to them and give them identity and continuity with their past, as well as the vision of a livable future.

Methodology

Clinical ethnography with rich description of sensations and responses of stroke survivors provides a meaningful method of studying the stroke experience. As the hallmark of cultural anthropology, ethnographic fieldwork has as its primary goal the collection of rich data leading to in-depth descriptive analysis of cultural phenomena. Because clinical ethnography focuses on the experience of human illness as well as biomedical disease processes, it is possible to attend to both personal and biomedical perspectives and the relationship between the two.

This research was interested in the progressive experience of bodily recovery following lacunar stroke (a small infarction in the brain that involves the occlusion of deep penetrating cerebral arteries) (Doolittle, 1990; 1992). Ethnography in the interpretive phenomenological tradition (see Benner, 1985; Benner & Wrubel, 1989; Geertz, 1973; Merleau-Ponty, 1962) was an ideal research strategy. Recording of the stroke recovery process in field notes, life histories, and interviews provided the text for understanding how individuals define recovery from stroke, how they experience their bodies, the meaning of the stroke experience to them, and how patients' views of recovery differ from the biomedical perspective.

Thirteen stroke survivors participated in the study (Doolittle, 1990; 1992). They were each interviewed within 72 hours of the lacunar stroke and during acute and rehabilitation stages of recovery. Two interview forms were developed for use in the study. The "Life History of the Body Interview" was used to collect information about the person's life history. The "Bodily Knowledge Interview" was used to gain understanding of the progressive experience of bodily recovery and practical knowledge of surviving with stroke. The participants were interviewed twice a week for the first 3 weeks poststroke. The frequency of the interviews was then tapered over several months. At the end of 6 months, 120 interviews had been conducted.

Interviews were read and analyzed from the beginning of the study as data were collected and transcribed. The text was read and reread as a whole and then searched via fine-grain interpretation for commonalities across recovery experiences. Major interpretive work began after 6 months of poststroke follow-up. First, the text was read for each participant across the entire 6 months. Next, the text was searched for similarities and differences at varying times poststroke.

Understanding the role of the skilled cultural and habitual body is central to understanding the experience of neurologic illness. Although clinicians may refer to the body as strict object, this is never an accurate account and is not reflective of the embodied survivor's experience. In extreme breakdown such as stroke, the person may objectify parts of the body, but even this objectification has limits because the cultural lived body is inseparable from the person. With weakness or paralysis there is loss of the skilled body. The stroke survivor is thus forced to relate to the world in new ways. In-depth ethnographies allow description of alterations in and regaining of bodily capacities and assist in understanding various adjustment patterns and stages.

They also enable understanding of responses and trajectories in recovery that occur secondary to interruptions of a survivor's particular set of goals and commitments.

As the following paradigm case illustrates, recovery for stroke survivors is not only recovery of the physical body but also recovery of the social body—a reconnection to concerns and social practices. This involves restoration of the member-participant self in the community. The negotiation of this depends on physical capacities, personal concerns and meanings, and the social context. Life before the stroke stands as a point of reference for recovery.

Paradigm Case

Mr. Rowland experienced a right lacunar stroke at the age of 66. My first encounter with him was one not easily forgotten. When I entered his room at the acute hospital, he was sitting in a chair in the corner, his limp left arm and leg propped up with pillows. Though he was awake, his expression and silence rendered him lifeless. His wife was also sitting in the room. Together the two sat in complete silence; there was a profound air of desperation.

At the time of his stroke, Mr. Rowland and his wife were ready to leave on a flight to the Midwest to attend their son's graduation from medical school. Two days prior to their scheduled departure, amidst the excitement of packing and preparing to be reunited with loved ones, Mr. Rowland suddenly developed severe left-sided arm and leg weakness. After several hours at home refusing to go to the hospital, he finally consented to a medical evaluation. His left-sided weakness continued to worsen over the next 48 hours.

> I was talking to my wife one morning, when all of a sudden I couldn't talk. My wife said my face was twisted. I was unable to walk. My foot became extremely weak. I stayed home from the morning to the afternoon. Hoping. But during the first 3 days in the hospital I became totally disabled. I could not move. I became totally dependent and very scared. I didn't know if I would ever get any movement back.

Mr. Rowland was deeply stunned and distraught over the stroke. The timing of it further magnified his discouragement. Through his sadness, however, Mr. Rowland had a new event to look forward to. The same son that graduated from medical school was getting married 2 weeks after graduation. Mr. Rowland's physicians told him that if he was strong enough, they would allow him to travel to the Midwest to attend his son's wedding. The possibility of this set the scene for an extremely dramatic recovery. Within 12 days, Mr. Rowland advanced to walking with a tripod cane.

Immediately following the stroke, Mr. Rowland had only a flicker of movement in his left arm and none in his left leg. But he was determined to walk onto that flight to the Midwest. He was solicited by his love for his son and his wish to attend this very important event.

He indeed recovered well enough to travel to his son's wedding. Upon his return he had many stories to tell:

> The therapists told me that I advanced too fast. But I knew I would not be able to leave [for the wedding] until I did real well.
>
> [At the reception] I was able to dance. I forgot that I was handicapped. I just wanted to dance and be a part of the celebration. I was listening to the band, and when I heard the music . . . the music was so nice. . . . The music was there. And then the audience started clapping for us and I realized I was dancing. And then the music came to an end and my feet stopped. And I had to stop. I also walked without my cane. I think sometimes you just do better if you don't think about it.

Up to the seventh week following the stroke Mr. Rowland made dramatic improvement. He kept his daily schedule articulately outlined in a little black book. He reserved a couple of hours each day for meals, 1 hour for bathing, 2 hours for a mid-day nap, and 6 hours for exercise sessions. He walked around the block for exercise and kept exact count of his steps. He was determined to recover his prestroke body through progressive, organized exercise. He was convinced that will power and sheer effort would bring his left arm and leg back to a strength that would exceed his prestroke ability. With sheer mental effort the weak arm and leg would ultimately become stronger than the unaffected side. His point of comparison was always prestroke life. Because of this, he was continually bothered by what his left arm would not do.

During the ninth and tenth week after the stroke progress was slow, and Mr. Rowland began talking about how degrading the stroke experience had been for him:

> I didn't want my friends to see me, I didn't want to see anybody, I just wanted to hide. I couldn't speak right, my arm and leg didn't work right, and I was only in a position of being pitied. And the one thing I couldn't stand was pity. Everything had closed in on me. I got so low I didn't want to live anymore. I would rather die than have this happen again.

Mr. Rowland spent the next 4 or 5 weeks groping with this plateau in recovery. It is notable that as a retired engineer, he consistently reported improvement in percentages and also regularly charted his progress with graphs made on engineering paper.

Although he was retired at the time of his stroke, approximately 4 months after the stroke he visited his former work setting:

> And I tried to meet all the workers. But I felt as though I could not tell them I had a stroke. I'm not proud of the progress I've made, not until I am like what I was before the stroke. When I was in the office before, I worked really hard. That's why I don't want people to know I've been sick.

At 6 months, Mr. Rowland continued to describe his walking. He continued to experience a very objectified body:

> When I start walking, things are normal. But then when I reach that other corner, it's as if I'm going back to the time when I think more about my left side. I have to instruct the arm [to swing]. That's what I've learned from the stroke. There must be some instruction coming from your mind . . . to do it . . . to walk erect. . . . In other words, my mind tells my body to do it this way or that way. I have to have the instructions, and then my muscles will follow.

Here the "mind over matter" metaphor comes through. Even with this attitude, in 6 months Mr. Rowland's bodily experience had not returned to the prestroke state. There was still breakdown with habitual bodily acts. His whole being was taken over by the stroke. His world and his body were rendered unreliable; the sense that diligent, hard work would facilitate better recovery made it very difficult for Mr. Rowland to accept his poststroke life.

This case illustrates Mr. Rowland's emotional and physical immobilization following the stroke. He was initially desperately frightened. His left arm and leg became passive objects under the control of his mind. He believed that effort and hard work would return the limbs to their prestroke state. He lived with a deficit view of stroke and was rarely satisfied with improvement. The work ethic remained a very dominant focus for him. He also experienced troubled social reintegration. He did his best to hide the fact that he had a stroke. He turned down social invitations because he wanted to be known as a strong, active, successful person. His stroke was the opposite of this personal and cultural imperative. The difficulty in his social reintegration mimicked his difficulty with bodily reintegration. Just as there was not a sense of smoothness in limb integration and interaction, social integration and interaction was awkward and constrained.

The Meaning of Recovery

Recovery of the Social Body

A view commonly held in rehabilitation settings is that motivated patients fulfill their recovery potential by becoming functionally independent (Kaufman & Becker, 1986). Functional independence is measured by physical, visible signs of self-care. For instance, putting on one's shoes is a level of functional independence. Health care workers focus on rehabilitation through the observation of physical, visible tasks and the achievement of objective goals. The completion of discrete tasks such as buttoning a shirt or brushing one's teeth is what counts.

This focus varies from the lived, habitual way humans perform tasks in their everyday lives. Although brushing one's teeth and buttoning a shirt are experienced as necessary daily activities, they are not sufficiently significant to provide meaning and identity. A focus on isolated functional capacities does not take into consideration personal meanings, the context of daily life, and activities important to the person. Progress with meaningful activities may go unnoticed. The biomedical view of rehabilitation has set functional independence as an optimal status. But for the person who has had a stroke, recovery is not lived as the completion of functional tasks prescribed by others. Recovery is the slow return to important activities and previously valued concerns that matter to the person.

Mr. Ward had a lacunar stroke of the internal capsule of his brain at the age of 54. The stroke affected the strength and control of his left arm and hand. Prior to the stroke Mr. Ward was an avid fisherman. Following the stroke, he judged his progress by how well he could fish. This progress was discussed in terms of reeling and casting with his left arm and hand. Fishing was Mr. Ward's point of reference for "total" recovery. For him, the ability to fish marked both physical recovery and the recovery of a social body.

For 6 months following his stroke, he lived and understood his progress through fishing experiences. With each interview, when asked his definition of recovery, he provided an update of his ability to cast and reel. As the months passed, the frequency of his fishing trips increased. He was finally able to walk the long distance to the end of the pier alone. Because fishing organized Mr. Ward's daily life, his recovery was measured in terms of it. Fishing was a focal practice that revealed possibility and progress to him.

For each person, the assessment of progress and recovery is based on possibilities within a context or within a situation. For each individual the social context may differ, yet the return to activities that matter marks recovery. Through involved recovery, people begin to understand themselves in terms of their possibilities instead of their deficits. A striking example of this was Mr. Rowland's attendance at his son's wedding. This activity was the focal point of his recovery the first 2 weeks after his stroke. His presence at the wedding and dancing at the reception dramatically marked recovery for him.

Return to Familiar Surroundings

The importance of the reconnection of the member-participant self in the community is exemplified by the individual who does very poorly in a structured rehabilitation program focused on physical functioning. Ms. Jones provides an example of this. For her, progress following her stroke was extremely slow. She had severe weakness of the left side of her body. Rehabilitation staff had to prod her to perform minimal activity. When she was finally discharged, there was a dramatic transformation. She was carried up the front steps of her home, and with great delight at being home again, stood alone and walked into the house, crossed the living room, and seated herself in her favorite armchair. What was so compelling about this was that Ms. Jones had not walked more than a few steps in the hospital setting. Upon entering her own living room, she was transformed by the familiar setting of home. Over the next few months she learned to walk again. Her husband provided her with tremendous incentive, insisting that she walk throughout the house several times each day. She soon was able to walk alone, unassisted, without even a cane. This situation is remarkable in that it illustrates the experience of solicitation by meaningful familiar surroundings of one's home.

Solicitation of the Body by the Familiar and Situational

Ordinarily, human beings experience movements as solicited by their situation (Merleau-Ponty, 1962). In the previous example, Ms. Jones was solicited by her living room and favorite armchair. Her experience of returning home was transforming. As discussed in the paradigm case, Mr. Rowland was solicited by the setting of his son's wedding to dance with his wife. In both situations mobility was returned to its familiar and habitual context; movement was much more than a decontextualized exercise.

The whole world is full of meaning of the touchable, the movable, and the approachable. Oliver Sacks (1985) and Dreyfus (1979, 1991) use the example of a glove. Anyone who experiences a glove actually experiences the solicitation of his or her hand into it. The glove just appears as if it is for our hand to slip into. The glove is always wearable to us, just as the chair is sittable and the doorknob is graspable. Another example is a light switch, which solicits the individual to flip it on or off. The body engaged in meaningful activity is always "on the way to" or moving, in order to grasp, turn off, pick up, and so forth. When one loses this involved, active capacity, what is left is an objective, calculating, functional capacity. It was the experience and solicitation of familiar surroundings that drew Ms. Jones' amazing response to walk.

This graspable world is also a source of despair; when stairs can no longer be climbed or painting can no longer be done, the person is faced with breakdown and deficit rather than progress and possibilities. As he or she becomes obsessed with what cannot be accomplished with weak limbs, a view of improvement and recovery diminishes. The person experiences failure at every turn. Although certain activities were not viewed as automatic and prereflective before the stroke, the person is left in turmoil because of this loss.

Sequential Focus

Certain parts of the body take their turn in terms of being the focus of attention for the person. For the first few months Ms. Jones focused intensely on her walking. She made marvelous strides with her left leg. For these first months she said virtually nothing about her paralyzed left arm. This was notable because her left arm was virtually useless. Her total attention and energy were focused on walking again. Suddenly 5 months after the stroke, as she mastered walking, her attention was drawn to her arm. Although this might be described as denial, the experience is better captured by sequential focus. Lived meanings and priorities changed over time for Ms. Jones. She had not denied the paralysis; she had survived the stroke and taken care of bodily priorities in an order guided by her situation. The phenomenon of sequential focus captures how the lived concerns of paralysis changed over time for her.

Bodily Set

Individuals have a bodily set that responds to the environment in terms of a sense of its own goals. Bodies recognize complex patterns in precognitive ways, thus allowing transparent access to the environment. An example is Mr. Ryan, who had a right lacunar stroke at the age of 87. One of his favorite hobbies was gardening. Prior to the stroke, he spent hours each day working in his backyard. He spoke of knowing his backyard, of walking across the uneven concrete and feeling it with his body:

> Well, the surface is uneven, but I'm so used to it. I know it. It's knowing it. . . . If it were a strange place I'd probably have trouble. But when you know your own yard . . . every dip, every turn . . . you get used to it.

With Mr. Ryan there was a bodily understanding of the very familiar setting of the garden. There was a precognitive, skilled, habitual, nondeliberative anticipation of broken and uneven concrete. His response to the demands of the situation and the setting was automatic.

When Hubert Dreyfus discusses the work of Merleau-Ponty (1962), he talks about bodily set—the body is always set to have certain experiences. However, these sets can change when the body gets surprised or when the bodily situation changes. The way things show up to us is correlative to our bodily set to them. The geared-into-the-world body is the background of everything. This is the body's habitual set. This background—the horizon or the atmosphere—is so pervasive that we never have ready formal access to it.

Another example of bodily set is the skilled capacity to climb stairs. Prestroke, the climbing pattern is integrated and smooth. The feet alternately "step up" and one's arm and hand automatically hover close to the railing. With stroke there is breakdown of this bodily set. This forces the survivor to learn new techniques, new rules. By memorizing new rules for movement, the individual may be able to perform the required motion. The problem with this, however, is that the movement is not the same integrated, smooth movement as before.

A Phenomenological Understanding of the Body

In daily life, human beings comfortably exist and are at home in the world in a bodily, nonreflective way. People turn doorknobs automatically without taking time to reflect on the doorknob as object. They also answer telephones, type, and drive in prereflective ways. But when a breakdown occurs in skilled know-how (Heidegger, 1927/1962), skilled practices and activities show up differently. With the paralysis of stroke there is sudden breakdown. This breakdown is actually close to our Cartesian understanding of the body as object. Paralyzed limbs no longer work. Movement that was once automatic suddenly ceases. The nature of the lived body has changed. The person must think about limbs reflectively.

Acute stroke presents people with fear, uncertainty, and a bodily experience of deterioration. The shock of sudden immobility and paralysis leaves them suspended in a passive, objectified body. They are immobilized by the stroke; they lose a sense of bodily wholeness, and their attention turns to the new object at their side.

The Work of Recovery

When I asked my arm to lift, it wouldn't. That was right after admission.
Now, when I command my arm to raise, it may be unsteady, but I can raise it.
In other words, if I say to myself right now, "Raise your left arm," I can raise
it a little. But if I say, "Raise it higher" . . . now that is hard.

Mind Over Matter

Immediately following onset of stroke, individuals concentrate very deliberately on getting and making movement. This is the work of recovery. It
is a conscious mental attempt to regain participation in meaningful activities.
They speak frequently of having to ask their bodies to do things, such as
asking one's leg to "step ahead."

> Before the stroke, I didn't think about things like eating, or feeding myself. I
> just did it. I just ate. I just let the right hand do whatever it wanted to do. Now
> I have to make it work.

The individuals consistently describe a "mind in control of the body"
experience. Purposeful effort is required for movement.

MR. BUTLER: It feels like my brain is saying to my left foot, "step forward."
Instead of doing that, my left leg says "I am too tired, your knee
is going to collapse, and you're going to go down."
INT.: So your brain is saying one thing, but your leg is talking back to you?
MR. BUTLER: Right. Exactly.

This is an example of executive orders being given to an uncooperative,
alienated, object body. Limbs are frequently referred to as "it" rather than
"my arm" or "my leg." The body becomes dense and unresponsive and the
affected limbs are treated as objects to be manipulated. This loss of bodily
continuity turns the taken-for-granted, smoothly functioning body into one
that fits the Cartesian description of the mind/body dichotomy and the
current biomedical view of body as machine.

> I learned that you think you can't do something but you can. You just have to
> try. You have to believe you can do it, too. Because if you don't, you can't. If
> I just sat here and looked at this leg, it wouldn't do anything. But I just pick it
> up anyway, and drag it.

The Cartesian view of the mind is that mental acts of intent or will can and
do determine action and bodily motion. During stroke recovery a struggle

ensues between the mind and the body. Participants believe that if they think long and hard enough, the act of thinking or of mental activity will empower the affected limbs to move again. There is a sense of the mind being in control of the body.

As spontaneous neurological recovery occurs, this mind-over-matter effortful striving is effective in propelling individuals through rehabilitation. A sense of directed effort organizes the adaptive task of recovery. The reward of effortful control of the body is visible progress. At the end of a day of strenuous work focused on relearning how to walk, any regained strength of an involved leg, for example, offers a sense of purpose and direction toward improvement. Total involvement in the work of recovery offers new possibilities.

But the possibilities inherent in the work of recovery change over time. Four or 5 months after the stroke, effortful direction of the body becomes less and less beneficial for the individual. This is because spontaneous recovery plateaus. There is less benefit from effortful striving and more frustration at confronting diminished recovery. Mind-over-matter mental operations cannot dictate the pace of recovery or hasten the return to valued activities.

Recapturing Bodily Knowledge

Although bodily skills are sometimes learned by following rules, when the individual becomes proficient at an activity, the sequence of original simple movements is left behind. A single, unified, smooth pattern of behavior remains (Dreyfus, 1991). The coarse, piecemeal elements of the beginning skill are absent from the smooth final skill. An example of this is swimming. The bodily knowledge of the swimmer involves know-how that cannot be accurately captured by rules.

Unfortunately, people who have had a stroke lose much automatic, prereflective movement. Following a stroke, the individual is still solicited by the sittable chair, by the graspable doorknob, by the flippable switch, and by the climbable stairs. But with paralysis, the sitting movement cannot be made, the doorknob cannot be grasped, the light switch cannot be flipped on, and the stairs cannot be climbed. For instance, Ms. Anderson was an avid bowler. She was fortunate in that following her stroke she was able to return to this activity. She described her bowling game 17 weeks after her stroke:

> During my delivery, I'm afraid I'll fall to the left. You see, when you bowl you do it the same way all the time. You just know how to do it. What I'm doing now . . . I'm just throwing the ball. I normally have a lift when I bowl. But I've lost that. I can't bend. Now I just sort of throw the ball at the pins.

Ms. Anderson had lost the sense of being with the ball. Before the stroke, she "knew how to do it." She had a very smooth, natural follow-through with the release of the bowling ball. With the loss of natural follow-through, her game became very awkward. She now had to think how to release the ball. She found herself "throwing" the ball down the alley. Before the stroke, she described "being one" with the ball and the pins. Following the stroke, she was separate from both.

Ten weeks after his stroke, Mr. Ward compared relearning activities following the stroke with learning to swim as a child:

> It just all came natural. It was part of our environment. Nobody really taught me to swim. I watched the others. Typically, they'd just throw you in and you had to do it. I got in the water and swam. I just did it. Just like the bicycle. I'd get on it, I'd fall off, but I'd just get on it again and keep trying. And you'd just pick it up naturally.

Once learned, the coordinated, rhythmic pattern of swimming cannot be reduced or decontextualized to fragments of limb movements. The automaticity and nonreflective pattern of coordinated bodily movement allows the person to remain afloat.

Throughout the experience of loss, the participants described a sense of recapturing bodily knowledge. This was evident in their discussion of stroke, when they realized the actual bodily capacities lost. Their poststroke frame of reference was evident in their comparisons of prestroke mobility with poststroke immobility.

The participants described several occasions when the body exhibited tendencies to act or move on its own. These acts were prereflective. The following exemplars illustrate these tendencies.

> Sometimes I forget about it. I go ahead and I'm driven to walk. . . . Then I remember and I have to stop and pick it up [the leg].

> Sometimes I just get out of the chair and walk across the room, and I forget about using my walker. I just walk.

This person had not thought about the walker or his need for it. What is remarkable about this comment is the surprise at the return of spontaneous bodily intentionality instead of consciously driven mental intentions to achieve certain goals and destinations. These are intriguing examples of the body as knower.

The person experiences inability and failure at every turn. Although the individual did not think about these activities as automatic and prereflective before the stroke, he or she is left in turmoil because of this loss.

The body is overlooked when it is functioning smoothly. It is only with breakdown of bodily set and automaticity that the body is openly addressed. There is a focus on bodily movement only after this breakdown, when the body is ill, because such focus was simply not required before.

Living with stroke goes far beyond living with physical impairment. For people who have had a stroke, life before the stroke stands as a point of reference for recovery. If health care providers are to assist and mobilize people to recover, they must have accurate and detailed historical knowledge of the daily concerns, values, and habits of the people they are caring for. Therapy strategies that treat personal concerns and meanings as paramount and that take into account social context will best assist the person to experience progress and recovery poststroke.

References

Benner, P. (1985). Quality of life: A phenomenological perspective on explanation, prediction, and understanding in nursing science. *Advances in Nursing Science, 8*(1), 1-14.

Benner, P., & Wrubel, J. (1989). *The primacy of caring: Stress and coping in health and illness*. Reading, MA: Addison-Wesley.

Doolittle, N. D. (1990). *Life after stroke: Survivors' bodily and practical knowledge of coping during recovery*. Unpublished doctoral dissertation, University of California, San Francisco.

Doolittle, N. D. (1992). The experience of recovery following lacunar stroke. *Rehabilitation Nursing, 17*(3), 122-125.

Dreyfus, H. (1979). *What computers can't do: The limits of artificial intelligence* (rev. ed.). New York: Harper & Row.

Dreyfus, H. (1991). *Being-in-the-world: A commentary on Heidegger's "Being and time," Division I*. Cambridge, MA: MIT Press.

Geertz, C. (1973). *The interpretation of cultures*. Basic Books.

Heidegger, M. (1962). *Being and time*. New York: Harper & Row. (Original work published 1927)

Kaufman, S., & Becker, G. (1986). Stroke: Health care on the periphery. *Social Science and Medicine, 22*(9), 983-989.

Merleau-Ponty, M. (1962). *Phenomenology of perception* (C. Smith, Trans.). London: Routledge & Kegan Paul.

Sacks, O. (1985). *The man who mistook his wife for a hat*. New York: Summit.

12

❖

Moral Dimensions of Living With a Chronic Illness

Autonomy, Responsibility, and the Limits of Control

PATRICIA BENNER

SUSAN JANSON-BJERKLIE

SANDRA FERKETICH

GAY BECKER

Asthma was a kind of neurotic, sissy. . . . [An asthmatic was] a weak person. "It's a weakness, not a disease, it's a weakness. It comes from emotions and it comes from maladjustment. It can also come from being too locked in on yourself. You're too concerned with yourself, you're emotionally immature in that you are unable to deal with your emotions. You allow them to get out of hand. You give in to them. You give in to yourself." . . . Then, of course, the great one, one of my brothers was real big on this one. "You get asthma from an animal, but if you go in a room and you don't know an animal has been there, you won't get asthma." That actually isn't true in my case. I researched it out,

AUTHORS' NOTE: The larger study on which this chapter is based was supported by a research grant from the National Center for Nursing Research, NIH (NR01536), to Susan Janson-Bjerklie, Principal Investigator; Patricia Benner and Sandra Ferketich, Co-Investigators; and Gay Becker, Research Associate.

and that's become one of my flagship statements. I've always thrown that into people, willy-nilly into conversations. If I go in a room like a motel or something, and they've had an animal in there before me, I'll get a violent asthma attack and I won't even know why, but I found out they had an animal in there before that. It is like I have this tremendous need to defend myself against this accusation. It is a sense of accusation. Asthma has always been in my experience a disease that is not considered a true disease. It is a personality defect that takes a physical form, and so I think that's one reason I never even talked about having asthma. . . . I never told anyone. If it had anything to do with breathing, or with any kind of physical weakness, it was a moral, character weakness, defect, and asthma was a part of that. It just wasn't like a broken leg or something.

(Sara, 47-year-old single Caucasian woman
who has had asthma for 30 years)

This narrative reveals how the moral emotions of shame, blame, and responsibility are engendered by the informal expectation that the person can control the body with the mind and how failure to do this is experienced as a threat to autonomy. Implicit in the above narrative is that entitlement to care is restricted to "real diseases," meaning diseases over which the individual bears no responsibility for causation or cure. Even more implicit is the way that the very existence of illness threatens the Western project to be autonomous, and the way that this project is tied up with our sense of what it is to be a moral agent (Nussbaum, 1986; Taylor, 1985, 1989). Body and mind seem to have mutual influence on the asthma illness experience. The attempt, however, to locate the "cause" in the mind heightens moral feelings of responsibility, shame, and blame.

The cause of asthma is unknown. The current medical explanation for the pathogenesis of asthma is multifactorial. It is linked to a hereditary tendency to have hyperreactive airways that constrict in response to physical irritants such as cold air, laughing, and exercise, inhaled irritants such as allergens and environmental pollutants, infections, and inflammatory reactions. Symptom perception, treatment, and emotional responses to illness episodes are shaped by personal concerns and social responses (Fritz, Rubinstein, & Lewiston, 1987; Janson-Bjerklie, Ferketich, & Benner, 1993; Janson-Bjerklie, Ferketich, Benner, & Becker, 1992; Janson-Bjerklie, Ruma, Stulbarg, & Carrieri, 1987; Jones, Kinsman, Dirks, & Dahlem, 1987). The older view that asthma is psychosomatic, that is, caused by disturbed relationships to the mother or parents, emotional dependency, or immaturity, has been losing credence as the mechanical and biochemical aspects of the disease have become better understood.

The interpretive study reported here is a secondary analysis of a larger study that combined quantitative and qualitative methods in a predictive design. This interpretive study was based on the assumption that coping is a form of embodied practical knowledge that relies on feelings, sense of salience, skilled embodied know-how, practical reasoning about present situations in terms of concrete past experiences, and an everyday taken-for-granted understanding of the world (Benner & Wrubel, 1989; Dreyfus 1979, 1991a, 1991b; Dreyfus & Dreyfus, 1986; Heidegger, 1927/1962, 1975; Kierkegaard, 1843/1985; Merleau-Ponty, 1962; Toombs, 1988). These taken-for-granted understandings of responsibility and causation of health and illness permeate the responses we have toward clients and even our structural arrangements for entitlement to and reimbursement of care. Seeking and receiving treatment may be delayed and health care systems avoided because of the common understandings of the nature of chronic illness exacerbations. Though four distinct self-described relationships to illness and body (discussed later in chapter) were uncovered, these may be collapsed into two broad self-described relationships with the illness: (a) an oppositional, control-oriented relationship and (b) a relationship of acceptance and care.

Asthma is an illness particularly well suited to illustrate the moral dimensions of psychological "determinism" common in North American culture because of its theoretical and folk history of being "psychosomatic" or "all in the mind," as illustrated in the narrative above. A causal model that locates the source of illness only in the mind or the body cannot adequately capture the mutual influences of mind, body, human world, and physical environment.

When one is well and performing fluidly, the body is experienced as oneself. In breakdown, the body is experienced as an uncontrollable dense other with a will of its own (Frank, 1991). All illness raises questions about the sense of self in relation to embodied existence. A chronic noncurable illness heightens and sustains these questions. Suffering with a chronic illness is further compounded by the heightened sense of responsibility for being healthy in the current wellness movement:

> The assumption [of the wellness movement] is that personal behavior will improve health, happiness, and longevity. The degree to which people believe they can control their health is striking (Crawford, 1984; Harris, 1981; Taylor & Brown, 1988; Weinstein, 1982). . . . Herein lies the paradox of control. People who are basically healthy worry about their health. Although they are

alarmed at the risk lurking everywhere, people overstate the control they feel over their health. (Brownell, 1991, p. 305)

Unrealistic expectations for personal control that confuse the healthy are even more confusing and troubling for the chronically ill. The quest to transcend the body and overcome frailty and suffering was led early in the tradition by Socrates' oppositional view of mind, spirit, and body. Rawlinson (1986) describes Western moral links to suffering as a disruption to the project of producing an autonomous subject. In this project suffering must have a sense, or particular meanings related to control and responsibility, in order for the autonomous subject to maintain that he or she owns the power to control his or her own ends:

> Having freed himself from the frailties of the body and having submitted his will to the guiding light of the intelligence, the philosopher, like Socrates who indifferently "marches barefoot in the snow" or maintains clarity of mind and person through a long night of drink, is the "happiest of all men" and does not suffer; nevertheless, the philosopher speaks authoritatively upon suffering, for he has the clearest view of the order of the ideal, and, thus, is best qualified to measure the kind and degree of suffering that attends the "fall." Suffering is both evidence and experience of a failure on the part of the subject or individual soul to assume its proper position in the harmony of an ideal order. Thus, no suffering is senseless; it is either deserved, or redemptive, or rewarded in the moment of death or judgment. Each specific case demands its appropriate response, but moral propriety is always determined by the goal of restoring the soul to its proper order. (Rawlinson, 1986, p. 40)

Indeed, senseless suffering assaults a sense of meaning and justice in Western philosophy beginning with Plato and extending through Kant and Christian Platonism (Benner, Roskies, & Lazarus, 1981; Rawlinson, 1986).

Data Collection

This chapter reports an interpretive phenomenological study of self-understanding, self-described relationships to the illness and body, and moral dimensions of illness based upon interview data drawn from a larger study (Becker, Janson-Bjerklie, Benner, Slobin, & Ferketich, 1993; Janson-Bjerklie et al., 1992, 1993). The 95 participants with physician-diagnosed asthma were interviewed three times over a 2-month period in 1987 to 1988. Initial screening spirometry at the first interview confirmed the diagnosis of asthma by at least 15% improvement in FEV (forced expiratory volume in 1 second) in response to an inhaled bronchodilator (Becker et al., 1993; Janson-Bjerklie et al., 1992, 1993). The sample included 36 men and 59 women with a mean age of 44.2 (±14.5 years). Ethnically, the sample was predominantly white (82 subjects), with the nonwhite participants including 2 Asians, 4 blacks, 3 Hispanics, and 4 others. The participants were primarily middle class and were primarily employed in white-collar and managerial positions. Twenty-nine participants had a yearly income of $20,000 or less, and 47 had a yearly income of over $30,000. The total sample experienced an average of 19 (19.4 ±12.2) episodes of asthma per month. Each participant was followed for 60 days with twice daily peak flow monitoring and was interviewed monthly for a total of three interviews per participant. This sample reflects the urban white middle class and may not represent minorities or lower socioeconomic groups.

The textual source was made up of three interviews. The first and third interviews were the Coping Interview, adapted from the Lazarus et al. Stress and Coping in Aging Study (Benner, 1984; Lazarus & Folkman, 1984; Schaefer, 1983; Wrubel, 1985). The coping interview elicited narrative accounts of actual episodes of asthma, what the participants were doing at the time, and what they thought, felt, and did as the episode unfolded. The interviews provide a detailed natural history of at least three actual episodes of asthma, in which the interviewer probed for practical knowledge, informal models of the illness, and actual self-care and coping strategies. During the second interview, in addition to the coping interview, participants were asked for the history (the story) of their asthma. These questions generated reflections on life experience with asthma, informal models of the illness, self-described relationships to the illness, and assessments of the impact of asthma on life choices and relationships to others. Taken together, the interviews focused on the participants' narrative accounts of particular asthma episodes and the story of their asthma from the beginning. The thematic analysis of the interview data was integral to a larger predictive analysis in which self-described relationships to the illness were examined in relation to morbidity, patterns of health care system use, and morale outcomes (Becker et al., 1993; Janson-Bjerklie et al., 1992, 1993).

Interviews for all 95 participants were coded using the Ethnograph computer program for qualitative analysis. For the purposes of this analysis, the ethnograph coding categories "informal models of the illness," "pivotal episodes of learning," "stigma," and "self-descriptions in relation to the illness" were read in order to understand the participants' narratives or stories of the illness, informal explanatory models of causation and responsibility, and sense of self and others in relation to the illness.

A thematic analysis of all three interviews yielded four different self-described relationships to the illness:

1. *Acceptance* ($n = 26$): Accepts illness and describes illness experience in terms that are neither highly objective—that is, personal experience and feelings are described—nor extremely subjective—that is, the illness is not described as internally caused by thoughts, feelings, or attitudes. For example, one young man explained, "I don't feel anything bad, or negative, or handicapped, or anything like that. It's like having a child almost. It's a responsibility you have. You take care of it. And if you take care of it, everything works out O.K. and if you don't take care of it, then you have problems."

2. *Transitional* ($n = 15$): The participant describes a changing relationship in which the self is less angry or rejecting of the illness and notes that the change is from a position of anger or other stance of "less acceptance." As one participant stated, "I am learning to accept the illness as part of myself."

3. *Nonacceptance* ($n = 35$): This is an either extremely objective or extremely subjective view of the disease as external to the self, or in the mind and thus controllable by the mind. For some, nonacceptance means that little space is given to the illness. As one woman described it, "I don't consider myself as being sick, it is just like having a headache."

4. *Adversarial* ($n = 17$): An angry, rejecting relation to the disease as alien and enemy, something that must be fought.

The total of participants in these categories was 93 (two of the cases could not be classified with these thematic categories). A comparison of the practical worlds of nonacceptance and adversarial themes shows a similar pattern of self-described relationships to the illness and similar illness meanings. Likewise, the transitional and acceptance themes demonstrate a similar narrative of change from earlier, less accepting and more control-oriented relationships to the illness. All themes demonstrate practical moral reasoning about the cause and sense of responsibility to control or care for the illness.

Rejecting, Fighting, and Controlling the Illness

In the nonacceptance categories (Categories 3 and 4 above), the disease is experienced as an outside entity apart from the self ($n = 52$; 56%). The self is considered to be separate from the body, and often a mistrustful or adversarial relationship exists between the self and body:

PART.: The hardest thing is just thinking that it won't go away. . . . Am I hanging on to it? Or do I want to believe that it can go away? Or am I hanging on, is it serving me in some way and all things? Sometimes I think it's bullshit and sometimes I don't know.

INT.: Do you think that it can go away?

PART.: I have a really hard time with that. It's like I really want to believe it can, but I don't know if I do, and that's really where I wish I could

> switch my mind to saying yes, I believe it can. It could be that I don't
> want to be disappointed. You read about cancer and how it can go away.
> I would like to really believe that, but I don't for some reason, I've had
> a hard time getting that. (Lina, a 34-year-old Caucasian married woman
> who has had asthma for 34 years)

The self as articulated in this stance is most closely associated with mind, will power, and personal control. The informal causal model that the illness is all in the mind or that the mind triggers or controls the illness is related to a sense of personal control in at least two ways. Sometimes psychological determinism is felt as moral blame: that is, the self is blamed for not controlling the body, allowing sickness to occur. This is the "moral weakness" described in the opening interview excerpt. At other times it can be a comforting thought that "asthma is all in the mind" because such an attribution creates the hope that the self or mind could take over and overcome the disease. The disease does not lie outside the self's control if "it" is all in the mind:

> I think about what my symptoms are and how expressions of my body for
> good or ill happen. Why they might happen and what that might represent. So
> I am not done with this task yet, that will be a long time. (Helene, a 37-year-
> old Caucasian married woman who has had asthma for 27 years)

Persons with asthma can experience swings from extreme subjectivism— "It's all in the mind"—to extreme objectivism—experiencing the illness as a capricious external force that assaults the object body. Both stances endanger the person with a life-threatening illness such as asthma because they interfere with developing expertise in managing the illness preventively and in emergencies:

> **PART.:** As I say, I see nothing to anticipate anything. I'm suddenly having
> these symptoms.
> **INT.:** Yeah.
> **PART.:** And, pyschologically, not because of anything I could possibly train,
> but just the way I've evolved and grown up, I am very—I would say
> academically detached—about any problems of any kind. If there is a
> problem I cannot handle, I do something else. (Joseph, a 65-year-old
> divorced Caucasian man who has had asthma for 6 months)

Extreme objectivism and subjectivism exist as two sides of the same coin, and typically participants shifted from one to the other depending on the circumstances. The desire to "control" the mind follows quite naturally from the assumption that the mind is the source of the illness; however, *how* to effect this control is not apparent, and participants had a variety of assumptions about how to go about this task. Often the approach was to not "think" about the illness:

> **PART.:** So I think it is psychological. It's in the mind. I mean asthma is a disease, but a lot of it is in the mind, from what I have heard.

[Later in the same interview, the interviewer is asking the participant to describe an episode when he was awakened out of a sound sleep.]

> **PART.:** See, that's another thing. Maybe it was psychological, because I left here, I was fine. Finally when I got some sleep I woke up and it was like, asthma, but like I said, it could have been a dream, or just in my mind. That's another thing I try to do is keep myself from thinking about, not totally . . .
> **INT.:** From dwelling on it.
> **PART.:** Right, dwelling, I couldn't have clarified it better myself.
> **INT.:** When you fill out these forms [daily peak flow readings and recordings of episodes] I can see how it really does make you aware of it. [Participant had stated earlier that the study made him notice his asthma.]
> **PART.:** Right, because I do have to face the fact that I have it. Basically, what I'm trying to do is tell myself I don't. That's all I'm trying to do. (Bill, a 24-year-old black single man who has had asthma for 24 years)

This participant attributes the onset of his asthma attack to his talking about his asthma during the previous interview, or perhaps his "dream." If the informal model is that "thinking makes it so," it makes sense to avoid thinking about asthma and to avoid noticing it when it happens. This same participant did acknowledge that keeping records for the study made him face his illness and take his medications, and that without the study as a prompt, he might have ended up in the emergency room again. By the third interview, a month later, he had cut down on smoking from two packs of cigarettes a day to one every 3 to 4 days, had eliminated other major allergic triggers, had begun to exercise, and was feeling better. At this point, he had stopped carrying medications with him and the illness once again assumed the ambiguous position of being all in his mind:

> I leave it [the inhaler] at home and I don't carry it. I think that was part of the psychological trip that I was relying on, this . . . [thinking,] oh, I can't leave without it. Theo-Dur, inhaler, Alupent, or anything. And so far it's been working. I haven't needed it. I almost totally forgot that I had asthma myself until I was going to log it in on my record every day. (Bill)

The objective measure of his asthma, his peak flow reading, was now 600, indicating that his acute episode was over. The fluctuation back and forth between an objective to subjective view of the illness can create coping patterns of vigilance and avoidance within the same participant, and both coping strategies can provide an increased sense of self-control. Vigilance can be experienced as a way of keeping the disease external to one's life, and avoidance or "not thinking about the asthma" may be experienced as a way of controlling the body by the mind. For example, another participant responded to an interviewer's comment about his self-care:

> **INT.:** It sounds like you do pretty much everything.
> **PART.:** Yeah, I really try to. I hate to think of it as controlling my life. It just really bothers me. If it's something that I have, I don't want it to take over my life. I need to control it, and I feel like so much of it is mind over matter. Not that I can control my attacks, but if I come into it with a positive attitude and know that I can take care of this. I am not going to let this control my life. I am going to work with it, then I can feel like I can do it. (Samuel, a 40-year-old married Caucasian man who has had asthma for 15 years)

Another participant illustrates this fight to set limits on the incursion of the illness on life projects in a similar way:

> [Not having asthma interfere], that's like a goal. Where I have it, but it's not part of my life. It's out, tucked away, and I can take care of it. Yeah, I don't want it to be up there as part of my life. (Maya, a 33-year-old married Native American woman who has had asthma for 13 years)

The disease and body are "other" in this stance, that is, something that is not self, an external entity that the self must control. To make accommodations to the illness is to lose the battle. Thus controlling the disease so that the disease does not control the self often means making as few concessions to the illness as possible. The participant quoted above states:

> I feel that I can, like I said, control it more. I can go to a house that has a cat if I do x, y, z. That has helped a lot. (Maya)

Circumventing and managing limitations imposed by the illness returns a sense of self-control. Here, medication is appropriated by the self to control the illness. One way to be "in charge" of oneself despite taking medications is to prescribe and manage the doses independently of the doctor's advice.

I've tried to basically prescribe the medicine for myself, what doses to take, and what to do to prevent from even feeling that way before. I get so frustrated with taking these [meds] all the time. I just totally forget what it was like for a few split moments—what it is like not to have air—and I just say, the hell with it. I can breathe. Soon as I can't, I take it back. I take it back. But basically those are the only times I get attacks. It's hard to face, but basically I bring them upon myself. Every time I've got one [asthma episode], it was my failure to take the medication. I bring it upon myself. No medication, or refuse to puff on the Alupent when I know I should. You know, even if it's maybe the wee bit of shortness of breath, I may just say, "No, I'm not going to do it because I don't want to have to depend on it." So all the times, I bring it upon myself. And, like I said, I'm new. I've had asthma all my life, but never had to have a prescription of medication to tame it. I'm not used to it. I'm new at it. [He had used only over-the-counter medications previously.] (Bill)

Deciding to take medication frequently creates a dialogue about self-reliance and dependency:

What I've found is if I take it sooner into the attack than later, then I can control. My problem in the past is that I would say to myself, "Don't worry about it, don't worry about it, I can deal with it." And I can't get a hold of it, and that's when I usually wind up going to the emergency room and stuff because I don't take any Theophylline. . . . I had a lot of denial going on. My husband said, "Well, I think that you need to go to a doctor," and I would say, "No, no, no, I can take care of it. I can take care of it." Until it got so bad that I turned *dusky* and everything and I had to go to the emergency room. That's when I decided that I had to take care of it right away. (Maya)

As evident in the above interview, the same participant may experience taking medicine as a way to gain control as well as a concession to self-control. This episode of "turning dusky" was pivotal for this person so that she reinterpreted taking medicine and even going to the hospital as a form of control. Now she relinquishes control so that she can regain control more quickly:

PART.: Before losing all my control [she refers to the pivotal episode of having to make frequent emergency room trips because she refused hospitalization] and now getting it back and getting it back more than I ever had it . . . you know, it definitely gave me a lot more confidence. When you have a lot of confidence, it's easier to give some of it up when you can't control it, saying you can't control it all the time. . . . [Referring to the pivotal episode] I don't know if I should say that [that she would be hospitalized if she had it to do over]. I take that back! I don't know

> if I'd be that rational at the time or if I would want to take so much
> control.
> **INT.:** But would you see that as a way of taking control, or is that
> relinquishing?
> **PART.:** A little of both. If I relinquish a little, I would get better a lot faster
> and I would get my control back. . . . I have learned to give up part of
> that control, and that was a very hard thing for me to do. It was very
> hard for me to give up the control of what I can do for myself . . . not
> like a weakness really, but maybe like a combination of weakness and
> an embarrassment. You don't want somebody to know about it. You
> know, I have learned that at least. As time has gone by and I am 5 years
> away from that incident . . . I have gotten better, so I give myself a
> little bit more leeway to take care of myself. . . . I would never let it
> go to the point that I did, and I watch the clock more if I have to take
> the drugs. . . . I don't OD [overdose] myself either. (Maya)

Shame and blame are inherent in the autonomous position of assuming responsibility for the existence and management of the illness while failing to acknowledge the limits of control. When the illness is severe, concessions must be made by seeking treatment and accommodating the illness. But taking medications is not a neutral task for the person who wants complete internal control; it symbolizes an acknowledgment of the illness and its demands:

> All right. I've got to start remembering that I have asthma. . . . I don't like us-
> ing medicine. I don't even use aspirin, not for a headache. Occasionally I'll take a
> vitamin if I think I ate real terrible that day but I don't use a lot of pills and so to
> use anything kind of eats at me. [first Interview] . . . I really wait to see if it's, I'm
> not, if you can tell, I'm not real anxious to use my inhaler. I'd like not to use
> it if I could. Like to not take anything. I'd like to not have asthma. (Elise, a
> 33-year-old married woman who has had asthma for one year)

Delaying treatment (a dangerous problem in asthma) is prompted by expensive, troublesome emergency care (Becker et al., 1993) and by the desire to win the "fight" alone:

> My worst fear is that I don't want to go back to the hospital. I think that's
> what keeps me out too. I am so heavy on not wanting to go there that I'm go-
> ing to try so hard. God forbid that I have any more [asthma episodes]. If I
> have another one, I am going to try until I know I cannot fight it anymore.
> That's why I wait to call a doctor, and I know that's wrong. It gives me a
> chance to prove to myself that I cannot do it or that I can do it. I was going to
> get rid of my machines, and my roommate said, "Don't do that." (Kevin, a 58-
> year-old single Caucasian man who has had asthma for 6 years)

The ideal is for the self to triumph over the body without dependency on machines or medicine. Another participant explains that she wants a cure rather than management through medications:

> **PART.:** The only ideal would be to not have the asthma. The ideal would be to have either a medical or a Western medical alternative treatment that worked, make it go away.
> **INT.:** [reflecting her earlier statements about not wanting to take medications] Yes, and preferably without medications?
> **PART.:** If it was medication, I would prefer that it produced a cure, not a management. (Emma, a 43-year-old married Caucasian woman who has had asthma for 4 years)

It is reasonable for anyone to prefer health to illness, but it is not only the illness at stake in these participants' ideal—it is also the ideal of self-control without medications. This participant's suffering is directly caused by the discomforts, inconvenience, and threat of the symptoms, but it is also a symbolic assault to her sense of autonomy. The problem with the informal model of mind over matter in its extreme form is that the person cannot switch to a place of acknowledging symptoms enough to care for the asthma. This is illustrated in the following excerpt, in which the participant steadfastly refuses to "give in" to her asthma, giving it as little attention or accommodation as possible. She has stated that other people, particularly her family, worry about her more than she worries about herself. The interviewer responds:

> **INT.:** I get that picture of you. You don't really, in your cycle, get concerned about your symptoms?
> **PART.:** No.
> **INT.:** Help me understand that.
> **PART.:** Well, I just—I don't know, I guess I don't worry about it. I just—
> **INT.:** How do you account for that in you? I mean, what is it about your history or who you are that makes you—
> **PART.:** Well, I've never been sick, and I've always thought I could do anything, and I keep going no matter what. And I guess I still—I have a hard time accepting the fact that I can't, that I just have to stop and sometimes I couldn't keep going no matter what. I could hardly take a step. Well, as I say, at this point in my life I look at myself, and I say, look, I've done most of the things I've ever wanted to do, you know, I'm not going sit around and worry about my health. If I have to do that, I'd just as soon be dead. So I'd just as soon go out and do things and if that's the end, that's the end. But I don't want to spend years sitting around thinking I can't do anything.

> **INT.:** Yeah, it seems to me as I hear you talk that you give very little space to it. . . .
> **PART.:** Seems like I'm giving a lot to it, cause I don't like it.
> **INT.:** Yeah, yeah. I mean not willingly.
> **PART.:** Yes, not willingly. (Elva, a 55-year-old married Caucasian woman who has had asthma for 4 years)

She is in an adversarial, oppositional relationship to her body, not accommodating her illness, and sometimes this backfires and her fighting makes her illness worse. She rejects the sick role. She has no middle position of adjusting her activity level or taking care of her illness. Anything less than her accustomed level of activity or complete self-determination feels like a loss of self and freedom and/or at least self-indulgence. She traces her approach to her family patterns around illness:

> **PART.:** Well we were never a family that stayed in bed all day when we were sick. Unless, maybe if you had surgery or something like that, yeah, and you were in the hospital—but otherwise, for just a cold, or flu, we always got up. Got dressed, stayed home, took it easy, took naps, but never babied ourselves by being waited on, staying in bed. (Elva)

With a strong preference for self-control, care of a chronic illness through long-term use of medication is not easily accepted. If "cure" is not possible, one is placed in the ambiguous situation of being controlled by the illness or being controlled or dependent upon the external resource of medication. Clearly cure or self-control of the illness by the mind are preferable. One becomes a therapist, trying to control thoughts and feelings in order to control the body; a physician, adjusting medication, making judgments about the seriousness of one's condition; and finally an active patient participant in recovery and cure, engaging in a never-ending course of rehabilitation. One assumes responsibility for causing the illness and for treating or curing it. Furthermore, one may take excessive responsibility for being the type of person who gets ill. This is illustrated in the interview with a 32-year-old white man who has had asthma since childhood:

> What I think is the bigger problem is that I feel responsible for it. . . . One of the things that I feel responsible for is keeping somewhat physically fit. If I don't go out (and I see this for people who aren't sick, of course), if I don't do my walk today or if I don't do my exercises today, if I don't go swimming today, I'm setting myself up to get ill again. But the fact is that lately I haven't felt well enough to go swimming sometimes, and so I skip it. And then I skip another day, and all of a sudden I'm really feeling like—now you're

really causing your problems. And then I miss a pill, for instance, then I know that it must be something really wrong. I wish I could get a better handle on that. If I don't feel well, I wish I had a way or a therapy in some way in which I could . . . This is obviously my next step. The treatment of asthma has improved so much. I think that even though it has taken me so far my whole life to understand it so that when something happens now, I usually know what to do next.

As soon as my medications stop holding me at a certain level, my sensors are out. Okay, how far am I dropping? How far am I going to allow myself to go? I'm more quickly on the phone now. I am more willing to talk and make judgments. I just have to be open to talking to the doctors, to the pharmacist even. I have to talk to my wife about it. Just trying to get enough information. I'm constantly renewing the information and reminding myself what the situation is so I can make a judgment. [In the past] I just let it take its own course. As far as guilt goes, I wish there was a similar program. I know how to deal with the medications now, but I don't know how to deal with my emotional stress. When I start feeling down a little bit, I don't feel as well. What is a good thing for me to do? . . . It's so bizarre because the medications aren't working, maybe I should start meditating. Or maybe I should do this. I have this little biofeedback instrument. The guy came to the asthma support group and I was his subject and he gave me this little thing. And it really makes a difference. And I feel guilty because I haven't done that in 2 weeks. Maybe I should do that instead of my Theophylline. It would probably work better. And I started thinking that things make no sense. . . . I still question my judgment and the judgment of my physician in the past. I wish I did have the same sort of mechanisms that would kick in and make me know what I should do next. (Everett, a 32-year-old Caucasian married man who has had asthma for 32 years)

In his own words asthma is "like a bad college roommate that I could never adjust to." He vacillates between objective external definitions of the "disease" to subjective definitions that require he manage his emotions and his body.

In summary, the nonacceptance themes reflect an implicit cultural understanding that the individual is responsible for being healthy by controlling the body with the mind and will. This is indirectly linked to the project of developing an autonomous self. It is this autonomous self that is considered to be morally responsible. This cultural expectation of responsibility is heightened when an illness is poorly understood or attributed to psychosomatic causes or assumed to be influenced by feelings.

Learning Acceptance and Self-Care Experientially

In contrast to this oppositional view of self and body, 26 participants described their relation to their illness and body as one of acceptance and care. The acceptance narrative was always described as experientially learned, a change from a control or adversarial narrative. However, acceptance was not described as a polar opposite to self-control or fighting the illness. Rather, it was described as an alternative understanding of responsibility and moral agency and an alternative understanding of the self in relation to the body. Acceptance is not a form of resignation or "giving in" to asthma or "losing the battle," as in the oppositional examples above. Rather, it is considered a positive movement towards coming to terms with living with asthma. The same participant whose interview excerpt introduces the chapter reveals that this "self-talk" begins in childhood:

> I said to myself [as a child] that maybe when I grew older I could, I could find some answer to what was wrong with me, and that it was more important to me to live. In a sense it was a choice of me as a person taking myself as a whole person, a total person, versus how I felt and uh, what was comfortable for me and sometimes perhaps not even what was sensible. And I link that to more to me as a body because my body seemed to be the main limiting factor at that time, and I just wanted to take myself as a whole person. I wanted to make that choice and keep myself as much in the mainstream of life. That was really important to me. . . . (Sara, 47-year-old single Caucasian woman who has had asthma for 30 years)

She describes a lifetime of fighting to be in control, not allowing her illness to determine her choices. She spent some time with sick people and did not like being in a sick group, and this pushed her further to define herself as healthy. Though emotions, feelings, and attitudes may influence asthma, this strong informal model of mind over matter precludes recognizing the multiple determinants of asthma, and variations in responses to treatment and the expectations to control the illness with the mind exceed practical knowledge for intentionally bringing about these changes. The frustration with this untenable project along with its attendant moral emotions of guilt, shame, and blame creates an impetus for forging an alternative self-understanding in relation to the illness. For example, a 35-year-old woman describes her transition toward acceptance:

> **PART.:** I went to a psychologist when I was about 22 or 23, and he related my getting asthma to being an angry teenager, like that's why I got it. [laughter] And so it took me a long time to figure out what a crock of B.S. that was. I mean, certainly my emotional state can affect how comfortable I am physically, but I doubt seriously if it had anything to do with its inception.
>
> **INT.:** Did you buy that for a while?

PART.: I probably did. "I'm an angry person. This is my punishment. This is the reward I get for being unhappy and not helpful and angry." Over the past 4 or 5 years, it's becoming clearer to me that judgment of myself has been an issue in my illness, maybe from a physical standpoint, I don't know, but surely from the psychological standpoint, when I don't accept what's happening to me, I have a more difficult time coping with it. Four years ago, I made choices about flexibility and clothing that were an effort to live with what I had, to not see it as something outside of myself, but something that's part of me that I can be more comfortable with it if I would make my schedule more flexible, buy clothing with elastic, surround myself with people that were willing to make changes and accept my limitations. And then it made it easier for me to accept my limitations as well. So now it is not as big an issue now to be labeled as it used to be. I have the clear definition of what asthma is for me and what I am as an asthmatic, and so it is not as important for me to have to be concerned about how other people see me. (June, a 35-year-old married Caucasian woman who has had asthma for 19 years)

She understands this transition as overcoming her sense of victimization rather than "resigning herself" to asthma. She sees her self-acceptance influenced by the expectations of her friends. She has made an effort to overcome the blame associated with psychological determinism and, in working through the blame, has come to a more accepting position of her self and her body.

PART.: I think I used to feel much more like a victim. I still sometimes feel like a victim. But that's a rare occurrence.

INT.: What do you think gave you the nudge or the insight or whatever to make that transition?

PART.: Well it just seems so corny to say, but it correlates with the time in my life when I began to accept myself more as well, just who I was and that I would find somebody who loved me just for who I was, and I didn't have to do certain things to become lovable. The asthma was like the last frontier, really. I mean, I've accepted so much more about myself before I got around to the asthma. I'm not exactly sure if there is any particular point in time, it just seemed to correlate with the time in my life when I became more accepting of myself.

INT.: For some people that doesn't change, so it is curious as to what makes it occur to someone that—

PART.: Well it is funny because I went to an acupuncturist for a while because I felt like the traditional treatments of medications and allergy injections and stuff. You know, I had no proof for me that they really worked except the inhalers. The acupuncturist said to me, "You really have to stop seeing this as something that attacks you, that you are a victim of something that is not part of you," and then he gave me this little passage from Jung, you know it was dealing with accepting yourself for who you are. I suppose that was sort of the core, beginning to realize that asthma for me was part of who I was. And that like I'd accepted other things about myself, I needed to learn how to fit that into my life in a way that wasn't negative because I think I also began to see my other parts of my life too, that the more negative I was about things, it didn't seem to work for me as well as some of the other ways you could approach life. And since [then] I started making changes. I get angry still about it and feel like a victim still, but it usually happens when I'm right at the low point of having an episode.

INT.: Could you summarize the changes you have made in the way you deal with your asthma over time?

PART.: Well, I'm still doing it. I'm becoming much more comfortable being labeled an "asthmatic" by others around me, and I use my medications in public. And I talk about having asthma and the restrictions that are placed on me, and I go to an asthma support group. Also I think that the people that I've chosen to surround me in my life are actually people that I think asthma has shaped the way that I have relationships as well. I think that I tend to gather around me people who are more tolerant than I might have if I hadn't had asthma, because I require that in my life. (June)

As this participant points out, the coping stance of acceptance is not an invariant, all-or-none position. She can still fall into anger and defeat over the limits of control imposed by the illness. But feeling the shame of victimization is now limited to her most vulnerable periods.

Another participant, a 42-year-old woman, describes her struggle with the ideology of choice rampant in the holistic health movement of the 1970s (see Lowenberg, 1989, for a critique and sociological analysis of this position) and the wellness movement of the 1980s (Brownell, 1991):

PART.: I used to be really defensive because coming to the '70s, it was very hard to have a chronic illness cause it was all in your head, or you could pray it away or psychic it away or something. . . . It was horrible. I cannot tell you how many times I was asked, "What did I do to give myself asthma?" I mean, over and over and over again. It came from health professionals as well as lay people. It was horrible, and at that time I was so confused. I got very defensive, and so I responded defensively. I finally really dropped the idea that asthma was purely psychosomatic caused. I learned that there might be a psychological component to it, but I really dropped the psychosomatic cause idea. . . . I used to deny my symptoms, yeah. Let's just sort of let it happen over there. Just let it go on in the background, but that is not very healing.

It's better for me to stay in my body [laughs] and feel what is going on and deal with it. . . . I began to try to see what might be a psychological component to it. But I really dropped that. I really and in truth, I believe and understood its process of disease process. I learned what it was, how it was, the side effects of medications, and how it might be caused, and finally got an answer. Well, this is one of the few times where doing the right thing got reinforced, because I got better.

INT.: Got better?

PART.: Yeah, but that's not usual. Usually you can do the right things and you still don't get better. So I guess from that standpoint, I mean, I felt good about what I did and it felt really nice to have it reinforced. It was almost a gift. It felt like a gift. You know, I don't know if I learned anything new, other than how nice it was to get reinforced. Yeah. (Susan, a 42-year-old Caucasian married woman who has had asthma for 17 years)

Even though she has increased "control" over her asthma through rigorous Western medical treatment, she experiences this change as a "gift" rather than control. The "gift" language may be seen as a relative contrast to the unrealistic expectations of complete control. Now that she experientially knows the limits of control, efficacious treatment is no longer experienced as a guaranteed contract but as closer to a gift. This is perhaps related to an earlier illness experience that did not respond to treatment readily, because she is describing a time when she was not "reinforced." Her acceptance of the illness relieves her from total responsibility for causing or curing the illness and gives way to the more realistic responsibility of following a reasonable self-care and medical treatment plan. She is freed from the moral burden and guilt associated with unrealistic expectations for controlling an illness that has limits to personal control.

Acceptance, as these participants describe it, means coming to terms with the reality of the illness and its demands for self-care. This "acceptance" is described neither as passive resignation nor as an enthusiastic embracing of the demands of the illness. These participants seem to be drawing on cultural meanings other than the oppositional self-in-relation to the body.

I think with these medications and with exercise and just coming to terms with my asthma, I make it—I try to live my life the best I can you know. It's like, I feel like I have a handicap. (Allison, a 29-year-old single Caucasian woman who has had asthma for 15 years)

The experiential learning required for this acceptance shows that an oppositional self-understanding in relation to illness is more accessible, more "natural" or taken for granted and has to be worked through in order to achieve an alternative relationship to the body and falling ill. This transition occurs over time:

> When I first got asthma I just freaked out. I said, "Oh my God, you can't control it." You know, you feel very defensive and there's not much you can do to control it, so it's very frightening. I would say in the first year of having it and not being able to deal with it. It's very frightening and you feel very defensive. So now I feel much more, I don't know if "confident" is the word to use, but I feel "Okay, I don't have to overreact about this. I'm going to really try and take it easy. I'm going to be fine, and these are the measures I'm going to take." You know, these steps. If I don't get well doing this, then I go to the emergency hospital. I really feel bad for people who, you know, get it and it's really hard to manage. That would be wonderful just having suggestions or guidelines for people to follow. Also, don't feel bad about the way you feel. (Maria, a 26-year-old single Hispanic woman who has had asthma for 3 years)

Accepting the "way you feel" frees her up from feeling defensive and, one can surmise, frees her up to follow suggestions and guidelines. All of the acceptance narratives indicate that absolution from guilt over personally causing the illness and relief from unrealistic expectations about controlling the illness perfectly are salient learning issues.

In the following interview excerpt, another participant describes his illness experience in terms that are neither highly objective (personal experience and feelings are described) nor highly emotionally charged with blame, guilt, anger, resentment, and bitterness. The illness makes unavoidable claims on his life. He responds to these claims in ways that keep the illness as much in the background as possible. He also has other concerns that set limits to his focus on the illness. He says:

> I don't feel anything bad, or negative, or handicapped, or anything like that. It's like having a child, almost. It's a responsibility you have, you take care of it. And if you take care of it, everything works out okay, and if you don't take care of it, then you've got problems. (Tim, a 31-year-old single Caucasian man who has had asthma for 26 years)

The relationship between the person and the asthma shifts so that the illness is not denied and the person attends to the illness. Self-care activities become less emotionally charged when they are no longer symbolically attached to self-recriminations for being ill. This transition is evident in the following account of the strain and effortfulness involved in trying always to act well and transcend one's illness even when ill:

I feel as if I tried. I gave it my best shot, and now it's not in my hands anymore. Now I will go along with the program, whatever it may be. I really gave it my best shot all of my life. I tried as hard as I could and did more. . . . [I] always tried to do as much as I could not to sink into the sense that I can't do this, or don't feel well, or, I don't have the energy. I really didn't have the energy, and I really was limited, and there really were things I couldn't do, but I just pushed myself and did anything that I could do that would make me have more energy, have more of a sense of well-being, be a little bit more clear-headed, be . . . more focused and directed. . . .

Before, I was looking at it from the point of view of, I will it, I will by my will power get well, and now I just feel like, well, I'll try to just take what comes and do my best with it. I don't rule out getting weller or that sort of thing. (Sara, 47-year-old single Caucasian woman who has had asthma for 30 years)

Later in the same interview, in response to reflecting on the interviewer's comment that the culture requires the person to be strong and independent, she states:

It does, but there is another way. There are two ways of dealing with it, and one is the way that I've taken and a lot of people take that way (the self-reliant, independent way), this sort of hardness on the one hand, and on the other hand, there is this sentimentality. So people can go the other way, which is to say, I'm so sick, you can't hurt me because I'm a sick person . . . [said in a whiny, victimized kind of voice]. I do think in other cultures there may be a more realistic attitude towards sickness. Just from little things I've heard, people are allowed to be human. They are allowed. And it's, you know, they are just allowed. [laughter] (Sara)

This patient's discussion depicts the extremes of the Cartesian view of mind over matter. The extremely objective stance is to unrealistically push the object body beyond its limits. The self-reliant stance makes no accommodations to the illness, whereas the subjective extreme is exemplified by engulfment and passivity in relation to the illness. These are polar opposites in the oppositional self-understanding that do not describe the ways the body can be experienced as integral to self, while not being wholly self or wholly other (Merleau-Ponty, 1962; Toombs, 1988).

In the last interview, this same participant talks about personal change toward taking better care of herself and accepting herself and her illness more—not fighting it so much. She states that she realizes from telling her story to the interviewer that she has "fought to be positive and to choose to be well." She now feels that she can take care of her illness without feeling too indulgent, dependent, or passive. Her relationship to others mirrors her relationship to her illness and body. She fears that they, like she, may give her too much help and make her an invalid, or she may disappoint them by not getting well and thus being a "waste of their time." For example, the following conversation was held in relation to not calling the doctor even though her peak flow readings were well below the level at which many people are hospitalized and even though she was feeling very ill.

PART.: I don't know when to call for help, and I don't know, I don't even know what can be done. I have this sense that it's very hard. I have a very powerful mind-set which says that, and that also was a coping thing to get away from blaming other people, or that it's my problem, you know, and I have to live my life. I'm responsible for my own life, ultimately, nobody else is.

INT.: Yeah, and so it means coming to terms with it in a way that getting assistance isn't letting go of your life or something.

PART.: Well, there are lots of things in there, you know. There's not wanting to be a drag; there's the feeling of, I will not, I cannot use other people's resources, wasteful. I will not. And there's the feeling of, there are people far worse off than I am, and I will not take time away from them. And there is always a voice in my head that says, nobody wants to hear your problems. People are going to get tired of you. They're going to think you're a drag or you're boring or you're not really sick. . . . I just always had the sense that it was my problem and I had to deal with it, and nobody really could help me much with it, and also there are other reasons, namely, that I never got well. And so when I've worked with people, medical people or people in the alternative health field, when they first see me, they are enthusiastic and then they discover that I'm not going to get well, and then they get depressed and disturbed and a little hostile, and I don't like that. I don't want to put myself in that position. I don't want to be a neurotic or a failure or whatever it is. So that's one of the things that I do to protect myself because I do not want other people having certain negative feelings about me because those are feelings that I have about myself and I don't want to encourage them. I don't want to feel them. . . . I do feel them, they're always there—Why am I such a terrible person in my very core, I've always been sick and never been well, and no matter what I do, I don't get better. What's wrong with me? And so I don't want, I'm very sensitive to other people's opinions of me and very protective of myself and have a real wall I put around myself. . . . I think my fear has always been that I'm sick because there's something sort of basically corrupt about me, and my mind, my brain, tells me this isn't true, but there is a very kind of primitive part of me that's very afraid, and so I think I've never been able to really understand that it's okay whatever it is, wherever it comes from, it's okay. (Sara)

Her illness experience has shaped her sense of self-worth. Self-acceptance is hard won if one is dependent and incurs intolerable debts by asking for and receiving help. For example, another participant talks about the problem of altering her schedule or planning ahead if she is sick:

> INT.: Yeah, we lead such planned lives, don't we? How easy or difficult is it for you to ask for help when you're ill?
>
> PART.: Well, if I can talk. [laughs] Well, no, I can ask for help. [In an earlier interview she had talked about getting a voice recorder that would request help from the emergency number 911 because she is sometimes so breathless that she has no air for an audible voice.]
>
> INT.: Does it occur to you to ask for help?
>
> PART.: No, I guess not. And I've tended to not like to call the doctor unless I'm really—I'm not the sort of person that goes to the phone and calls the doctor. [inaudible] Maybe I should, but . . . the first sign I keep thinking it will get better or won't be so bad, or I'll call him when I think he's going to be there.
>
> INT.: Yeah. Who's likely to be most helpful to you?
>
> PART.: Hum? Well, no, but other than the doctor I don't think anybody has really helped me.
>
> INT.: Okay. The least helpful?
>
> PART.: Well, I would say people who don't generally understand this disease. Well, I think sometimes you say to people—you know, I couldn't come, or I was late because I had to do this because I was having an asthma attack, sometimes they just sort of look at you like, oh, come off it. What sort of an excuse is that?
>
> INT.: Yeah.
>
> PART.: Which I can understand.
>
> INT.: If you had heart trouble and you said, "I was having angina . . ."?
>
> PART.: People would understand. (Elva, a 55-year-old married woman who has had asthma for 4 years)

This participant echoes other participants' sense that asthma is a stigmatized, low-status illness, not as legitimate as a social excuse for assuming the sick role. If it is all in the mind, one should be able to control it if one wills it strongly enough or has the right attitude. Asthma is not considered the same as a broken leg or angina, both of which are considered "real" diseases, beyond personal control. This is similar to the understanding of responsibility, shame, and blame in the time of Hippocrates (Reiser, 1985; Williams, 1993). Reiser (1985) points out that in early Greek medicine

> One might not, for example, be blamed if illness was the result of uncontrollable forces such as heredity, a factor that was thought to play a role in certain indispositions. . . . But even in some cases of illness produced by

hereditary forces, the possibility for prevention existed. Consider, for instance, the matter of cheese. . . . Those who know this truth [that some bodily constitutions do not tolerate cheese] should be able to forestall the events caused by eating this food. (p. 8)

Early in the Platonic tradition, people were held responsible for causing, treating, and recovering from illness, but then, as now, certain illnesses were more blameworthy than others. In this tradition, illness and culpability are woven into our social relationships. Turning to others is easier if one accepts the self and illness, as illustrated in the following interview excerpt:

PART.: The other thing is, if I'm real wheezy and my husband massages my back, and just really gets me to relax and concentrate on my breathing, so that I don't hyperventilate or, you know, just become tight just from being nervous, that helps a lot. But I think that a lot of the things that I've learned have just come from past experience, and I think that I used to just hyperventilate a lot and just really be tense, so once that I really learned . . . and the other thing is that once I learned that the hard part isn't getting air in, it's getting it out and so I wasn't going [hyperventilates] so much, I was concentrating on slowly breathing the air out so that my lungs were getting smaller so that I could breathe it in. But before I was always going [demonstrates] and I wasn't. . . .

INT.: You learned about that through, primarily, by trial and error?

PART.: No, actually one of the nurses or doctors where I went one time for an attack told me. . . . She said that the hard part wasn't getting it in, it's getting it out. And that's helped a lot! I do the . . . I just do the [demonstrates breathing], and then I can take one in even if. . . . I can always do a long breath out, but even if I can do just short little ones, at least I'm getting something out, and that also makes me feel that also getting oxygen in, so . . . don't panic!

INT.: When you are having an episode of asthma, are people likely to be a help or a hindrance?

PART.: Well, I think that when people hear me wheeze, you know, they worry about me, but I've never had anyone, I don't think, be uncomfortable. I've had people give me strange looks. . . . One time that we had to pull off the highway when I was wheezing was outside of [a major city], and we pulled up to this gas station and they had an outlet in their hallway by the bathroom, so I just plugged it in and started using it and Dan explained something to the attendant, saying, "Oh, my wife has asthma"—he asked if there was anything that he could do. So people's attitudes generally have been pretty good.

INT.: How easy or difficult is it for you to ask for help when you are ill?

PART.: I guess it's like I know in the back of my mind I have to get myself to get help, and if no one else is around I'll ask a neighbor. There was one time when I was having an attack and my car wouldn't start [laughs] . . . just one of those little things that make you panic, and I was thinking, "Oh, shit!" So I kind of knocked on my neighbor's door and go, "Jim! I'm wheezing," and he took me to Hospital X and dropped me off. I know that I need to get help and to get myself there, and I just do it. Just gathering my strength is getting up off of the bed and getting to the phone. (Linda, a 36-year-old married Caucasian woman who has had asthma for 11 years)

She is no longer engaged in fighting or avoiding her asthma and she is open to learning from experience. That she experiences little or no shame or guilt is reflected in her ability to ask for help and her comfort level in publicly disclosing her illness. She is freed to attend to the symptoms without experiencing additional emotional and moral burdens about *having* them..

Interpretive Commentary:
A Phenomenological Perspective

The participants in this study reveal a hidden cultural dialogue about self-reliance, falling ill, dependency, and self-respect. Opening up this hidden dialogue can clarify and liberate people when they fall ill, enabling them to respectfully take care of themselves instead of rejecting the natural contingent vulnerability associated with being embodied and finite. Fatalism, resignation, engulfment, and passivity are enemies of self-respect and self-care. Even a positive acceptance of an illness may cause the person to adapt to a lower level of wellness than necessary. Our proclivity to both excessive dependence and dangerous self-reliance is increased when we hold an either overly objective or overly subjective view of illness and responsibility for health.

The informal belief that asthma is controlled by the mind is, as Rawlinson (1986) suggests, linked to the Western project of creating an autonomous self in charge of one's own ends. This view of autonomy since Kant is inextricably linked to our modern sense of moral agency. For the participants in this study, asthma becomes linked with unconscious or conscious motivations. The limits of control are overlooked, and the person becomes wholly subject, in control of his or her object body. This position is contrasted with a more relational and situated position of acceptance and acknowledgment of the illness as related to self, experience, and the situation. In embracing acceptance or peacemaking with the illness, these participants sought neither to will nor to deny their asthma. Their position seems to be closer to that of the pre-Socratic Greek poets combined with an ethic of care and acceptance.

Their practical moral reasoning about their illness offers an alternative to a Kantian view of responsibility and agency. The early Greeks questioned the limits of reason for creating a good life, as pointed out by Nussbaum (1986):

> For it is their instinct that some projects for self-sufficient living are questionable because they ask us to go beyond the cognitive limits of the human being; and, on the other hand, that many attempts to venture, in metaphysical or scientific reasoning, beyond our human limits are inspired by questionable ethical motives, motives having to do with closedness, safety, and power. Human cognitive limits circumscribe and limit ethical knowledge and discourse; and an important topic *within* ethical discourse must be the determination of an appropriate human attitude towards those limits. (p. 8)

Frustration and suffering are heightened by expectations for control that go beyond the cognitive limits of control. False systems of public and private shame, blame, and guilt are set in motion. Choices made only in the service of self-control preclude the richness of risky human commitments and relationships. As Rawlinson (1986, p. 4) points out: "We are always 'at risk' and subject to loss in precisely those ways in which we are open to and immersed in the world." Nussbaum (1986) and Williams (1993) both point to practical reasoning about necessity, luck, and agency in early Greek thought:

> If an agent ascribes intrinsic value to, and cares about, more than one activity, there is always a risk that some circumstances will arise in which incompatible courses of action are both required; deficiency therefore becomes a natural necessity. The richer my scheme of value [or notions of the good; added comment based on author's footnote], the more I open myself to such a possibility [conflicting goods]; and yet a life designed to ward off this possibility may prove to be impoverished. (Nussbaum, 1986, p. 7)

This stance toward the limits of personal control and reason allows for a discussion of competing goods instead of assuming that choice making and control can always determine one "right" choice (Becker et al., 1993; Benner & Wrubel, 1989). Self-determination is at odds with multiple commitments and being related to others. Addressing the possibilities and limits of control and personal meanings related to taking medications soon after diagnosis can facilitate learning to live with the illness. Assisting persons with articulating unrealistic aspects of autonomy and personal control may enable them to attain more humane self-reliance and interdependence. Feelings can be experienced and worked through without becoming alienated aspects of the self that the self must control—that paradoxical relationship to the self that leads to feeling bad about feeling bad. Expectations for cognitive control of the body through pure intentional thought or will power exceed our knowledge and capacities. We may affect our body through habits, practices, rituals, meditative visualization, turning to others, and all the ways of caring for the body and living in our world, but even the most efficacious of these cannot be considered cognitive control. Furthermore, healing practices and rituals seem to be undermined when they are taken up in a purely instrumental fashion. We may always offer inappropriate blame or praise for the success of well-being and health promotion activities for effecting a cure because we simply do not know how they work when they work. Health and well-being are gifts to the extent that we cannot fully will or control them, and, as one participant stated, successful outcomes from effective medical treatment can also feel like a gift. Schmidt, referring to Luther, has called taking full credit for one's recovery and health "glory theology" (cited in MacIntyre, 1993, p. 15). The logic and possibilities of health and wellbeing promotion practices are radically different from a technical understanding of controlling the object body with the mind. This is a critique of a particular understanding of the mind-body relationship, not an argument against the healing influence of states of mind and body. Nightingale's (1860/1969) notion of putting the body in the best position for healing and recovery is more respectful of the body's own recuperative powers and the finite limits to those powers.

If health care professionals are attuned to the common struggle to maintain a sense of autonomy and the experiential learning required to manage self-care, they will be in a better position to understand the common problem of delaying taking medications and help-seeking. Open discussions about the self-adjustment of medications can increase skill and safety in making these adjustments rather than pretending that doctor's "orders" are followed as given.

The Cartesian view of the body as a possession or resource that the mind controls, directs, manages, makes sick, or heals exceeds the realistic limits of cognitive control and generates a discourse about power and entitlement. The body becomes one more potential that the mind exploits, realizes, and controls (Foucault, 1975). This dualistic position contributes to the swings from an overly subjective to an overly objective understanding of the self in relation to the body and inevitably leads to a moral view of sickness. One becomes "responsible" for one's sickness by "bringing it on the self" or by being too "weak" to control the body with the mind. Responsibility is individualistic with little acknowledgment of environmental, social, economic, or public health issues. Illness becomes a moral burden, and asking for help is done at the expense of one's sense of self-sufficiency. One must not "burden" others with one's illness; one must "take responsibility" for being healthy. This view sets up a high likelihood of "blaming the victim."

The two extremes of "psychological determinism" or complete subjectivity (a private conscious self causing an object body to be ill) on the one hand and a view of disease as a simple mechanical failure (caused by an objective, alien, unrelated germ or biochemical reaction) on the other leave out the alternative perspective exemplified by the participants in this study with acceptance perspectives. Both have their aspects of truth, but neither view allows for a middle ground of situatedness where one's embodied experience is situated in relationship to others in a social and environmental milieu. Persons who have come to terms with caring for their illness and who have experientially learned to accept the inherent limits to control present an alternative moral vision for responsibly caring for one's illness instead of the vision of excessive responsibility of absolute control that leads to paralyzing guilt, shame, and blame.

Like the early Greeks, modern Westerners still have a sense of moral responsibility for staying well and for being self-reliant. This tradition works well if the expectations for self-reliance and prevention are commensurate with realistic possibilities for managing and preventing the illness. But as the Greeks also taught, inherent in each virtue lies the seeds of misuse or vice. Self-reliance works well when the limits of self-reliance are acknowledged. However, unrealistic expectations for cognitive control create blame and shame and govern social relationships involved in seeking and receiving help.

Help seeking and receiving remain closely linked with an oppositional understanding of the relationship between the mind and body. It is not easy to change one's paradigm, and usually the change is uneven. Helping another or receiving help in oppositional individualism (utilitarian individualism) costs the one giving because it is at the self's expense, and receiving help costs because one is made dependent and indebted. These participants point to a cultural alternative to a self and illness acceptance that promotes taking care of oneself while decreasing the moral emotions of guilt, shame, and blame.

Sullivan (1986), in a historical analysis of the similarities and distinctions between Cartesian dualism and the dualism in modern medicine, draws on Foucault's (1975) analysis of the modern clinical gaze of medicine. This gaze stems from the introduction of autopsy to study tissues and organize clinical findings into a coherent disease theory. This approach to pathological anatomy allowed

the eye of the physician to replace the words of the patient as the measure of similarity and difference between diseases. . . . Disease thus begins to be autonomous from patients' experienced sense of disability. An individualized and spatialized disease is a disease that occurs not as much within society as within the body. And it is by means of the dead body that it is found there. Medicine can thus be construed as a purely natural science studying disease, now a purely natural object. . . . Both Descartes and Bichat treat the known body as entirely external to the consciousness which knows it. . . . Knower and known are epistemologically distinguished with the physician assuming the position of knower and the patient/corpse the position of the known. . . . Only a clinical inquiry which anticipates confirmation or disconfirmation at autopsy could find "subjective" evidence of disease deficient. Only at autopsy is it possible to bypass completely the "subjectivity" of the patient. (Sullivan, 1986, pp. 337-345)

The separation of knower from the known, and the relegation of the body as dense *other* rather than as an embodied knower, has health care policy implications. It sets up a discourse of suspicion that fuels an entitlement discourse in relation to disease treatment. "Subjective" is understood as private and idiosyncratic and therefore unknowable by another. Skilled embodied intelligence that may have much in common with others' experiential learning about the illness is overlooked. The physician questions: Is the patient a reliable reporter or observer of his or her body? Do the patient's emotions, character traits, or history distort his or her understanding of what is really going on at the tissue or cellular level? This is mirrored in the patient's own discourse with questions of "How sick am I?" Do the bodily sensations and symptoms warrant attention or care? Or are they merely "in the mind" and not truly in the objective body? If they are truly in the objective body, can the mind overcome them? If they are in the object body, where has the executive managing mind gone wrong? Is such a defective mind (a) not accurately perceiving the disease and/or (b) causing the disease through lack of executive self-control and self-management? Suspicion and doubt about the ability of the knower to know his or her own body, accompanied by the pervasive moral directives for the mind-self to control the body as other and thus to be "independent" of others' care of the body, fuel an expensive and nonhealing discourse about only "real" disease, namely, that which is documented at the cellular or organ level, being worthy of and entitled to treatment. Anything that cannot be so objectively determined must be "all in the mind" or caused "by the mind" and thus be a moral weakness or defect rather than a legitimate disease. The suspicion and the entitlement discourse are rampant in the clinic, health care bureaucracies, insurance companies, and an individual's mind as he or she evaluates symptoms, trying to decide if they are "worthy" of treatment, that is, if they are substantial evidence of "real" disease.

The entitlement discourse is further fueled by treating health care as both a right and a commodity in a free market. Because it is a right, the boundaries of the right have to be equal and administration of the right must be fair and just. Because it is a commodity judged in purely economic terms, the buyer is offered an array of goods and services to be bought and sold. Both set up public debates about individual responsibility for health that may exceed the individual's capacity. The ethics of rights and justice are not sufficient to address and shape our health care according to our notions of what constitutes a good life and what social policies foster good health.

References

Becker, G., Janson-Bjerklie, S., Benner, P., Slobin, K., & Ferketich, S. (1993). The dilemma of seeking urgent care: Asthma episodes and emergency service use. *Social Science and Medicine, 37,* 305-313.

Benner, P. (1984). *From novice to expert: Excellence and power in clinical nursing practice.* Reading, MA: Addison-Wesley.

Benner, P., Roskies, E., & Lazarus, R. S. (1981). Stress and coping under extreme conditions. In J. E. Dimsdale (Ed.), *Survivors, victims, and perpetrators: Essays on the Nazi Holocaust* (pp. 219-258). Washington, DC: Hemisphere.

Benner, P., & Wrubel, J. (1989). *The primacy of caring: Stress and coping in health and illness.* Reading, MA: Addison-Wesley.

Brownell, K. D. (1991). Personal responsibility and control over our bodies: When expectation exceeds reality. *Health Psychology, 10*(5), 303-310.

Crawford, R. (1984). A cultural account of health: Control, release and the social body. In J. B. McKinlay (Ed.), *Contemporary issues in health, medicine, and social policy* (pp. 60-103). New York: Tavistock.

Dreyfus, H. L. (1979). *What computers can't do: The limits of artificial intelligence* (rev. ed.). New York: Harper & Row.

Dreyfus, H. L. (1991a). *Being-in-the-world: A commentary on Heidegger's "Being and time," Division I.* Cambridge: MIT Press.

Dreyfus, H. L. (1991b). Heidegger's hermeneutic realism. In D. R. Hiley, J. F. Bohman, & R. Shusterman (Eds.), *The interpretive turn* (pp. 25-41). Ithaca, NY: Cornell University Press.

Dreyfus, H. L., & Dreyfus, S. E., with Athanasiou, T. (1986). *Mind over machine: The power of human intuition and expertise in the era of the computer.* New York: Free Press.

Foucault, M. (1975). *The birth of the clinic* (A. Sheridan, Trans.). New York: Vintage.

Frank, A. W. (1991). *At the will of the body: Reflecting on illness.* Boston: Houghton Mifflin.

Fritz, G. K., Rubinstein, S., & Lewiston, N.J. (1987). Psychological factors in fatal childhood asthma. *American Journal of Orthopsychiatry, 57,* 253-257.

Harris, P. R. (1981). *Health United States 1980* (USDHHS Publication No. PHS 811232). Washington, DC: U.S. Government Printing Office.

Heidegger, M. (1962). *Being and time* (J. Macquarrie & E. Robinson, Trans.). New York: Harper & Row. (Original work published 1927)

Heidegger, M. (1975). *The basic problems of phenomenology* (A. Hofstadter, Trans.). Bloomington: University of Indiana Press.

Janson-Bjerklie, S., Ferketich, S., & Benner, P. (1993). Predicting the outcomes of living with asthma. *Research in Nursing and Health, 16,* 241-250.

Janson-Bjerklie, S., Ferketich, S., Benner, P., & Becker, G. (1992). Clinical markers of asthma severity and risk: Importance of subjective as well as objective factors. *Heart and Lung, 21*(3), 265-272.

Janson-Bjerklie S., Ruma, S., Stulbarg, D., & Carrieri, V. (1987). Predictors of dyspnea intensity in asthma. *Nursing Research, 36,* 179-183.

Jones, N. F., Kinsman, R. A., Dirks, J. F., & Dahlem, N. W. (1987). Psychological contributions to chronicity in asthma: Patient styles influencing medical treatment and its outcome. *Medical Care, 17,* 1103-1118.

Kierkegaard, S. J. (1985). *Fear and trembling* (A. Hannay, Trans.). New York: Penguin. (Original work published 1843)

Lazarus, R. S., & Folkman, S. (1984). *Stress, appraisal, and coping.* New York: Springer.

Lowenberg, J. (1989). *Caring and responsibility.* Philadelphia: University of Pennsylvania Press.

MacIntyre, R. (1993). Sex, drugs, and T-cells: Symbolic meanings among gay men with asymptomatic HIV infection. Unpublished doctoral dissertation, University of California, San Francisco.

Merleau-Ponty, M. (1962). *Phenomenology of perception* (C. Smith, Trans.). London: Routledge & Kegan Paul.

Nightingale, F. (1969). *Notes on nursing: What it is, and what it is not.* Philadelphia: J. B. Lippincott. (Original work published 1860)

Nussbaum, M. (1986). *The fragility of goodness: Luck and ethics in Greek tragedy and philosophy.* Cambridge, UK: Cambridge University Press.

Rawlinson, M. C. (1986). The sense of suffering. *Journal of Medicine and Philosophy, 11,* 39-62.

Reiser, S. J. (1985). Responsibility for personal health: A historical perspective. *Journal of Medicine and Philosophy, 10,* 7-17.

Schaefer, C. (1983). *The role of stress and coping in the occurrence of serious illness.* Unpublished doctoral dissertation, University of California, Berkeley.

Sullivan, W. M. (1986). In what sense is contemporary medicine dualistic? *Culture, Medicine and Psychiatry, 10,* 331-350.

Taylor, C. (1985). *Philosophical papers* (Vols. 1 & 2). Cambridge, UK: University of Cambridge Press.

Taylor, C. (1989). *Sources of the self.* Cambridge, MA: Harvard University Press.

Taylor, S. E., & Brown, J. D. (1988). Illusion and well-being: A social psychological perspective on mental health. *Psychological Bulletin, 103,* 193-210.

Toombs, S. K. (1988). Illness and the paradigm of lived body. *Theoretical Medicine, 9,* 201-226.

Weinstein, N. D. (1982). Unrealistic optimism about susceptibility and health problems. *Journal of Behavioral Medicine, 5,* 441-460.

Williams, B. (1993). *Necessity and luck.* Berkeley: University of California Press.

Wrubel, J. W. (1985). *Personal meanings and coping processes: A hermeneutical study of personal background meanings and interpersonal concerns and their relation to stress appraisals and coping.* Unpublished doctoral dissertation, University of California, San Francisco.

13

❖

The Ethical Context of
Nursing Care of Dying Patients
in Critical Care

PEGGY L. WROS

M any patients die in critical care units, and nurses provide care to dying patients and their families in that setting. Given that the ICU has unique characteristics, including its goals, environment, and work structure, it would be premature to assume that nursing practice in caring for dying patients in critical care is the same as nursing care for dying patients in other settings. This phenomenological study was designed to describe nursing care of dying patients and their families in critical care. An understanding of the moral aspects of nursing practice evolved from the data, giving dimension and meaning to the bedside practices of nurses described and observed during the exploration of this domain of practice.

The Ethics of Everyday Practice

Critical care nurses are constantly faced with multifaceted ethical responsibilities when confronted with human needs and wants in the complex critical care environment (Pierce, 1989). Patients, families, and health care professionals too frequently find themselves caught in moral dilemmas, in which there are conflicting opinions of right and wrong. Advocates of the traditional, rational approach to ethical decision making indicate that ethical situations should be approached using formal reasoning in an attempt to arrive at the ideal solution. Within this model, decisions are based on identified ethical principles such as autonomy, beneficence, nonmaleficence, and justice (Krekeler, 1987). However, the "correct" solution could vary according to the principle cited. For example, Weir (1989) describes a continuum of principle-based positions from extreme "pro-life" options, in which abatement of life-sustaining treatment is never justified, to extreme "right-to-life" options, which allow intentional killing as a moral and legal alternative. Critical care nurses have been encouraged to become more educated regarding formal, theory-based resolution of ethical issues in order to participate in informed, logical, and consistent decisions in the clinical setting (Catalano, 1991). Although it can be argued that people's behaviors are based on some underlying ethical stance, an alternate perspective seems more compatible with the phenomenological tradition.

More central to this study than ethical positions is the moral notion of the good described by MacIntyre (1984). In his critique of the salient charac-teristics of contemporary moral disagreement, rival arguments are concep-tually incommensurable (the arguments cannot be weighed against each other; all arguments are logically valid), paradoxically emphasize rational decision making, and are based on decontextualized concepts that have changed in meaning over time.

MacIntyre (1984) makes two additional relevant contentions about morality. First, he asserts that "the narrative in which human life is embodied has a form in which the subject . . . is set in a task, in the completion of which lies their peculiar appropriation of the human good" (p. 175). Morality is revealed through narrative describing human action embedded in culture rather than rational examination. Second, MacIntyre views morality in practice as follows:

> What is distinctive in a practice is in part the way in which conception of the relevant goods and end which the technical skills serve . . . are transformed and enriched by these extensions of human powers and by that regard for its own internal goods which are partially definitive of each particular practice or type of practice. (1984, p. 193)

An individual's search for good is conducted within a professional and personal tradition. In this interpretation, the notion of the good inherent in a profession is embodied in excellent practice (MacIntyre, 1984).

Bishop and Scudder (1990) have incorporated MacIntyre's conception of morality into a description of the ethics of nursing practice. They believe that sound nursing practice has an integral moral sense that fosters the good of the patient by excellent nursing care. Nursing is primarily concerned with bringing about its inherent good in the world, not by applying science and technology but by the practice of caring. Because a practice is founded on the good it is designed to achieve and makes no sense apart from it, nurses "become aware of the moral sense of their practice only when it is replaced or challenged by goals other than the good that health care is designed to achieve" (Bishop & Scudder, 1990, p. 33). Because nursing is a practice with an inherent moral sense, much of nursing ethics is integrated into everyday practice and comportment and is not labeled as moral decision making.

The current study searched to understand the notions of good underlying caring practices seen in excellent nursing care. These moral aspects, though difficult to articulate, were revealed in skilled behaviors and reflected the notions of good inherent in the personal and professional beings of nurses practicing within the culture of critical care units.

Description of the Study

The purpose of this phenomenological study was to describe and understand nursing care of dying patients and their families in critical care units. The specific study questions were:

1. What are specific caring practices of expert nurses caring for dying patients and their families in critical care?
2. What are the interpersonal concerns and background meanings that shape expert nurses' caring for dying patients in critical care, including moral beliefs and issues?
3. What are the interpersonal concerns and background meanings of bereaved family members related to nursing care during the time the patient is dying in critical care?

The key study informants were 15 critical care nurses from five critical care units in two hospitals with experience and expertise in nursing care of dying patients and their families. These key informants were nominated by nurse managers for participation in the study. The study was carried out in four phases. In phase I, key informants were interviewed in groups about their experiences in caring for dying patients and their families in critical care. In phase II, key informants were observed in clinical practice as they cared for dying patients and their families. Eight observations were completed. An additional six nurses participated as secondary informants and were observed during this phase. In phase III, the nurses who were observed in phase II were interviewed about the particular episode observed as well as about their personal beliefs and values related to nursing care of dying patients in critical care. In phase IV, bereaved family members of patients who died in critical care were interviewed. The family members were recruited during observations and from phase I group interview data. Eight bereaved family members were interviewed.

All interviews were taped and transcribed verbatim. Field notes were kept during observations and supplemented by taped commentary and a personal journal kept by the researcher. Data were analyzed using interpretive analysis, or hermeneutics. This analytic process incorporated the following overlapping strategies: reflective interpretation of data, identification of major themes, coding and retrieval of data according to an interpretive plan, and reflective writing based on paradigm cases and exemplars explicating the major themes and issues.

Moral Aspects of Nursing Care of Dying Patients in Critical Care

The data contained many narratives describing practices and concerns socially embedded in the moral culture of nursing and specifically related to caring for the dying patient. In an effort to capture the complexity of the moral tradition shaping nursing practice, a paradigm case that summarizes many of the meanings, concerns, and issues is presented and followed by an interpretive analysis. Supportive exemplars are added to further illustrate and expand understanding of the moral aspects of this domain of nursing practice.

Paradigm Case: "Do No Harm"

This account describes the group practice of several nurses caring for Sharon, a young woman dying of complications of cancer treatment. After many months in and out of hospitals, the patient was hospitalized in the critical care unit for several weeks. She was on a ventilator, receiving kidney dialysis, and desperately ill. The patient's husband, Mark, who was a health care professional, was very involved in the supervision of medical and nursing care. This was not usually allowed and initially caused controversy among staff. However, as the hospitalization stretched on, a core group of nurses assumed the care of the Sharon and her husband. Several of them were involved in the storytelling.

> **N1:** After about 2 weeks, I was drawn into their stream of things.
> **N2:** And I found it really rewarding and interesting and a major challenge to take care of her.
> **N1:** And him.

N3: Well, you get so invested. It seemed for me I got so invested in it that I, even on my days off, I mean it was all I thought about. And part of it was because there were particulars about it that once you got involved with it and knew, it was easier to do because you knew him, you knew her, you knew the situation.

The nurses described the type of care that was required as they came to know and understand the particulars of the patient and the family.

N3: I took care of her from the time she was first admitted. And before she was intubated, we did talk. She had this very soft sweet voice and she would say my name. And she was a real people person. She knew your name, knew who you were, wanted to know about you and she connected with you right away. And so every time I'd see her before she was intubated, she remembered who I was and when I'd come into the room she'd say my name. She'd say, "Shelley, I'm so tired, I'm just so tired. I've been through so much, you know." She'd talk but it would tire her to talk. She didn't talk a whole lot. And then after she was intubated, she would write notes up to a point and she liked just little comfort things. At first she wasn't a real touchy feely person but toward the end she was much more. Wanted to hold your hand. Sometimes she was just scared and I'd say, "Are you scared?" Just wanted to hold your hand, wanted to hug you, wanted to touch you.

N1: She was constantly reaching up for your hair and holding it up to your face, and she didn't want to be alone. She needed somebody to touch.

N3: And in that way I almost thought of her as a child in certain ways. Because she was very small and petite anyway. And then that need, you just knew that she needed that comfort and reassurance. [She and her husband] weren't very demonstrative at all. At the end they were more so. But at first they weren't, and you'd kind of want to fill in the gaps, so to speak. And so that's how I got connected with her right from the beginning in speaking with her and knowing that every time I came in the room she always said my name. . . . And sometimes you could not comfort her. She would be almost psychotic. She'd be desperate, frantic and fighting for every breath and wasting so much energy that she'd make herself worse. And I could never turn my back on her. I could never just walk out of the room and turn my back on her and leave.

N2: I always tried to figure out how to tell her that I really cared. Like little things like she couldn't stand certain TV shows. And she couldn't stand rock and roll. . . . And every morning I'd come in and there'd be this rock and roll station on. So finally I put up this little sign that said, "Classical only." And little things like that. Just trying to help make it as pleasant as we could.

N3: We spent one afternoon, I swear, an hour. She loved cooking shows. Trying to get her so she could see that dang TV. Well it wasn't just quite right and her glasses weren't quite right and then her position today wasn't quite right, and I thought, you know, for who else would I spend this much time trying to get the dang cooking show. But those little things were so important to her to be able to have that piece of her day. And when we got her all situated, it was probably at least three quarters through the show and she could really see it. Well, then she fell asleep. But she was happy. She got to get in the right position. Thank God she's asleep!

The nurses also described how they learned about Mark, the patient's husband, and integrated his needs and concerns into their care while still tending to the patient. For example, the nurses were very concerned for the patient's comfort and wanted to use drugs for pain management. Later interviews with the patient's husband, however, showed he believed that medications might have been overused and preferred that they would have used other strategies such as holding her hand or distracting her with television or radio.

> **N3:** Little things, like he didn't want her to have Inapsine, didn't want her to have any allopurinol or any of that stuff because she had reactions to it. And other doctors would say, "Oh, she didn't have that bad a reaction. Oh she really didn't have that." Well, but you know it got to the point of why fight with him about it? There's other things that we could use, that we could try. He'd even find stuff. He wanted her on Serentil, not on Haldol. And really when it came right down to it, it's that tug-of-war, that control issue, but it really shouldn't be that. What it came right down to, it was just as fine for her to get the other drug. And he wasn't wrong, you know. And once she did get Inapsine, that did have a strange lasting effect.
>
> **N2:** I had a hard time because I would, I perceived that she was in a lot of pain at times. And one day I'll never forget, her husband just said, "Pain isn't an issue."
>
> **N3:** He was always afraid of her being addicted to anything.
>
> **N1:** And he did not want her to be knocked out by it. He didn't like that. Because then she couldn't be her.

The nurses understood that, from Mark's perspective, a certain amount of pain was acceptable, and preferable to loss of his wife's ability to respond. They came to understand and learn to deal with Mark's needs as well as Sharon's.

As the nurses became more certain that Sharon was going to die, they also became more fearful of what the death event could be. They described their approach to decision making.

N3: We made the physicians have care conferences every couple of weeks because they didn't want to talk about it. They didn't want to deal with it. Anyway, her oncologist is kind of an optimistic kind of guy. He kept saying that there is this 1 percent chance that she could survive. But her husband would hear that 1 percent and he couldn't withdraw. He couldn't stop things. So in care conferences we would spend a lot of time dealing with the what-ifs. And the biggest what-if that scared everybody was what if she coded and what if her husband was there. She was so tiny and frail.

N1: Are we going to break her ribs, are we going to pounce on her like we normally would do?

N2: It's the ethical dilemma that I had. I kept thinking, I don't want to hurt her, and if her heart stops I don't want to push on her chest and crack a rib. And I cannot ethically do this. And I couldn't sleep for a couple of nights until we finally had a care conference and made her "no chest compressions," because I didn't feel I could do it.

One nurse further explained the process involved in making this decision, which occurred about a month before the patient died.

N2: I finally contacted the ethics committee and talked [to one particular member] about this particular case. He really helped me get things more systematic. He helped me figure out what was causing my distress. And I was able to focus on what was causing my stress, and it was fear of harm. And this is an ethical principle, and I hadn't really had the time or the knowledge to figure this all out. In that I didn't know what was bothering me, but something was bothering me really bad and I didn't know what to do about it. And he helped me get it down to fear of harm and what it is that we can do about that. There was a conference the next day or two, and I brought up the ethical situation of the fear of harm and how I arrived at it, and that's when we made the first "Do not do chest compressions." And I felt this major relief, albeit temporary, that I wasn't going to have to pounce on her. And then after a few days of that and she's still lingering, then the stress kind of built up again because I was fearing, I didn't want to shock her even and then the fact that we kept having these little talks every week. Then I would have something to focus on.

As the patient continued to decline, it became emotionally more difficult for the nurses to continue to care for her.

N2: And you know, one thing that sort of kept me going with her too, since I didn't know her [before she was ill], was that I heard what a feisty gal she was. I had a hard time with my own feelings because I would think, "Well now, if I was her I would want people to just let me go," but then I'd think, "Well now, wait a second. She was her own person. She's been married for so many years, and it's not my choice or my decision on what's going to be done. So I'm going to take the role of what can I do to make the situation as good as it can be." Because I'm not in charge of the decisions other than it's important for me to communicate what's happening and what I've seen. But that kept me going too. . . .

Int.: So she wanted to keep going too?

N3: We had to believe that of her husband and also her attending that everybody communicated that was always her wish. Cause when it got to the point where she really couldn't communicate with us anymore, you didn't know how much she could understand, and I had to keep remembering that too. Because it came to a point where if this were me . . . and I thought that every day. If this were me I would not want this, for me to live like this.

In the end, the nurses believed that the patient had died with dignity and that her care was the best they had ever given.

N2: When she finally died she did surprise me. I mean I knew for weeks that she was going to die, but it was like when they finally die you can't believe it's really happened. She went asystolic. Her husband and I were shooting the breeze about something. And he said, "Oh no." And it was quiet. It was so quiet. The doctors they came in. We just all came in and we just . . . it was not violent. We did drugs, atropine, but she had just died. And Mark was just standing there and he didn't raise his voice. He just said, "Is this everything? Is there anything else that we can do?"

N1: He stood back in the anteroom and just took his glasses down on his nose and he just looked.

N2: And the doctor just said, "No." And that was it. It was very peaceful.

The nurses went to the patient's funeral, and described their personal grief after she died.

This paradigm case was similar to many other situations described by nurses in the study in that Sharon was desperately ill and unconscious for much of her stay in critical care. She was connected to a multitude of technological supports. Mark's vigilance in supervising her medical care was an extreme case of "standing guard," which occurred with other families studied. His protectiveness could be understood as a response to her vulnerability, their experiences with medical care prior to this hospitalization, the nature of their relationship, and his background as a health care professional. This particular situation was different from some of the other cases described because of the length of time Sharon was a patient in critical care and the degree of involvement of the core group of nurses. The situation was very powerful for these nurses, perhaps in part because the patient was herself a young health care professional.

This situation incorporated recurring themes found in many of the stories told by the participating nurses. The interpretive analysis of this paradigm case includes a description of (a) characteristics of an ethic of care, (b) the role of judicial ethics in decision making, and (c) specific moral concerns expressed by nurses.

Ethic of Care

The values embedded in this paradigm case are centered on caring and relationship. The discourse was characterized by its subjectivity, flexibility, and contextuality. Words describing the care include *invested, involved, connected, cared, needs,* and *particulars.* The focus of the story was relief of suffering and maintaining dignity.

The relationship described between Sharon and the nurses was one of interdependence and reciprocity, in which the patient, when able, was involved in sharing personal experiences. Sharon knew the nurse by name and wanted to know about her as a person. A similar kind of relationship evolved with the patient's husband, Mark, for whom the nurses developed understanding and compassion. Respect for relationship was shown by valuing and preserving the history and essence of the marital relationship, for example, by facilitating his involvement in her care and respecting their ways of interacting. The nurses were able to describe particular characteristics and needs of Sharon and Mark on which the moral context of caring turned, for example, her need for touch and his need for his wife's unsedated presence. The empathy that the nurses felt for the patient generated the moral distress they felt for the patient's suffering, which they worked to minimize through careful attention to detail and continuity. However, even in their involvement, the nurses maintained an understanding that this was not their struggle. Gadow (1980) describes this relationship as "fellow feeling," in which the nurses participate in the patient's suffering, but do not suffer themselves. This distinction in focus between fellow feeling and emotional identification is important in preventing nurses from overidentifying and confusing their needs with the patient's, which can contribute to emotional depletion.

The theme of relationship was further played out in the ongoing discussion of issues between physicians and nurses. The nurses insisted on regular conferences. The process of maintaining a dialogue and sharing perspectives was seen as vitally important in the quest toward a positive outcome. The nurses acknowledged that their role was not as a decision maker but as a communicator, and they struggled to maintain open communication. However, much of the communication seemed one-way, and the nurses did not always feel supported by physicians as they sought answers to the difficult questions. Rather, they trod thoughtfully—for example, asking for advice from an ethics committee member regarding how to approach resuscitation questions. During the patient's 3-month illness, working relationships between nurses and physicians, family and physicians, and nurses and family were maintained as each approached concerns from his or her own perspective.

The moral agency of the nurses was heard in interpreting and particularizing the moral choices surrounding end-of-life issues. Although they did not see themselves as responsible for decisions, their issues and communications were the focus of regular team conferences at which decisions were made. For example, the nurses did not take a stand on discontinuing Sharon's life support but asked the questions that shaped the resolution of how she would die. In this and other situations described in the study, the nurses explored patient/family values and wishes and sought to understand the plan of care from the viewpoint of the physician. They introduced moral concerns based on involvement in the situation and assumed an active role in communicating, coordinating, interpreting, and translating between the patient/ family and the physicians. This role was based on the spirit of caring and advocacy and went beyond aspects of the "in-between" position described by Bishop and Scudder (1987, 1990), in which nurses skillfully facilitate communal decisions while representing the interests of patients, physicians, and the organization. Although cooperative decision making was recognized as the best situation, it was not always possible in the clinical context. Rather than equally representing the patient, physician, and hospital, the nurses relied on their knowledge of the system and medical practice to clarify and facilitate the needs and wishes of the patient/family.

The nurses' involvement and relationship with Sharon and Mark informed the nurses' moral struggle surrounding continuation of life support. Despite their own concerns about the appropriateness of continuing, they trusted Mark's interpretation of Sharon's will to live and understood that he could not discontinue medical treatment. The moral essence of this young couple shaped their continued fight for Sharon's survival. Suffering was not primary, and there was a willingness to endure suffering for life. Consistent with Mark's courage to fight, the notion of hastening death by discontinuing life support (or choosing to die) was inconceivable for him. The nature and character of this practical moral stance that a person should fight to live is qualitatively different from death avoidance or denial, which implies an inability or unwillingness to face death.

Based on this understanding of the lived experience of this particular family, the nurses' concerns focused not on whether to withdraw life support but on to how to create a peaceful death within the circumstances by anticipating the "what-ifs." Mark and the physician did not withdraw treatment or life support, but they did agree that there would be no aggressive measures administered at her death. Other potential issues of control were subjugated to concerns related to relationship and suffering, for example, regarding pain management. Although the nurses had conflicting views with Mark concerning the patient's pain, they were able to understand his concerns for his wife's mental and physiological responses to sedation. They worked with him toward a compromise, using drugs that he suggested and incorporating strategies besides sedation to control her discomfort when possible.

The primary moral concern in this narrative was the patient as herself, as opposed to ethical principle. The driving force behind her care was not patient rights and autonomy, as seen in other narratives and described by Gadow (1980) as the basis for advocacy. Sharon's personal wishes regarding continuation of treatment were really unknown. Her husband and primary physician said that although typically she would initially refuse some procedures, she would consent with encouragement. In the absence of specific knowledge of the patient's view, the nurses' understanding of the patient's notion of the boundary between harm and benefit was assumed through embodied knowing grounded in relationship (Gadow, 1989). Her suffering was understood through her bodily responses, particularly later in her illness when she was unresponsive. They struggled with a concern that they might have gone too far by continuing treatment, but despite this discomfort, the patient was not abandoned. One nurse talked about not being able to turn her back on the patient when she was in need of comfort. The concern was with her ongoing suffering and her dignity. Morale was dependent on the ability of the nurses to provide this care. Even in the context of unresponsiveness and high technology, the patient was not dehumanized. Instead, the effort at playing her favorite music and tuning in her favorite television show reflected the particularities of the patient's life. These practices support the notion that care is needed to temper the technology (Cooper, 1991). Gadow (1990) goes even further in her assertion that efforts at cure without care are immoral.

The care was contextual not only in that it was responsive to the particular needs of the patient and husband but in that the rules and norms of the unit were, in some sense, irrelevant and cast aside. In the most obvious example, Mark was permitted and even supported in supervising medical and nursing treatment for his wife. The demands of the situation drove the action, rather than rigid and external expectations.

In the final analysis, the nurses were satisfied with the care they had given. Beyond giving good physical care, they were responsive to the particular demands of the situation. Relationships were maintained, and the patient died without having to undergo additional suffering that would have resulted from resuscitation attempts. This expression of satisfaction supports conclusions drawn in a study by Condon (1988) that when nurses felt that they had been caring, they felt fulfilled and self-actualized, having achieved the moral ideal.

Role of Principle-Oriented Ethics

As in the larger data set, this narrative focused primarily on the clinical ethic of care but also incorporated some reference to abstract moral principles. This tradition, as understood in contemporary philosophy, "is built on a model in which reliance upon rules and principles is primary in moral action and justification. Moral choice involves a consideration of competing principles" (Cooper, 1991, p. 23). Contrary to values arising from an ethic of care, which describe involvement and relationship, values underlying the principle-oriented model arise from detached principles, rules, and rights.

In one section of the narrative, a nurse described her fear of hurting the patient, who was frail and depleted, by using aggressive resuscitation measures. Her feelings motivated her to contact a member of the ethics committee, who helped her to translate her emotional turmoil into the language of principled ethics. She invoked the principle of nonmaleficence, or "do no harm." Using this language, she was able to approach physicians at a care conference and exercise the principle to support her case not to do chest massage if the patient should have a cardiopulmonary arrest. At a later date she used the same strategy to prevent defibrillation. It is notable that even the language in the nurse's description of the situation changed as she switched perspectives from a feeling to a cognitive approach to her concern. In discussing her actions after the ethics consultation, the words that the nurse used to describe the situation changed from caring/relational language to rational language. Words such as *dilemma, systematic, principle,* and *knowledge* showed up in the narrative. Gilligan (1982) contends that it is impossible to see both moral perspectives at one time; "instead, a shift in orientation denotes a restructuring of moral perception, changing the meaning of moral language and thus the definition of moral conflict and moral action" (Cooper, 1989, p. 12).

This interplay of contrasting approaches to ethics is interesting in that although both played a role in the final outcome, formal ethics language was deliberately used to communicate to physicians in this situation where the stakes were high. Although the physicians may have in fact responded to the naive expression of the nurse's fear of causing additional pain and suffering to this woman who had already gone through so much, the use of formal principles may have been a more powerful tool when confronting the issue within the medical paradigm.

The appearance of both types of ethics in this narrative can be interpreted in different ways. Davis (1986) contends that medicine and nursing arise from different ethical/philosophical convictions. Medicine, along with other health care professions, is concerned with specific and circumscribed needs of patients. On the other hand, nurses view patients in their wholeness, in their integrity as persons. As such, the two professions should adopt different forms of ethical thinking: relational ethics for nurses and rights-based ethics for physicians. Davis, however, does not discuss whether these approaches are mutually exclusive.

Cooper (1990, 1991) asserts that nurses use both, primarily relying on ethical rules and principles initially in their care of a patient. As the nurse becomes more involved with the patient and the particularities of the patient's experience, the moral perspective broadens and tension develops between the abstractions and the caring response to the situation. Callahan (1988) describes the need for both emotion and cognition, as human traits selected through evolution, in comprehensive ethical decision making. In fact, often the emotional experience is primary, in that it brings the issue forward for consideration, energizes the quest, and motivates perseverance in finding the right answer. In the paradigm narrative, the nurse's feelings stimulated discussion of the nonmaleficence issue. Her continued discomfort ensured subsequent discussion until all the "what-if" questions were answered. As such, the ethic of caring, represented by nurses, and the principle-oriented ethic, represented by medicine, are equally important in clinical ethics.

Skilled Ethical Comportment

Dreyfus, Dreyfus, and Benner (1990) offer an alternative explanation for the interface between caring and principle-oriented ethics that is based on their model of the development of expertise. Their understanding is focused on a phenomenological perception of ethics that is concerned with what is good as opposed to what is right. In this conception, ethical theories and judgments are dependent on expertise in everyday skillful ethical comportment, which is defined as "embodied, skilled know-how of relating to others in ways that are respectful and support their concerns" (Benner, 1991, p. 2). The novice nurse comes into a situation with some ethical and relational skills as a result of growing up in a shared culture. Skills of involvement and connection are modified and extended through clinical practice and ethical theory to meet the demands of nursing. In the novice stage the nurse relies primarily on rule-governed behavior—for example, following guidelines offered by theories on therapeutic relationships. As nurses gain experience, they gradually compile a background of clinical situations in which the rules for interacting as a nurse with patients are grounded in experience. Some situations may particularly stand out because the nurse feels better or worse (Benner, 1991). The practitioner experiences directly what "the good" feels like and looks like over the course of many situations. One nurse described a situation early in her career in which she learned about involvement:

> I remember once when a 15-year-old was dying of leukemia that I was really uncomfortable taking care of her. And I avoided it, took care of all her physical things, I kept everything taken care of, but there was more lacking. You know, she confronted me. I was blown out of the water. I didn't know what to respond. And finally I realized what was going on was that she was younger than me and dealing with the ultimate. [When she confronted me] I broke down, as I am right now [crying]. She was able to understand and she allowed me the space that I needed. But by the same token I was more able to be there for her later because of it.

This nurse learned about the moral value and obligation of connectedness through the challenge given to her by her young patient. Through her own feelings of shame and discomfort at not being present with her patient, she learned to respond to the moral demands of each situation. This patient needed her, and she was later able to respond based on her new understanding.

The skilled ethical comportment of the expert nurse incorporates many of these background situations, and the nurse develops an ability to respond immediately to the demands of the particular situation. Acting ethically in a situation is automatic and nonreflective. The following narrative is the account of a nurse responding to the needs of a mother to touch her dying child. This teen-aged girl had tried to commit suicide and was now brain dead and maintained on a ventilator.

> The mother was so distraught that she couldn't touch her daughter. And she just kept telling me, "If I can hold her, if I can just hold her one more time." So I put the side rail down and she went up and laid her head on her daughter's chest and just kind of held her, and so then I just scooted her to the side

of the bed so her mother could get up and crawl in bed with her and just kind of hold her daughter. And I felt really good about that. Letting the family come in and be with her and her brother was able to come in as well and just kind of hold her and get close to her, you know, while she was still warm.

Some nurses might not have heard the plea of the mother or understood her need. Others would have dismissed her request as impossible given the technological environment or the rules of the unit. The nurse could easily and truthfully have responded that "we don't do this," believing it not to be possible. But this nurse both heard and responded from a framework that values caring and connection, and she responded immediately, sensitively, and morally by making room for the mother next to her daughter. Understanding that all families would not want or request this kind of intimacy during dying, she nonetheless responded in this situation to the mother's particular needs. She felt very good about what she did and remains open to this type of "risky practice" in the future. This is an example of skilled ethical comportment.

Consistent with this novice-to-expert model, rational deliberation is only necessary in the case of ethical breakdown or in the case of conflicting or competing values. Principles are unable to produce expert ethical behavior, and falling back on them may produce inferior responses if context-based understanding is available (Dreyfus, Dreyfus, & Benner, 1990). In a situation in which intuition does not produce automatic responses, an experienced practitioner can make a good decision through involved deliberation of the intuitive expert in a familiar situation. "In familiar but problematic situations, therefore, rather than standing back and applying abstract principles, the expert deliberates about the appropriateness of his intuitions" (Dreyfus, Dreyfus, & Benner, 1990, p. 28). In contrast, the detached deliberation of an expert in a novel situation produces inferior responses. Principles are unable to produce expert ethical behavior. In this conception, intuition is primary in both moral comportment and problem solving.

For example, in the paradigm case, the nurses were confronted with the collision of two competing but key values, those of preventing needless suffering and upholding the family's right to make decisions about medical treatment. The nurses were concerned that they were causing Sharon to suffer. The patient and her husband wanted to face death by resolutely choosing survival within reason. Discontinuing all treatment would have violated this moral concern. Each of these values would direct the nurses' responses to the situation in a different way. To prevent suffering they would be compelled to push for withdrawal of life support; to protect the family's right to decide would direct them to fight for the patient's life tenaciously until the end. In many situations these values did not conflict because patients or families requested that their suffering be ended by termination of life support.

Although the nurses understood that Sharon was both dying and suffering, they continued to care for her, based on their understanding that the patient would have wanted to continue on. This situation did not feel right to some of them, who began to ask the "what if" questions that finally resulted in the patient's peaceful death. One nurse in the paradigm case deliberated about the appropriateness of her fear that she would harm the patient, not about the competing principles at stake. The nurses' involvement and intimate knowledge of the patient and family, their experience with similar cases, and their understanding of the possible interventions and outcomes guided questions they asked at care conferences, which were specific to the situation. In the end they were able to sustain both values by preventing further suffering inflicted by useless resuscitation procedures but not removing life support.

Moral Concerns

Moral concerns, understood as what the nurses believed to be good or right in the particular context, showed up in how they focused their practice as well as in situations of breakdown, when the smooth functioning of practice was disrupted. Several concerns were expressed by the nurses that were based on the caring values of involvement and connection, including comfort and respect for others. Those expressed in this narrative include (a) relief of suffering, (b) patient involvement in choice/wishes respected, (c) priority of family needs, and (d) maintaining dignity. Other concerns expressed in the study data but not included in the paradigm case are (e) differential treatment of patients and (f) acting as the agent of death. Exemplars will support the addition of these concerns to the list.

Relief of Suffering. Relief of suffering was a concern throughout the paradigm case. Nursing care focused on pain management and control of air hunger but also, in a broader sense, on providing some distraction from the technological space in which the patient was imprisoned—for example, by finding a comfortable position to watch a cooking show. The nurses tried to make the situation "as good as it [could] be," finding less painful ways to perform procedures such as catheter irrigations and being with her when she was afraid or lonely. The nurses were concerned about their own role in not wanting to inflict pain or prolonged torture by providing aggressive resuscitation measures. They were concerned and struggled with their role in prolonging her suffering, and their morale was, in part, dependent on their ability to act in ways that would minimize her pain and suffering.

Patient Involvement. The nurses were consistently concerned, in this and other narratives, that the patient should be involved in decisions regarding their care. They did not agree with assumptions that being severely ill and medicated, or even unconscious, in critical care precluded participation in care or decision making, and they were enraged when patients were overlooked or overridden. Sometimes nurses solicited patients' concerns; others responded to verbal or nonverbal cues at the bedside. These understandings of the patients' wants/choices formed the basis for the strong advocacy role assumed by the nurses. In some situations described in the study, nurses voiced the patient's concerns at care conferences.

In the paradigm case, Sharon was directly consulted regarding pain management while awake, then later understood by interpretation of bodily responses. Treatment was negotiated with her husband. They were uncomfortable that they had not directly spoken with the patient about how far she wanted to continue with therapy, but they respected Mark's interpretation instead and did not push the issue of withdrawal of life support (as they did in other situations in which the patient/family did not want to continue).

Family Needs. The nurses were concerned with maintaining the integrity of the family as much as possible given the technological space and the demands of the situation. They were also concerned with the primacy of family needs over the demands of the institution or even the physician. In the paradigm case, the nurses extended their view of the patient to include her husband and modified their approaches in consideration of his needs. They incorporated his suggestions in giving care. In this situation as in others, families of dying patients were allowed, even encouraged, to visit whenever and as long as they wished. This kind of flexibility was sometimes seen as risky practice, which might not be approved of by other nurses in the unit. However, the primacy of patient/family needs over those of the organization/physician were inherent in this type of expert care. Mitchell (1981) discusses the moral distress nurses regularly experience when their loyalties to patient/family and physician/organization are in conflict. If they cannot be consistently trustworthy to either, they are unable to maintain their integrity and become dissatisfied. There was evidence in this study that the nurses put forth much effort to oppose the physician or the system when the situation demanded, reaping their personal rewards from an outcome that they perceived as positive and/or the gratitude of the patient/family.

Maintaining Dignity. The nurses were concerned with maintaining the patients' dignity. This was in part related to prevention of suffering and supporting their right to direct their care but also involved the importance of privacy and respectful care of the body and the personhood of the patient. For example, playing rock and roll was interpreted as disrespectful of the patient's personhood and a violation of her dignity.

Several nurses remarked about the indignity of being restrained during dying. One nurse described a situation early in her career in which an elderly man who had experienced a heart attack became confused and combative.

> This man we had tied down in four-point restraints and he was fighting with us and he was a heart attack person and a real old person. My thoughts were that must be just the most awful way to die. To have your body tied down, fighting and we're tying you down for your safety as well as so you don't beat us up. And I felt real guilty over his death because of what he must have experienced within himself, with being tied and then dying. And being captive.

Dignity was also maintained by the attitudes of others toward the dying patient. For example, it was seen as a violation of dignity if staff talked over patients as if they were not there or if uninvolved staff made derogatory comments about patients. One nurse discussed her outrage when others would react insensitively to a patient she was caring for:

> I would get so involved in it, and I would get really mad sometimes. IV nurses, for instance, would come up. "Oh I just hate working on her." "Oh I just hate sticking her." "Oh she was so deadly when she was on the floor." And "I hope she dies." Or the old, "This is so cruel."

Gadow (1985) describes commitment to the protection and enhancement of human dignity as the ultimate goal of caring. Dignity is embedded in the meaning of the experience for the individual patient and diminished by reducing the person to the status of objects. External interpretations such as those above negate the patient's integrity and violate dignity. This is unconscionable within an ethic of caring.

Differential Treatment. Two additional concerns expressed by nurses in the study were not represented in the paradigm case. In several different stories, nurses expressed their concern with differential treatment of patients. One nurse described a morbidly obese patient with an acute abdomen whom the physicians could not take to surgery because of her weight. The nurse believed that the patient did not want to be taken off the ventilator, basing her belief on the patient's physiological responses to bedside talk about discontinuing life support. The woman's family was of lower socioeconomic status and was not able to travel to the hospital to be with her. The nurse believed that the possibility existed that eventually the infection could have walled itself off, but the woman could not survive without ventilator support. Because of her perception that the patient wanted to keep trying, the nurse wanted the physicians to keep trying. The woman was disconnected from the respirator and died, and the nurse commented:

> I don't know what to think. Are we at a point where if you don't listen or take care of a patient as well when the family members are not there looking out for them? Or, and in addition to that, when we have simple people come into our high-tech environment, are they also not treated as well? Those are my two unresolved questions.

Other patients that were identified as at risk for less than optimum treatment (versus "going to the wall" or "full court press") or for not being involved in their own decision making included unconscious or incompetent patients without families, persons with AIDS, and drug abusers.

Agent of Death. In the most common scenario related to the withdrawal of life support, the physician wrote an order to extubate the patient and keep the patient comfortable as he or she died. The medication order was usually a liberal sedation order for morphine or Valium, giving the nurses the latitude to titrate the drug intravenously if the patient seemed to be suffering or struggling. The physician then most often left the unit, and the nurse proceeded to withdraw the life support. In general, they viewed their role with dying patients as positive and themselves as facilitating the end to the patient's suffering or a peaceful death.

Although it was understood that the patient's illness or condition caused his or her death, there were feelings expressed by some nurses about being the agent of death. The nurses were most often the health care professionals responsible for disconnecting the breathing apparatus and giving the sedation. It is important to note that many of the sedatives routinely ordered for comfort also cause respiratory depression, and the difference in dosage for either purpose varied between patients. Although patients usually received small doses titrated to symptoms frequently, many times the patient's death occurred shortly after a sedative dose. In those situations, the nurses were all aware that the medication most likely precipitated the patient's final cardiopulmonary demise. Although most nurses denied that this was a problem for them, others struggled with the notion. The subject came up frequently in interview and observation data, where they sometimes referred to "killing their patients."

> **N1:** I'm thinking of specific situations that I know of. We're extubating, but can they do it on their own and, you know, try to progress from there. So are you keeping them comfortable or are you suppressing their respiratory drive?
>
> **INT.:** It's a fine line.
>
> **N1:** I think 23 [dosage of morphine] is over [more than] fine.
>
> **INT.:** An act of commission as opposed to an act of omission?
>
> **N2:** Yeah, it's really on the line between active and passive euthanasia when you're turning that drip up.
>
> **N1:** You know, chances are that person would have died anyway. But which caused it?
>
> **INT.:** So that's a routine thing?
>
> **N1:** Not a routine thing, but it's something that happens. It's not necessarily that bad.
>
> **N3:** A morphine death looks a lot prettier than a nonmorphine death. From our perspective.
>
> **INT.:** And do you feel comfortable doing it?
>
> **N2:** It depends.

Although individually nurses acknowledged that their sedative injections most likely contributed to death, that was not universally acknowledged or discussed within a moral context among involved health professionals. It would be erroneous to assume that nurses carry a moral burden because of their role in the timing of the patient's death, but the data point out that some nurses struggle with the concern. In a study by Wilson, Smedira, Fink, McDowell, and Luce (1992), both physicians and nurses verified that they ordered and administered sedatives and analgesics when life support was withdrawn to hasten death, although that was never the only reason. This was deemed ethical if the intention to relieve the suffering was primary rather than an intent to hasten death.

A concern related to assuming the responsibility for the death revolved around the perceived lack of concern and participation of the physician during the dying time. One nurse expressed her feelings:

> I get so sick of those "extubate patient and keep comfortable" [orders] . . .
> And a lot of times it's not even, they're not even in the unit writing it. It's
> over the phone, or whatever. And then they leave. They're either not there or
> they write it and they leave. And it's not even, it's not even thought that they
> would be in the room or participating in the death. And so that's where you
> struggle sometimes with that. You know, "look what I've done" and whatever.

Although the nurses seemed to relate the absence of the physician to devaluing of the dying patient (or dying itself), there are other explanations, including fear, feelings of guilt or failure, or unfamiliarity or discomfort with the dying vigil. It is important to point out that although several nurses struggled with the absence of the physician, others were comfortable being in the situation alone. Among those who were concerned, they did not want the physician to take over the withdrawal and subsequent vigil but to be available and validate the significance of the event.

As nurses became more experienced with the process of discontinuing life support, the details became less of an issue and did not show up in their narratives. But the nurses expressed continued frustration that when the patient was dying, the physician left the bedside. One nurse told a contrasting story, in which a physician coached the family through withdrawal decision making, then helped the nurse extubate the patient.

> **N1:** Usually the physician will come in and write the order and leave, which I'm used to. And I've had to go in the patient's room, extubate them by myself and then proceed with whatever orders to keep them comfortable and the family and everything else. But no, this doctor, what he said was, he looked at me in this conference room and he said, "Will you help me?" And I tried not to look too shocked in front of the family. Only I thought, "You bet I will." And I'd get him out in the hall and like go "whoa." So he went in there with me and he actually, literally, hands on, untaped the endotracheal tube while I got morphine and suction, and we together extubated this patient.
>
> **N2:** I've never seen that happen!
>
> **N3:** Never, never seen that happen.
>
> **N2:** Banner over his office. *Dr. Extraordinaire.*

Nurses considered the care for dying patients as an area of practice that has long rested within their domain and that they do not want to give up. However, what they seemed to be asking for was some recognition that this is in fact an important area of practice that is valued by both nurses and physicians.

Summary

Values and concerns describing the moral foundations of nursing are embedded in nursing practice. Involvement, caring, and relationship were strong moral themes throughout the narratives. Major ethical concerns focused on relief of suffering, patient choice, priority of family needs, maintaining dignity, and nondiscriminating treatment of patients. Because the nurses were most commonly responsible for the actual discontinuation of life support and sedating the patients as they died, issues and feelings about the nurse as the agent of death also stood out as a major concern.

From a clinical perspective, expert ethical practice is embedded in everyday situations and may not be recognized unless situations arise that are new or that spawn conflicting values. In situations where the patient, family, physician, and nurse communicate and respect and understand each others' values, ethical concerns are not brought forward for examination. However, when these situations do occur, nurses have a legitimate moral role based on their understanding and familiarity with the patient/family, physician (and usual medical practice), and organization. Given this understanding, the nurse is responsible for coordinating, communicating, interpreting, and translating from the position of caring and advocacy. Excellence in this role is a moral obligation because the nurse's expertise in this role affects the decisions made and the outcome of patients' illnesses. Nurses are able to act morally despite overwhelming obstacles, sometimes engaging in "risky behavior" by confronting physicians and breaking organizational rules such as visiting policies.

Nurses often feel that their role in moral decision making is not legitimate or important because they are not skilled in the language or processes of formal (principle-based) ethics. However, nurses in fact have their own unique role that serves the very important purpose of balancing the detached, abstract perspective that is the cornerstone of traditional ethical theory. The involved, caring perspective of the nurse often brings forward situations that are not right, not in the sense of not adhering to principles, but rather in the sense of not fitting the values or particular demands of the situation. This involved stance propels and persists until a solution is found that fits the situation.

These understandings of the inherent moral sense of nursing, the role of the nurse in decision making, and the legitimacy of that position must be incorporated into contemporary nursing theory. Further study of everyday practice is needed to continue to identify and refine the scope and depth of the moral tradition of nursing.

References

Benner, P. (1991). The role of experience, narrative, and community in skilled ethical comportment. *Advances in Nursing Science, 14*(2), 1-21.

Bishop, A., & Scudder, J. (1987). Nursing ethics in an age of controversy. *Advances in Nursing Science, 9*(3), 34-43.

Bishop, A., & Scudder, J. (1990). *The practical, moral, and personal sense of nursing.* Albany: State University of New York Press.

Callahan, S. (1988). The role of emotion in ethical decision-making. *Hastings Center Report, 18*(3), 9-14.

Catalano, J. (1991). Critical care nurses and ethical dilemmas. *Critical Care Nurse, 11*(1), 20-25.

Condon, E. (1988). Reflections on caring and the moral culture of nursing. *Virginia Nurse, 56*(4), 23-27.

Cooper, M. (1989). Gilligan's different voice: A perspective for nursing. *Journal of Professional Nursing, 5*, 10-16.

Cooper, M. (1990). *An interpretive analysis of the moral experience of the critical care nurse.* Unpublished doctoral dissertation, University of Virginia, Chapel Hill.

Cooper, M. (1991). Principle-oriented ethics and the ethic of care: A creative tension. *Advances in Nursing Science, 14*(2), 22-31.

Davis, D. (1986). Nursing: An ethic of caring. *Humane Medicine, 2*, 19-25.

Dreyfus, H., Dreyfus, S., & Benner, P. (1990). *Acquiring ethical expertise in nursing.* Unpublished manuscript.

Gadow, S. (1980). Existential advocacy: Philosophical foundation of nursing. In S. Spicker & S. Gadow (Eds.), *Nursing: Images and ideals* (pp. 79-101). New York: Springer.

Gadow, S. (1985). Nurse and patient: The caring relationship. In A. H. Bishop & J. R. Scudder (Eds.), *Nursing: Images and ideals* (pp. 31-43). New York: Springer.

Gadow, S. (1989). Advocacy with silent patients. *Nursing Clinics of North America, 24*, 535-541.

Gadow, S. (1990). Covenant without cure: Letting go and holding on in chronic illness. In J. Watson & M. Ray (Eds.), *The ethics of care and the ethics of cure: Synthesis in chronicity* (pp. 5-14). New York: National League for Nursing.

Gilligan, C. (1982). *In a different voice: Psychological theory and women's development.* Cambridge, MA: Harvard University Press.

Krekeler, K. (1987). Critical care nursing and moral development. *Critical Care Quarterly, 10*(2), 1-8.

MacIntyre, A. (1984). *After virtue* (2nd ed.). Notre Dame, IN: University of Notre Dame Press.

Mitchell, C. (1981). New directions in nursing ethics. *Massachusetts Nurse, 50*(7), 7-10.

Pierce, S. (1989). The critical care nurse: An ethicist by trade. *Critical Care Nursing Quarterly, 12*(3), 75-78.

Weir, R. (1989). *Abating treatment with critically ill patients.* New York: Oxford University Press.

Wilson, W., Smedira, N., Fink, D., McDowell, J., & Luce, J. (1992). Ordering and administration of sedatives and analgesics during the withholding and withdrawal of life support from critically ill patients. *Journal of the American Medical Association, 267*, 949-953.

14

❖

The Ethics of Ambiguity and Concealment Around Cancer

Interpretations Through a Local Italian World

DEBORAH R. GORDON

Between the conscious and the unconscious lies the most critical domain of all for historical anthropology. . . . It is the realm of partial recognition, of inchoate awareness, of ambiguous perception, and sometimes of creative tension: that liminal space of human experience in which people discern acts and facts but cannot or do not order them into narrative descriptions, or even into articulate conceptions of the world; in which signs and events are observed, but in a hazy, translucent light; in which individuals or groups know that something is happening to them, but find it difficult to put their fingers on quite what it is. . . .

(Comaroff & Comaroff, 1991, p. 29)

AUTHOR'S NOTE: I am deeply grateful to the many people who participated in the researches reported here. Patricia Benner's influence, including her essential insights on many parts of this interpretive puzzle, is a constituting, pervasive background for which I am profoundly grateful. Her caring, challenging, and inspiring contribution to our intellectual, professional, and patient communities is a true paradigm case—a very strong instance!— of what it means to be human at its very best.

Many sincere thanks to my patient interlocutors, in particular Allaman Allamani, Eugenio Paci, Guido Miccinese, Mariella Pandolfi, and Antonella Venturini; to Professor Spinsanti and his collaborators in the bioethics courses; to Eugenio Paci for his continued support of my research; and to C.N.R., The Italian National Research Council: Project ACRO contract number CNR 92.02385.PF39, and A.I.R.C. for the funding of the projects upon which this chapter is based.

279

A moral reaction is an . . . affirmation of a given ontology of the human.

(Taylor, 1989, p. 5)

Communication practices around cancer are extremely contested in Italy today and as support for more explicit and complete communication directly to patients increases, what once was a relatively homogeneous practice of nondisclosure grows increasingly diverse according to specialty, hospital, age, gender, class, and relative cosmopolitan, regional and local influences (Cattorini, 1992; Comitato Nazionale per la Bioetica, 1992; GIVIO, 1986; Spinsanti, 1992; Tamburini et al., 1988a).

Ethnographic and survey research, however, shows that the traditional practice of physicians and family members not to communicate cancer diagnoses and prognoses directly, explicitly, or completely to the patient but rather to mask or communicate partially, ambiguously, implicitly, or indirectly still survives in many contexts in Italy. Cancer is still silence (Paci, 1993). Such nondisclosure may be practiced even with a very curable diagnosis[1] or clear indication by the patient that he or she wants to be informed. Consensus remains much stronger for noncommunication of diagnoses with bad prognoses and, in turn, of bad prognoses themselves. (Thompson, et al., 1993)

Family members often lead in "don't tell the patient," arguing, like physicians, that communication could "destroy hope," "make the patient agitated," "be psychologically damaging," or "cause useless suffering." But the family is not alone. Not infrequently patients who are being diagnosed for possible breast cancer keep the process a secret from their family members until the last moment, and some never inform their own parents, even if the latter are relatively young and healthy. People who apparently do not know that they have cancer or are dying will suddenly pronounce an oral will or make a gesture a few days before they die indicating that they undoubtedly knew what was happening but said nothing.

On the other hand, we hear much about people "knowing and not knowing" they have cancer, people who know "inside themselves," *dentro di se*, but "in their minds" believe something else (Gordon, 1989, 1990), people who apparently "don't want to know" or who "will believe anything you tell them just so it's not a 'bad' diagnosis," people who ask few questions and accept few explanations, people who are clearly dying but who speak as if they will go back to work tomorrow. We also hear of many who do prefer to be informed about having cancer or who want to know more but are not told

(Cantoni, 1992; Moscone, Meyerowitz, Liberati, & Liberati, 1991; Paci & Venturini 1989).

We have, then, a world of many silences and secrets, of much cultivated vagueness and manipulated hope, of institutionalized "middle knowledge" (Weisman, 1972), in which the fact of cancer, a possible impending death, and many of the emotions triggered by them are excluded from speech and shared public space.

Notwithstanding the diversity of perspectives in the present situation (Gordon & Paci, 1993) and the irreversible thrust toward change, the voices of tradition will be privileged in this chapter. In particular, I consider areas of consensus in this local world through triangulation of the perspectives of physicians and health professionals in general, patients, and family members in an effort to understand how cancer, communication of bad news, and knowing or not knowing potential terminality are lived in this traditional context. In so doing, I hope to articulate some dominant and enduring concerns and ways of being that can help us understand what is at stake (Kleinman & Kleinman, 1991) in a situation of change and thus what is most resistant to change. For example, though recent medical and bioethical codes give greater recognition to the individual, a "rights" discourse, and support for informed consent of the patient, we still hear a stipulation for "serenity," the legitimizing of masked, vague, or minimizing language, and the sense that it would be "inhuman" to "leave someone without hope." According to the Italian Medical Deontological Code (Turin, Italy, 1989),

> The physician has the duty to provide the patient . . . the most serene information about the diagnosis, the prognosis, and the therapeutic perspectives and their consequences. . . . The physician might evaluate . . . the opportunity not to reveal to the patient [the diagnosis] or to mitigate a serious or lethal prognosis. In any case it will have to be communicated to the family. (cited in Surbone, 1992)

And according to the Comitato Nazionale per la Bioetica (1992),

> In justifying the dismissal of being completely explicit about "important pathologies," it is necessary to speak to the patient of an "important illness," of the "seriousness of the situation," of the necessity of "particular, delicate exams," of therapies that can "carry some risks." (p. 10)
>
> When the diagnosis is incurable, communication is to be precise, but using terminology that is "nontraumatizing" (preferring, for example, terms such as *neoplasm, tumor pathology,* or *atypical cells* rather than *cancer* or *malignant tumor,* and so on). . . . (p. 10)
>
> The traditional role reserved for family members in the sharing of information and in consent is being questioned ever more frequently today. . . . The

committee holds that even in situations when the family asks that the patient not
be given information about his or her condition, . . . one must behave with the patient according to the general rules (exact news but lacking dramaticality, and
characterized by a composite of elements that may leave the patient with the possibility of hope for the future, which it would be inhuman to deny. (p. 11)

In this chapter I explore some dimensions of the background or "world"
that makes practices of silence and ambiguous communication around cancer
show up as the ethical thing to do, with particular attention to what kind of
subject one must be for these practices to be lived as ethical and to "work."

By background, I do not mean a "whole culture" of which we are seeing
only a manifestation. Nor do I imply a holism or determinism of Italian or
Mediterranean, European, or even Tuscan cultures. Clearly, this is an open
cultural field (Comaroff & Comaroff, 1991), and in fact history and
contacts with other cultural orientations and practices are pushing the situation toward increasing international homogenization of disclosure, as there
once was homogenization of nondisclosure (Comaroff & Comaroff, 1991).

Rather, the approach taken is that "human being is a kind of space in which
coping with certain kinds of beings becomes possible" (Dreyfus & Wakefield,
1988, p. 275). Things show up through a background, which in turn consists,
according to Heidegger, of social practices.

The shared practices into which we are socialized provide a background understanding of what counts . . . as human beings, and ultimately what counts as
real. . . . Heidegger calls this background understanding of what it means to
be, which is embodied in the tools, language, and institutions of a society and
in each person growing up in that society, "understanding of Being." . . . This
understanding of Being creates what Heidegger calls a *clearing* in which entities can then show up for us.

The clearing . . . is a context that both opens up and limits the kinds of objects we can deal with . . . what things can show up for us, . . . for example,
. . . as a person. (Dreyfus & Wakefield, 1988, p. 275)

Merleau Ponty compared this background to the illumination in a room
(Dreyfus, 1991; Merleau-Ponty, 1962).

After describing some practices and self-understandings of those involved
in "not telling" cancer patients their diagnosis, I argue that these concealment
and ambiguity practices as well as those of not knowing clearly extend
beyond the cancer situation, and that many people in the local world of
study—Tuscany—are socialized into them even from birth. These practices
form part of a network of related practices and understandings—similar to
an "equipmental whole"—that make sense together (Dreyfus, 1991; Heidegger,
1962). More specifically, we may consider the practice of ambiguous or

concealed communication around cancer as belonging to a network of related situations, such as

1. Communication between an authority and a dependent
2. Dealing with separations, death, and change in general
3. Dealing with suffering, specifically the avoidance and minimization of suffering and protection from suffering
4. Living with uncertainty
5. Covering over potential social rifts

Practices such as these—of which a few examples will be proposed in the second part of the chapter—constitute the everyday background of many people raised in this local world and among other things serve to eliminate or cover up possible ruptures—separations, differences, changes, conflict—in the social and individual fabric, while maintaining the status quo, unity, and hierarchy in the social world. Habitation—official and nonofficial—of what Pandolfi (1990, 1991) calls "inbetween spaces," spaces between consciousness and unconsciousness (Comaroff & Comaroff, 1991), or knowing and not knowing, through silence, shadow, ambiguity, and indirect communication, is an important way of being and knowing in this relational context.

Embodied and projected within these and other practices are local understandings of Being, of what it means to be a person (Benner & Wrubel, 1989; Dreyfus, 1991; Rubin, 1988)—to be human or "inhuman." More specifically, we find a very social way of being in the world and of understanding being, in which being, reality, truth, and language are lived as relational, contextual, and embodied; in which people are differentiated, some being stronger and more powerful, and most being basically fragile. On the other hand, one hears relatively little of an objectified self or a self of possession (Sandel, 1982; Taylor, 1989).

The temporality of subjectivity in the noninforming stance often shows up as living very much in the present while being anchored in the past. An open future that is taken for granted and in the background rather than in the foreground as an object for goal striving, appears to be essential for well-being and hope in the present. Life is to be lived now, in the everyday, rather than earned and delayed until tomorrow. Taken for granted within this stance is that there are distinct limits to our capacity to know, predict, and control life events and that problems, suffering, death, and misfortune in general are inevitable and basically capricious. Tomorrow is less a beacon of progress or a resource to cultivate, but perhaps a new unexpected problem that challenges the continuity of today.

In this way we consider how an ethical practice such as nondisclosure around a cancer diagnosis is embedded not only in the biomedical world but in the everyday local world. Selfhood and the good, specifically the good life, are inextricably intertwined (Taylor, 1989, p. 3, 1991).

An Evovling Dialogic Study

Because I am an American anthropologist living in this Italian context, this research was clearly dialogic, sometimes implicitly, sometimes explicitly. It began in 1985 in the United States in preparation for research in Florence, Italy, on the care and information "desires" and "needs" of patients with terminal cancer. When I arrived in Italy I was in for a shock, for I learned that the very explicit, elaborate interview questionnaire I had developed was useless because none of the patients had ever been told their diagnosis. Thus I entered the world of silence and ambiguous, indirect communication around cancer, feeling as if I were newly blind and trying to touch things with a long stick instead of with my hands. I learned that research assistants, young physicians themselves, were especially prepared by a psychologist for dealing with this very sensitive subject (Gordon, Belloni, & Allamani, 1990). I was challenged to understand a series of apparently contradictory phrases I would hear over and over again:

> If you tell, you remove all hope. It's like giving a death sentence. It's as if it's all over.

> But most usually know anyway.

My first reaction to this noninforming was moral outrage— whose body and whose life is it anyway? As I tried to understand this practice, however, I came to understand that not telling had much to do with caring and not just power and ownership. I thought back to how some patients in the United States come to treat themselves objectively as "cases" and wondered if there was any less "illusion" or "denial" involved—whether in the United States feeling in control was a way of feeling better and a basis for hope. Despite my beginning understanding of the Italian approach, I was struck by how not knowing did not feel like an existential and perhaps cultural possibility for me, not because of the often-mentioned need and desire to control one's care but because I felt that my having cancer would be part of who I was, and not knowing that would be not living my life in some fundamental way (see Gordon, 1991, for further discussion).

Since then I have been studying this topic formally and informally through a number of research projects at the Center for the Study and Prevention of Cancer in Florence, Italy. [2] Furthermore, residing in Florence, I have lived through situations of cancer, death, and health care involving close friends, acquaintances, and myself.

The exploration of parallel practices began through everyday experiences. Having a child brought me into the world of infant and child care practices and exposed me to many of what I hypothesize to be some continuities of features we find in medical adult ethical practice.

These practices and assumptions are now being explored more explicitly and widely through more intensive ethnographic study as well as through a questionnaire survey (Gordon, in press; Gordon & Paci, 1993). The latter consists of statements and case examples—mostly drawn from ethnographic research—about communication practices and background understandings and was piloted with 239 participating health professionals—physicians, nurses, and others in a course on bioethics offered to health professionals throughout Tuscany, Italy. Selected results from this pilot study are presented in the Appendix of this chapter and are referred to throughout the text by "(Appendix, Q#)."

Some Notes on the Context

Many factors contribute to the particular practices of informing around cancer: the epidemiology of particular types of cancer (e.g., stomach cancer is particularly prominent in Japan), the political economy of cancer treatment (Good et al., 1990), the health care and economic systems, and local history, to name but a few.

For people in these studies, public medical care was readily available and essentially free, and thus the possible costs of being ill and cared for were not major factors people had to consider. Technologically, the level of care available is high by international standards, particularly for breast cancer, which is at times state of the art quality. In general, experimental treatments and the chance to participate in clinical trials are significantly less available locally than in a comparable city in the United States. Other than at a major and socially visible specialty cancer center for prevention, diagnosis, and follow-up, treatment generally takes place in general public hospitals and clinics rather than specialty oncology centers; similarly, only a minority of health professionals involved are oncologists. The major cancer treatment center in Milan is an authoritative point of reference for physicians and patients alike, but local practice follows national and international protocols.

Though there are beginning signs of change, medical contexts are clearly hierarchical and authoritarian. Even the department is named after the chief, the *primario*, with decision-making power concentrated in his hands and the succession of medical strata. Nurses are clearly under medical authority, and health care decisions remain primarily physician decisions, with little choice presented to patients, even in cancer centers. Though the law states that patients should be informed, practice still rarely corresponds.

A city admired internationally for its glorious past, works of art—noted for their balance, humanism, and perspective—and physical beauty, Florence and surrounding Tuscany share a strong and positive cultural and historical identity that includes being a cosmopolitan center.

Though attendance at church is steadily decreasing, the impact of the dominant Roman Catholic religion is still pervasive. Many of the people in the age groups studied attended church (Roman Catholic) as children (Gordon & Paci, 1993) and describe themselves as Catholics. Most grew up in Tuscany itself and at most changed only city of residence.

Economically, along with the rest of northern Italy, the area has enjoyed relative economic prosperity since the war. The two world wars, however, remain alive in memory and outlook.

Ambiguity About "Ambiguity": Some Notes on Terminology

It is difficult to find the right terminology for describing types of communication and understanding cross-culturally, in part because of the insider/outsider dimension but also because of the difference between what is said and what is understood. Obviously, implicit, symbolic communication that does not explicitly state the topic may be lived and understood as very precise and clear communication. The term *tumor* when used in Italy usually means one has cancer and is perhaps less ambiguous than might be the case in a context where *cancer* and *malignant tumor* are more frequently used. Similarly, the tendency is to assume that very technical, explicit communication is very clear communication, but we know very well from patients that this is often not the case. For some people in Italy, the word *carcinoma,* though precise, may allow and actually be used for misunderstanding. The word *cancer* in Italy constitutes clear, unambiguous communication.

Furthermore, we must distinguish between, on the one hand, being vague or ambiguous about the future (prognosis), masking, reassuring, or giving partial information, and, on the other hand, offering clear, certain communication of uncertainty, that is, the uncertainty of whether someone will survive or die (M.J.D. Good, 1993). Further, although in the American context ambiguity is now most present around the prognosis (Barnes, Koenig, Mirande, & Davis, 1993; Good et al., 1990; Orona, Koenig, & Davis, in press), with the diagnosis being generally disclosed clearly and correctly, one still senses that this ambiguity is already within relatively clearly communicated parameters. For example, ambiguity may be around how long one may expect to live, but already within a context in which the patient is told he or she has a terminal illness.

In the Italian context, though implicit communication may be very clearly understood, much is made and said about the difference between "telling" and "not telling," "knowing" and "not knowing," even though this fails to capture differing forms of communication and knowing that are operative. Local self/other descriptions, however, do distinguish broader communication styles and emphasize that in Italy the preference is for communication that is "soft," "sweetened," "gradual," "personal," "metaphorical," "nuanced," "indirect," "implicit," and "nonverbal." This is in contrast to communication that is "brutally honest," "explicit," and "matter-of-fact," which may be experienced as "cruel" and "harsh." This is the difference I wish to capture, and although communication and understanding may be quite precise without words attached, or through other words, for ease, I use the term *ambiguity* to refer to communication whose meaning is not fixed, clear, and singular and that consequently allows the listener some space for interpretation. This does not mean that understanding is necessarily ambiguous.

Exemplar of a Nondiscloser and the Relationships Between Foreground and Background

Let us enter the story of foreground and background through the examplar of Dr. J, a male physician born in 1946 to a merchant family with long roots in Florence. His regular practice is to not explicitly inform patients of their cancer diagnosis.

I first interviewed Dr. J in 1987 when he was an assistant in a department of medicine in a public hospital in Florence as well as a family physician in the community. As described by Dr. J, the regular practice followed in that department, which treated a large number of patients with lung cancer, was nondisclosure. I also observed him briefly in practice and in meetings around the care of dying patients, for which he was a local promoter, and interviewed a number of family members and some patients with whom he had worked. I interviewed Dr. J again in 1989, and once more in 1993, when he had become an "associate physician" in the same hospital department. Following are some excerpts from our interviews:

INT.: Do you inform patients explicitly that they have cancer?

PART.: To tell you the truth, I have never told anyone who has a cancer, who in any case is at the end of his life, that they have cancer.

INT.: Why not?

PART.: Without a doubt there is difficulty on my part, and I think for everyone, in giving a sentence. I have difficulty in making someone suffer, in causing someone sorrow, a *dispiacere*, that I can cause in telling him. That is, there is always on the part of the physician the need to make a person feel better, feel good; even I can say nothing, he [the patient] can understand everything, but I didn't say it, I didn't give it precisely the official stamp. In the meantime, the patient wants to have the confirmation. . . . But this confirmation is difficult to give because it closes everything, closes all possibility, hopes, hope to participate in life, in everything. If he knows, there is no more hope.

INT.: The danger of telling is so great?

PART.: The danger is very great because it takes away from someone all possibility of experiencing a more serene, more tranquil period in the very moment when he needs that instead of knowing the truth. I do not, however, tell lies either, saying to the patient, for example, "It's nothing," and giving them a slap on the back.

INT.: What do you say about a difficult prognosis?

PART.: I always say that the illness is not curable, always. I have never said that one will be cured from this illness, but I also tell them that even if the illness is not curable, the patient will feel better. Thus it is true information but at the same time, often not true.

INT.: Who makes decisions about treatment?

PART.: I think that the patient never has anything to say. The choice is made by the physician, . . . and if the physician knows how, the patient will accept any therapy that he proposes. If I tell a person, "You must cut off your arm and then your leg because it is important," this one has his arm cut off and then his leg. . . . My experience has shown me that patients will do the most incredible things . . . according to how one proposes the things to them.

Dr. J recounted the death of his father as a "good" death. He was the physician responsible and made all the medical decisions regarding his father's care alone: "As in all situations, it is the physician who decides." He never told his father he had a lung tumor:

PART.: He didn't know because no one ever told him, but inside of him, *dentro di se*, he knew, that is as always happens, he knew . . . because a week before dying, before his children, he made a kind of oral will. When he realized that the illness was going ahead, he stopped asking me questions, I didn't give him any more answers, and little by little he understood alone. My mother was told only at the end what my father had, a month before he died. Even if she understood earlier, she didn't let us understand that she had understood because if she did we would have felt bad, but she understood without a doubt. . . .

INT.: What happens if someone suspects or knows?

PART.: What terrifies is not so much the fact that one must die, because this I think everyone knows they must die, it is the fact of the deadline, the *scandenza*. For example, I have a patient now, a young man with a malignant lung tumor with metastasis. His wife asked me and the other physicians not to tell him anything, but he continually asks questions regarding his illness. When he comes to the clinic I reassure him and he leaves feeling much more secure and tranquil. . . . I never told the patient he had a tumor or a metastasis, but that he had a tumor that was not malignant, but not benign either, in other words, intermediate. . . . About the metastases I told him that a wound had formed near where he was operated on that was pressing the nerve and thus giving him pain. . . .

It's classic, this discourse that each person has the right to know about his life. But this person is going on: he was operated on a year and a half ago for the tumor, had metastasis to the bone. If you look at the statistics, a person so young as this with metastasis to the bone should not live a year and a half as he did. So . . . if I had told him, "You have a malignant tumor, you were operated on but you have metastasis to the bone and you have a probability of survival of 6 to 8 months . . . " it would have been very difficult for me and above all for him to live this time without tormenting oneself continually with this . . . deadline. Instead, the facts have demonstrated that I was correct. . . . I am convinced . . . that I give him great security. Maybe his fear passes, maybe only for 3 or 4 days and then we need to rethink it again because the pain returns. In other words, the reassurance that I give him makes him pass a relatively tranquil period. He makes projects, it pushes him to keep up a realized life also for the others, not to close himself up in his problem.

The experience with my father also demonstrated to me that even if you don't tell someone that they will die in a month or two, they know themselves, when that time comes they know alone. Thus I tend not to inform them. [from interview in 1987]

Dr. J said he has changed his practice in the last 5 years. Now he is less inclined to follow the family's requests; now he tries to tell the patient the "most possible," still not using terms such as *cancer* or *malignant tumor* but rather expressions such as "It is a problem of a thickening of a branch of atypical cells." He starts with this and tries to make the person understand.

INT.: Why have you changed your approach?

PART.: I am ever increasingly aware of the "right to know." I have grown too. I have worked more on my own these last years, with less support, and I have worked with more patients. I am now realizing that knowing is not *that* dramatic. Finally, patients are increasingly making more demands, more criticisms, and the law is entering the picture even more. . . .

The term *cancer,* however, frightens both the physician and the patient. It remains difficult for me to say, loaded with so many mean- ings— an illness that makes you suffer. I have a certain modesty around illness, a certain reserve. It's private, like one's problems; you don't want to involve others in this.

INT.: How was cancer, and illness in general, dealt with in your family?

PART.: Illness was not talked about, it was dealt with privately as long as possible, when it would be finally discussed only because it could no longer be avoided. This was in order not to disturb us, but also out of modesty. Cancer was never talked about, it was avoided.

Going back in time, we hear a story that well prepared Dr. J for the practice of not communicating the diagnosis of cancer to patients. In fact, one hears how not telling and not clearly and publicly knowing were very common ways of being in his family of origin.

"Words," Dr. J went on to say, "were of extreme difficulty in my family, it was not just a reserve about illness." For example:

- "Talking about sex was a taboo."
- "Anger was expressed with silence."
- "Everyone held his strong emotions inside; at most, he supposed, his mother may have confessed to someone at church."
- "If someone had a problem that bothered him, we were brought up to keep it inside, to not say anything about it, because you are sorry to involve others in this suffering, especially if there is nothing they can do about it, this is egotistical because you only make them feel worse."
- "There was little [verbal] expression of love. You showed your love through caring surveillance; there was no doubt about it, however."

"There were many secrets. My mother hid not only her feelings but also her religious sentiments from my father. She was a fervent Catholic and always went to church, hidden," because Dr. J's father was an atheist and very much against this. "Did your father know about this?" I asked. "Certainly he knew, but he said not a word. It was a tacit agreement." When I asked if this was not like the situation of people with cancer, he said, "Of course."

He said that his father was one who tried to completely evade facing problems, and not saying and not knowing, along with joking, were the main ways he did this.

As a child, Dr. J and his sister were protected from difficult things, from illness, from death. When his grandmother was dying of cancer, for instance, he and his sister, who were both over 12 years old, were told only that she had the flu. "My mother was trying to protect you every moment without your even being aware of it; she was invisible, like an angel."

His family was authoritarian and he and his sister learned early not to speak of certain things. But they also learned quickly that "following father's rules" really meant never saying anything about the prohibited behavior more than not doing it. "I learned not to tell the truth, that this would only cause my father to suffer." However, this is different from lying, he stressed. Lying was not acceptable.

Though Dr. J could not remember precisely how separations were handled when he was a child, when I mentioned the common practice of parents waiting to leave until a child is distracted or using little lies to cover up or ease a separation or pain, he said, "Yes, yes, they teach you early on to lie, from childhood. That sounds right! I learned that's how it is. You mustn't say things as they are. You are better for it, I am better for it!"

Dr. J's biography is of course particular, but it draws upon common cultural and social resources shared to varying extents by people of the same age, gender, class, city, region, country, continent, and religion that intersect to constitute the cultural field of this local world and echoes themes heard repeatedly in other accounts (see Gordon, 1989, 1990, 1991, for fuller discussion and examples).

Dr. J's description of his communication with and treatment of the young man with lung tumor and metastasis was used as a case example in the bioethics questionnaire. Of the 239 respondents, 51% of physicians (who included only a few oncologists) and 29% of nurses and other health professionals in a bioethics course that openly supported patient autonomy agreed with his behavior and reasoning (referred to in the tables as "traditional" as opposed to "nontraditional" (Appendix, case example, Q2.2).

One major recurring theme mentioned by the physicians in the traditional stance is that informing means giving and receiving a death sentence (Appendix, Q3.1), a "condemnation" that could destroy all hope and make it be "like it was all over," a statement that we may interpret through a number of interacting dimensions.

First is that despite many changes in the curability of some cancers, many, including physicians, still feel on a "gut" level that cancer is incurable (Appendix, Q20.3) and causes certain death and suffering (Cantoni, 1992; Gordon,

Venturini, Rosselli Del Turco, Palli, & Paci, 1991). In fact, as speech about death has receded from the social scene, cancer and morbidity have taken its space as social symbols of death (Cantoni, 1992).

Second is the power and in turn responsibility that physicians such as Dr. J sense they have towards and on patients and the parallel dependence, "suggestibility," and "fragility" they perceive in patients. Many such as Dr. J feel that if the physician is effective, the patient will do what he says (Appendix, Q1.4). In general, "reality" is clearly understood by these health professionals to be socially constructed: "If they see me tranquil, they will think, if he is so tranquil, why do I need to worry!" (Appendix, Q12.2). Patients often corroborated this feeling:

> I trust very much in those around me, be it my son or the doctor who reassures me. So I am tranquil even if I do feel a little bad. . . . If my physician tells me, "Signora, be tranquil," I am tranquil. Obviously I have faith in my physician, he is a person that I esteem very much and who truly gives me serenity. (Mrs. Teresa, 65 years old, with advanced breast cancer)

Third, one senses a pervasive way of living language in which language is lived not only as a transmitter of information but also as capable of invoking the very thing to which it refers (B. Good, 1993; Taylor, 1985). The power of the physician, together with this way of living language, sets the physician up to feel as if he is "condemning to death," not just being a messenger of bad news and transmitting the "sentence" already in the cancerous cells, as an American oncologist might feel (M.J.D. Good, 1992, personal communication).

Another theme in this exemplar is the importance of the uncertainty of the "deadline" for living and for hope. Knowing that one will die within a relatively bounded time frame or a "deadline" is regarded by many as unacceptable. Death itself, according to many, is not something one can ever really accept (Appendix, Q9.2). Professor Z, a chief of pulmonary medicine and a noninformer, repeats this theme in an interview:

> **PART.:** Life is made in such a way that one does not know when one is born and when one dies. If a subject knows exactly when he will die, I do not know if his life, so ordered, is worthy of being lived. So, we are not people with the ability to determine the date of death, ever. . . .
>
> You need to think that life is an unrepeatable good, this is the basic idea, it is not a pair of shoes that one can throw away and buy again. Thus the idea of accepting that life can end and knowing when one will die, is, according to me, unacceptable . . . but fortunately in each of us is the hope that we will continue to go for a walk with our children.
>
> **INT.:** Is it unacceptable even if one knows that one has a year of life left?

PART.: And with 1 year? One goes to the seashore this year with one's children, next year I will no longer be able to go to this beach. I will no longer have them, how can I live this year in a tremendous spasmodic waiting for death? Death is not an acceptable situation. . . .

We have here a very strong statement of how not knowing when one will die is essential for the good life, as if knowing this would be a violation of order in the universe. Uncertainty is essential for life. Further, we hear how knowing one has no future cancels out one's present.

Another theme is the strong ethic against causing suffering in another person, an ethic in which all are involved: the son doesn't tell the father the diagnosis, nor the mother, in part to avoid causing them suffering, and the mother doesn't let on that she knows because "she knew that if we knew that she knew we would feel bad." This shared responsibility contributes to keeping the knowness of the cancer diagnosis officially from the public arena.

"Patients understand anyway, there is no need to say it [the diagnosis or prognosis] explicitly" is another theme. For many, implicit communication and understanding are not only sufficient but preferable. They seem to be considered more relational, warm, and open, whereas explicit, complete, precise communication is considered cold and mechanical, closing off relationships—as if relationships depended upon ambiguous, open-ended communication and exact communication stood outside of relationships.

Open, frank communication was often interpreted as quick, irresponsible, impersonal communication, as dumping on the patient, and inevitably, as giving specific time prognostications of how long someone will live.

> Informing on the part of the physician is telling someone how long they have to live, shaking their hands, and saying thank you very much!
> Informing feels cold and mechanical, as if it will end all relationships.
> Informing is like shoving their noses in it.
> Informing is easier for the health care provider; it is refusing to carry out one's responsibility.
> To say it is a tumor is to end collaboration with the family and the patient, whereas telling the patient it is "grave and chronic" is a good base for future questions. . . . I almost never use the terms *cancer, tumor,* or "carcinoma." To say so explicitly is mechanical; usually the patient understands. . . . It is enough to understand that the patient understands. (medical oncologist, male, in his 40s)

The important issue for many is not so much what is said or whether the patient knows, but the relationships the person has with providers and family (Appendix, Q2.5; see also Feldman, 1992).

As Dr. J noted, a "rights" discourse is definitely increasing as the official bioethics stresses informed consent (Comitato Nazionale per la Bioetica, 1992), but this discourse played a minimal role in discussions of traditional professionals, superseded by a discourse of protection or the "right" to hope.

Finally, we hear the importance of serenity and tranquillity (Gordon et al., 1990; Appendix, Q1.5, Q2.2). In fact, no qualities are mentioned more often as important for patients and people in general than these. As we will soon hear again in a narrative of Professor L, serenity is the basis for a "good life" and a good death; worry and agitation make for bad living and a bad death.

We hear how Dr. J, as others have noted, learned early to distinguish what one should say and what one should not say, and with whom (see Carroll, 1987). This is not "honesty is the best policy."

Because living without knowing about one's life and about many things in life is a background possibility with which many people have experience, not knowing and not telling are dominant possibilities. It is clear that there is less suffering and more serenity in not knowing; it is clear that the teller has much more responsibility in the impact of telling. It was a choice; there was a possibility not to tell.

In this exemplar, we also see how concealment, ambiguity, and vagueness are not just practices of protection from death and illness in the health sector but a way of keeping problems (Appendix, Q11.9) and deep emotions (Appendix, Q16.7) "private" and out of the social arena; of avoiding conflict, disobedience, and punishment; of asserting autonomy for the dominated (Crapanzano, 1990; for example, Dr. J's mother said nothing but continued to practice her faith); of avoiding facing problems or painful topics; and of expressing love and protecting another.

We see how Dr. J was well prepared for the practice of not communicating explicitly the diagnosis to cancer patients, that he was very skilled in keeping disruptive news to himself through his family and professional socialization, and that he had a strong background familiarity with this practice (Dreyfus, 1991). In any case we see how biomedical ethical practices repeat, support, and partake of practices more extensive in everyday life.

The Ways and Meanings of Knowing

How does knowing one's diagnosis appear to caregivers in this traditional stance? In the following exemplar, Professor Z offers a narrative about being informed that tells us more about what he and others who share his stance consider good and bad living and dying.

Exemplar: "People Who Know Die Worse"

In my experience I find that people who know die worse—in the sense that
this is an illness, especially lung cancer, that allows for long intervals of well-
being, and if the subject knows, he continues to think about his illness and not
live his normal life, but he has this anxiety, this problem that devours him.
Thus anxiety and moral pain exceed by a long shot the physical pain. If the
person does not know, these long intervals of well-being give him hope, make
him live moments of happiness with his family, with the environment, with
his normal work, he can often return to work and thus live a life presumably
normal, as would be the case for all other subjects who have nothing. And I
saw those who did know stay there thinking, thinking, wearing themselves
out, being'agitated, asking for sedatives, "but I have these pains." "No," I say,
"it's the thought, the torture. . . . "
    Let me give you another example that has even reinforced my convictions.
About 10 years ago I received a patient in the clinic at my home who came
from Denmark . . . a civilized country with few religious convictions. Thus, I
was led to believe, it is the common habit that all must be informed of their
destiny. He came to Italy once a year to buy ceramics. He came to me and
said, "Look, I go around the world every year and I must have a point of reference in two or three countries. I need one in Florence because I come often to
Italy. Three years ago a tumor was found in my lung, the diagnosis was certain." This is a very civil person who speaks with much intelligence and
logic. . . . "Three years ago they removed the tumor from my lung and for 3
years I am well, but I want a response to these questions: Are there any local
recurrences of the tumor? Are there any metastases to the other lung? Are
there any distant metastases? . . . I am here a week, you can do all the exams
you want. . . . I want to know these things." I did them all and they were all
negative. He came for 2 years and did the same thing. The third year I didn't
see him because he died.
    He lived well, this man with these problems in his pocket, or did he live
poorly? A civilized man of a civilized nation who knows everything, to whom
you say everything to his face. He traveled the world and wanted answers to
all his problems. But he, with these worries, with this waiting, with this unnerving waiting that one of these exams would be positive, did he live well or
did he live badly? For me he lived badly.

For this physician, for whom the most important thing is to enjoy and live
as presumably normal a life as possible with his family, with as little
suffering and worry as possible, this way of living with cancer was "living
poorly." Professor Z clearly questions this so-called "civilized"—and we
may say "modern"—way of living and knowing and "seeking answers to all
his problems." For him, for whom knowing is not necessary and in fact

negative, living while knowing one has a tumor is "waiting," "unnerving waiting," living with "worries." It denies one potential life and creates unnecessary suffering. Professor Z does not perceive the possibility of knowing moving into the background, or of being able to live life even serenely and with more freedom with death in the foreground.

Further, one hears—from this physician who is used to knowing things that patients do not know—a sense of presumption in knowing: God (like physicians) knows things that humans (patients) cannot—and should not—know.

Another frequent way in which knowing shows up in this context is as "courageous" (Appendix, Q4.1). We may interpret this as meaning that knowing is understood as a choice and less as a vital existential necessity because not knowing is still a "live option" (Dreyfus, 1991).

We find different ways of knowing, different interests in knowing, and and differing meanings of knowing among patients (Gordon, 1990). Here let us briefly describe common ways of knowing and being with cancer that I observed among women with breast cancer.

Though there is good indication now that many women in Italy with breast cancer want to be informed of their diagnosis and treatment (Cantoni, 1992; Moscone et al., 1991), a number of things are striking here: (a) the acceptance of minimal information and middle level awareness and understanding; (b) the minimal use of warnings and preparation; and (c) the nonpragmatic uses of knowing. Some of these themes show up in the experiences of Mrs. M and are recounted in the following exemplar.

Exemplar: "It Was 'Carcinoma,' Not a 'Tumor.'"

Mrs. M is a 70-year-old, widowed, middle-class, Florentine woman who still works as an independent salesperson and has two grown-up children, one with a family of her own. She was initially diagnosed through a screening program and was told clearly that a tumor was highly suspected. Because a relative was the head of a department in a private hospital, he "took over" her care in a traditional manner and offered her little information. Her surgeon, known locally for his skill and relative frankness, and his associates communicated the essentials of the diagnosis and operation. After she had come into contact with other breast cancer patients and learned more of what her relative did not tell her, she was very angry, especially at not having understood that her lymph glands would be removed. She wanted and needed to be informed, she said, especially because she is alone. Her narratives for the first 2 years focused on physical symptoms and experiences, and the implications for managing everyday life.

She was remarkably calm about the discovery of a second lump, almost more so than the surgeon who operated on her the first time or the physician who diagnosed her, both of whom were bothered by the recurrence. She had been forewarned that she would probably lose her breast this time because it was on the same side and was told again that the histological report showed the lump was "suspicious." The word *carcinoma* had been mentioned to her.

She went through her operation with extraordinary calm and good nature, joking about things, relieved she had no allergic attack this time. The day after her operation the surgeon had open office hours at 2:00 p.m. for patients and family members. He had already passed by in the morning and had told her that he was able to do another conservative operation. They thought it was *in situ carcinoma* but they took another sample of material surrounding the lump for study to make sure it was not of the infiltrating kind. If in fact it was, she recounted, he said he would have to reoperate (this physician is quite unusual in giving such warnings before the results are in). Mrs. M tried to recount this to me and her son, not understanding well and saying that it was "carcinoma," not a "tumor." The son repeated this distinction, so I suggested that they should check about this with the physician. We stood outside the physician's office at 2:00 p.m., at which time her cousin arrived. Mrs. M. and her cousin began chatting and then decided to go down the hall to wait where they could sit down—I assumed only until the physician came. The son and I stood outside the physician's office and went in alone when the physician arrived. The physician repeated what he had said, saying that there was some concern that the surrounding tissue contained infiltrating cancer cells and that if that were the case they would need to reoperate right away. Given that the surgeon was leaving the next day for vacation, the son asked if the reoperation could wait until he returned. The surgeon discouraged this, saying that it was best to move quickly in such cases. This was relatively shocking news for the son.

The son left the office and returned to his mother. Calmly she wanted to hear what he said, and she listened attentively as he basically repeated what the physician had told her that morning, leaving out the urgency of it and adding that the surgeon did not expect this to be a problem and was very hopeful. Though the son was a bit tense, he performed rather automatically, editing out the important but unpleasant information and emotion and augmenting the positive. His mother quickly and naturally returned to the story she had been telling her cousin about what happened in her room the preceeding night, how the woman on one side of her bed was doing this and the other over there was doing that, how she couldn't sleep at all, but laughing all the way about the absurdities of the situation. I was reminded of a number of other women who did the same and I was struck how easy it would have been for this woman to complain, to have been angry—"the idea of it!"—none of which reactions were present. How little she seemed to live in her mind about how things should be, how easily she went with the flow of life. Making the most of the situation and enjoying life were the dominant modes here, rather than problem solving, wishing it weren't so, thinking how things should be, or worrying about the future.

The woman returned home from the hospital and was "as serene as could be," "like a newborn." After a few days, however, she was called by the hospital and asked to come to a meeting in the next days with Dr. X, her surgeon's associate. Both sons were gone on vacation, and she went alone and received a tremendous shock: she was told that infiltrating material was found and they wanted to reoperate right away. When she told this to her son, he said he had known of that possibility and that maybe he should have told her earlier, but he didn't want "to fill her head just in case it wasn't necessary." She said no, she agreed with him. "Why should I worry about something like that if maybe it won't happen?"

But Mrs. M was absolutely dumbfounded at the idea of having another operation so soon and also extremely displeased at the idea of losing her breast, even if she had been somewhat warned about this for the second operation. She refused to do anything until she spoke to her relatives and until the chief returned from vacation. She was extremely upset and closed herself up in her house "with my problem," not speaking to anyone, for a few days until she arrived at some acceptance of it. Those were very black days, she described, where she preferred to be alone.

Though Mrs. M appreciated being told directly by her physician on his rounds in the morning, she clearly did not understand what he said very well, nor did she struggle very hard to do so. It was fine that her son would go in and hear what the surgeon had to say, but even so, although she was interested in hearing what he had to say afterward, she listened and then went on, without any further questions, to her storytelling, as if it were irrelevant to how she felt then.

A number of things stood out for me as I was present through this story. Like other women I have observed, Mrs. M, though clearly wanting to know what she had and what the physicians were doing, really wanted basic knowledge and outlines rather than detailed, forward-looking, thorough knowledge. Though she asked questions, there was not an active push for clarification, for examining the options of treatments and insisting on more information from physicians, or for wanting to choose which therapy to undergo. Mrs. M., like many others, did not evidence a burning desire to know and control everything. Many clearly want to know and follow what is happening to them. But in the end, it is as if the specific details are not so very important and do not determine their lives very much.

The result is often, as in this case, vague general knowledge or blatant misunderstanding, and middle awareness. On her second operation, both Mrs. M and her son thought that the second tumor was carcinoma, not a tumor (by *tumor* she meant malignant tumor).

Warnings were often kept to a minimum with the reasoning, why cause people unnecessary worry? In fact, we find a strict economy of worry: One deals with what one has to when it happens. With the limited use of warnings comes a bumpier ride with more sudden shocks and more unexpectations. This in turn nurtures a common sense of life as being unpredictable and uncontrollable (Appendix, Q13.2).

Third, I was struck by how automatically the son edited out the unpleasant parts of the physician's report, focusing on and augmenting the positive and the known. Even though he was uncomfortable and, as he later told me, unsure of what to say, he acted quite naturally, as if he, like Dr. J, had had much experience.

The approach toward knowing one's diagnosis and prognosis appears to change significantly when it concerns a very serious prognosis or a metastasis. Here we found that even women who were staunch crusaders about "wanting to know everything" readily accepted a different diagnosis offered by physicians and chose to speak and focus only on symptoms and getting well rather than their diagnosis and the possibility of their dying. As people get sicker, "the truth" begins to appear more irrelevant, clearly secondary to how one feels and to one's relationships, as we hear in the following story of Mrs. Teresa.

Exemplar: "I Don't Know If They Are Telling Me the Truth or Not."

Mrs. Teresa was diagnosed very late with advanced breast cancer. She had always kept herself informed of her situation and insisted on being told what she had. After several metastases had developed, including to the lung, she became sicker and sicker, bothered most by a continuous cough. She was given radiation treatment for symptom relief. More than a month after she finished the radiotherapy, with her cough still constant, she said that her doctor still attributed it to the radiotherapy. This was of course far-fetched, and she said very wearily, "I don't know if they are telling me the truth or not, whether in fact this is from the illness, but for the moment it makes me feel a little better [to believe her doctor]."

There seems to be a living in the in-between spaces, in which one knows and doesn't know, one knows without a name, one knows the general parameters of one's life and what is important for one's life, such as whether one can pick up heavy objects and clean the house alone because one is a widow—this is what matters more than the objective clinical narrative, the name of the illness that is so clearly associated with a terrible death.

The more certain the terminality of the situation, the less negative is said, the more comforting the communication, as if not adding insult to injury. One senses—and here I refer to those situations that appeared to "work" for all involved—that by speaking hopefully and of cure, one guarantees feeling better in that moment, being together in a sense of hope rather than a sense of despair, as if the despair is taken for granted. Knowing about one's fate and the direction one's life is taking is implicit—one knows how one feels, one senses how others feel, on an embodiedlevel. On a level of middle awareness or middle knowledge (Weisman, 1972), people share, in an embodied way, the same reality. Words do not need to confirm, explicate, or reflect this deeper reality; rather, they can and should be used to make people feel better. Boosting each other's spirits and minimizing the situation are fundamental ways of expressing caring and love.

The hope is to stay together, to maintain continuity, to have nothing change. This hope is enacted through the intense presence and protective care of the person (Paci, 1993). A public announcement of the diagnosis, on the other hand, evokes the anticipated future separation in the present and creates an individuation of the individual, so that it is the separation that is lived together instead of continuity and connection. The hope offered here is the sensation that nothing has changed, that life goes on as normally as possible (Gordon, in press).

The effort that this takes on the part of everybody must be considered not only protective of self and other but also an expression of love and commitment, as if a demonstration that they will not let a person go.

The point is not to construct overt endings (Good, 1990) but to keep the narrative open and maintain life and the everyday narrative to the last moment. A good ending is not felt or acknowledged as an ending but rather lived as if life continues as normally as possible until the end arrives (Appendix, Q9.4; Cantoni, 1992). In this way, no life is lost through anticipating or preparing for an ending.

Background/World

In this part we consider two dimensions of this interpretive story. First we briefly describe a network of practices that contributes and intersects with others that may provide necessary background skills involved in communication practices around cancer. Second we consider the understanding of being—of the individual, the social, the natural, the supernatural, temporality and in salvation, and in their possible relationships to the ethical preference for ambiguous, concealed communication around cancer.

Habitus and Network of Related Practices

To spell out what exactly background or world looks like in this traditional context is of course impossible theoretically and practically. But, as the story of Dr. J shows and as we know from other studies, many biomedical practices are not exclusive to medicine but reflect local culture, so that people raised in this local world often learn the skills—a type of habitus—involved in ethical practices at an early age, in their families and communities of origin.

Following are a few representative examples of common practices observed with children around separation, uncertainty, suffering, language, and truth that may constitute formative skills that later contribute and support practices active in the biomedicine and health care.

1. Contestation, giving courage
   - The very common habit of countering depression, sadness, and crying can be observed even in the hospital nursery, as day-old babies are told, "Courage, courage" (*"Couraggio, couraggio"*) when they cry for food.
2. Distraction, no acknowledgment of the source of suffering
   - A child who is just learning to walk falls down and hurts his knee. He is distracted immediately and somewhat urgently by having his attention diverted to a new shiny object nearby. Essentially no acknowledgment of his fall is made.
3. Distraction as cover-up, avoidance of confrontation with separation and suffering; training in living with uncertainty and unpredictability.
   - A young child is left at day care for the morning. With no need for coordinating discussion, his parents wait until he is distracted and then take leave, with no acknowledgment to the child. When their absence is discovered, the child is told that his mother just went out to get some bread and will return in a moment.
   - The G family deliberated at length over the idea of telling their 2-year-old child explicitly that they were leaving instead of waiting until she was distracted, asking themselves whether they were asking their child to deal

with something she was not yet able to deal with, whether it was asking too much of her.

4. Distraction through "invention" or lying

- A baby cries, and the "grandmother" quickly takes him to look out the window: "Look, look at the cat!" she says in an excited, urgent voice. The child looks for the cat. So do I, who have been watching from a distance. I see no cat and, fearing failing eyesight, ask the grandmother where it is. "There is none!" she whispers back.

5. Distraction; suffering is a community concern.

- A child cries loudly on the street, and despite his noise and that of the passing cars his attention is drawn to a building across the street, up on the third floor where a woman claps her hands to attract his attention.
- A very young child cries in the supermarket. A number of people rush up, asking/scolding him, "Why are you crying? You shouldn't cry!"

6. Avoidance

- As mentioned by Dr. J, children are often excluded from death, funerals, and contacts with people with serious illnesses.

These practices, which form part of an aesthetics around suffering that people learn early in life (Desjarlais, 1992), embody and communicate understandings about the nature of suffering: painful emotions are not to be shared, if possible not to be felt, not to be talked about; they are frightening to others, they make them uncomfortable and embarrassed, and it is not kind to express them. Words may be used freely to resolve a situation and to make a person feel better.

Suffering is a social embarrassment, even the suffering of very young children, and is to be stopped immediately. We see direct continuities among these practices with those observed and experienced by adults. In fact, keeping suffering out of the social and personal arena and feeling suffering not accepted in it are recurring themes in both medical and nonmedical arenas.

- Very few newly discovered breast cancer patients publicly cry during the diagnostic process (contrast this to the situation described in Canada by Taylor, 1988). Those who do cry are sometimes scolded as if they were behaving like children.
- Many women with breast cancer often do not feel free to express their sad and worried emotions with their family, in part not to "weigh them down" and in part not to be met with the inevitable wall of negation and minimization (Gordon, 1989; Paci & Venturini, 1989).
- A husband recounts the tremendous effort it took him to control his emotions with his young dying wife. If he showed himself calm, she too would feel calm and feel the situation under control. If he cried with her, the situation would only be worse.

- The most common attempt is to try to diminish or take the suffering away through "trying to pick up another's spirits," minimizing or denying that there is a problem, being "light" and changing the topic (Appendix, Q10.5).
- A woman with serious breast cancer bursts into tears in the courtyard immediately after the funeral service of her beloved friend, who also died of breast cancer. Her circle of mutual friends (most of whom also have breast cancer) all rush to stop and comfort her as she apologizes and suggests they change the subject and talk about where they are going to go. They do just that.

Speaking about problems (Appendix, Q10.7) or crying together about something (Appendix, Q10.6) are only considered to make the situation worse. Notably absent is a language for talking about suffering. But nor is there usually a problem-solving approach to it or its cause. Rather, social support for its removal in the moment is the major strategy.

If the expression of suffering is not allowed into the social scene, where does it go? Much appears to be lived privately, "inwardly," referred to as *"dentro di me"*; and it appears to be expressed through the body (Pandolfi, 1990, 1991).[3]

These practices also embody social ways of being and the strong value of the social:

- The social field is used almost like a magnet to pull someone away from suffering.
- Suffering is a public concern. It is the very strong obligation and responsibility of each person not to cause suffering in another (Appendix, Q16.3) and to relieve it when it is present.
- Emotions are regarded as very social. They are not just the private, insulated possession of an individual; they are basically contagious (Appendix, Q10.8).
- The expression and feeling of suffering appears to be experienced as antisocial, almost selfish, something that serves only the person expressing it but makes others feel bad. It can keep a person more inside and private than outside in the world. It ruptures a smooth social surface.
- Bad news and separations are excluded from the social field.
- Suffering does not necessarily belong to a person but can be taken over by another, and it is the responsibility of others to do this (e.g., women, physicians).

Understanding of Being: Understanding of Human Being

In this section, I consider some preunderstandings and assumptions of this stance that may contribute to the preference for ambiguity and concealment of a fatal diagnosis being lived as the good and ethical thing to do. It must be stressed that the strokes used here are very broad and general, unable to capture the diversity of human lives that one finds in this as in other contexts. It is hoped that those lines of analysis may be explored more extensively in future case studies.

The dominant understanding of Being that comes through in these accounts is relational, part of and in harmony with a larger whole.[4] One is a being in context, open to context and social influence. One is rooted in one's past, a part of it, as one is of one's present. This is an "indexical self" (Gaines, 1985), self-defined by involvements (Appendix Q152), and open to what others say, a self who may "catch" the emotions of the context.

I hypothesize possible parallels among the following understandings of being and practices that may go together:

- a relational/contextual understanding of the person
- agency: much outside of self, in a social field, in those above, in God and destiny
- a temporality located in an embodied present continuous with the past, with the future in the background
- a relational/contextual understanding of words and communication
- a relational/contextual understanding of truth
- goods as relational goods, such as harmony, acceptance, protection, responsibility, serenity, and tranquillity
- hope to remain connected, to maintain continuity with the past, of being cared for
- preference for ambiguity and concealment of fatal diagnosis

These harmonious, contextual, relational, united ways of being in and understanding the world contrast with more essentialist and oppositional understandings and relationships (Ruddick, 1989): the individual as discrete and prior; the past as adversary; the future as a distinct foreground; relations between mind and body self/illness, man/nature as oppositional; words as autonomous; and preference for the explicit and for complete knowledge. They contrast with a technological understanding of personhood, in which people, one's self, one's life, and one's future are objects to control, author, and direct according to one's own desires, and in which information is a fundamental tool for this control.

Understanding of Being Human: Relational Being in a Hierarchical and Differentiated World. The understanding of relational being in this local world shares much with that described by Caudill (1976) for Japanese mothers he studied, who experienced their babies, already within the first months of life, as part of themselves for whom they acted. In contrast, the American mothers, he felt, approached their babies from the outset as separate beings and interpreted the world for them. Family members and physicians act for the patient rather than trying to translate for him or her—ergo the little importance attributed to patients' expressed wishes.

The world is also fundamentally hierarchical (Dumont, 1970), marked by differentiation. Beginning with the distinction between God and humans, there is always someone, something higher than oneself and lower than oneself. One maintains throughout life two positions, moving fluidly between them. One is always a child in life—in the face of God, one's parents, one's elders. And this means that in situations such as illness, one is looked after or taken care of. Others share or have total responsibility for taking care of you. People who know more than you act for you, so you do not have to figure it all out and do it all yourself. You can relax and live life as well as you can while others worry for you. In fact, throughout life, people can "ask for help" from a higher source.

Being vulnerable, lower, weaker, or younger means being respectful, dependent, humble, obedient, and —important to our argument here—in the dark or ignorant about certain matters. Knowledge is central in this hierarchical world. One of the distinctions between God and humans, for example, is that only God knows our destiny. Humans cannot know this and should not know this. In this way, because knowing one has cancer means for many knowing more or less when one will die, this amounts to knowing something one should not or cannot. This is presumptuous, futile, and wasteful, causing more suffering and a loss of real living.

On the other hand, one is responsible for others, especially for those weaker or younger or more vulnerable than oneself—for maintaining their well-being, for not causing them suffering, for deciding and acting for them, for taking care of them. People are basically fragile (Appendix, Q15.4).

Movement back and forth between the strong and the weak, the higher and the lower, the cared for and the caring for is fluid but continues throughout life. This contrasts to more linear understandings and practices, in which the understanding is that one moves from child to adult in a relatively linear unidirectional way.

Relationships tend to be more mediated than direct in this local stance: social relationships, to be sure, but also the important relationship with the supernatural, which until the 1960s was in large part a mediated relationship through the priest because the main rites were conducted in Latin, a language known by only a few.

The term *social,* it should be noted, applies most strongly to one's family, one's local group of trust, which may be a large corporal body where unity is stressed. Here we see great predictability of everyday life, perhaps a defense against the unpredictable forces of change. One is prepared for thriving in and managing this social world which, though complex, is considered basically controllable and trustworthy within small circles.

Thus, in terms of agency and responsibility, much is in the hands of others, and one is socialized into this from the beginning. One may have little control over your life; one is a member of a particular family in a particular locale, and one's identity is strongly defined by this, not just or primarily by what one has oneself accomplished in life. Growing up, one is responsible for few decisions in one's life. Most are in the hands of others (Gordon, in press), and one learns to live with these decisions, to accept them, and to expect them. The individual is not solely responsible for his or her own tranquillity around illness; this is taken care of for him or her by healthy and stronger others. Nor is one considered in large part responsible for one's own cure, or for "working" or "willing" to get better.

Where one's being and identity and possibility are so socially determined, controlling one's destiny and in turn choice are not world defining (cf. chapter 12 of this book) in this context. Knowledge is not necessarily vital for self- determination because one is not considered to determine oneself. In fact, such a view would be considered rather naive because it is felt that people are determined in large part by forces much bigger than themselves.

In fact, many feel that close others would be able to know better than they do what their resources are at the time of a serious illness. This derives not only from a lifetime of being cared for but also from being deeply anchored in a long past—in some cases feeling oneself actively related to the Greeks. The issue of controlling one's destiny, cancer care, and death looks very different within a subjectivity that includes the ancient Greeks and family members. When one's identity is so firmly defined, defining oneself through control and through illness parameters is less crucial.

Understanding of the Good Life. In this context, the relational goods that show up are social unity, familial duty and loyalty (Appendix, Q16.6), and "staying together" (*stare insieme*); a smooth social and individual surface, embodied in the explicit qualities of "tranquillity" and "serenity" and continuity or "maintenance" (*il mantenamento*); respect and responsibility; and protecting others from distress, from *dispiacere.*

Living in harmony with life, accepting life and others, and having respect for others, specifically for authority, are important social values, and many common expressions capture this way of being: the approach is more to go with life, to "arrange oneself," to "accommodate," to accept, to "resign oneself," to "make peace with" or "content oneself" with one's situation (see also Singer, 1988).

The good life, the good way of being, is most often spoken of in terms of "tranquillity" and "serenity"; typical answers to questions such as "How are you?" "How is life?" or "How is your child?" are "Tranquil" or "Tranquil, everything is normal." Obviously within this is the sense that trouble could happen at any unpredictable moment, but that at least for now everything is all right.

A person who is emotionally upset is spoken of as being "agitated" or "nervous" and is urgently implored to "be calm!" This aesthetic of tranquillity and serenity also has parallels in the artistic heritage of the city and region.

Understanding of Relationships With Nature, Illness, and Technology. In contrast to a known, relatively predictable, controllable, and trustworthy small social group is a relatively untrustworthy, unpredictable, uncontrollable, and unknowable "world" or "life" out there, where the adversary is located. Misfortune is basically capricious (Gaines & Farmer, 1986); the good and bad happen through no fault of one's own (Gaines & Farmer, 1986, p. 302), or, as the expression goes, "cancer pardons no one." Many events are basically outside of individual and even human control; they are determined by destiny (Appendix, Q13.1) or God's design.

Illness and nature are relatively independent capricious forces on their own. One faces and deals with illness when it comes (Appendix, Q14.3) more than one goes out to prevent it, meet it, fight it, catch it, or control it. The relationship to illness is less an oppositional relationship than a peaceful one: tranquillity and serenity are the states health professionals try most to instill in patients rather than a combative spirit (Appendix, Q1.5). Faith, compliance, serenity, physician expertise, and family protection are the dominant means here, more than will, work, technology, and partnership (Good et al., 1990; cf. chapter 12 of this book). Basically there is a sense that illness, and nature in general, escape human control, and consequently there is no great expectation that medicine will cure all.

The greatest faith here appears to be in the social, the family, and the supernatural rather than in human ability to control nature and the future. The known, social world "runs interference" (Miller, 1987) on the natural, distant world and constitutes the fundamental reality and basis of truth. This is a world wherein words are tied less to correspondence with an "objective" world, as in the Enlightenment tradition, than to a social world and its purposes (Appendix, Q8.2). On the other hand, the spoken word may be experienced, as mentioned, as having power to invoke realities.

Further, there is a strong lived sense of the limits to knowledge and control. There is much mystery in the world, much that we cannot know—ever— (certainly the church emphasizes this), and consequently there are sharp limits on how much we can predict and in turn control.

Fundamental for keeping this social unity and hierarchy is social and psychological use of a shadowy in-between space of ambiguity. Where social possibility is limited and the demand for unity strong, it provides more space to maneuver in words and desires and unofficial activities.

One wonders—and this must be further studied—how much the belief in destiny is a sense that something is already written for each one of us and that although what we do in this life is important, we are living stories that are already basically predefined. When people say "telling is informing people of their destiny," do they mean that it is informing them of something already "written," already determined?

Temporality, Salvation, and Death.[5] Temporality appears to be in an engaged living in a present that is continuous between past and future. The relationship to the past is openly constitutive, continuing, and harmonious rather than adversarial. It is not a past that one must supersede or from which one must liberate oneself through objectification, disengagement, and change. It is a past lived, embodied, accepted as part of one's self and in which one's self is rooted.

Nor is the future supposed to be so different from the past; it is not clearly objectified as separate from the present. Rather one lives in a river that is continuous between past, present, and future. There is more a notion of eternity of time, as described by Kierkegaard.

Living in the present, however, does not mean that one does not have a future or that the future is not important. Rather, in this context, the future is taken for granted as something that comes to one, that is revealed, that has its own reasons and forces that are unpredictable. It is not a future that stands out on the horizon in the foreground—a future that is a project to be authored, that holds the promise of better times and progress, that one approaches to actively design, that one cultivates as a resource. This future is less seen, more assumed and experienced as background.

Learning of a terminal diagnosis brings this future into the foreground so that one confronts it face to face. For people who already live predominately in the present, this offers few positive possibilities: they have already lived and appreciated life in the now, in contrast to those who have delayed "living" in order to do what they want to accomplish, to define themselves and their lives, or to complete their life's project.

In this local world, time is lived less as linear—working hard for rewards, waiting to live in the future, living by delayed gratification, in which there is no time for things today, only a hope that things will get better in the future and a faith in the future as positive. Open and unpredictable. Ergo, live now while you can.

Basic to understanding this temporality are preunderstandings about life and salvation. Traditional within the Catholic religion is the meaning of life as a divine gift to be lived and appreciated. This gift of life is already given; life and a future salvation do not need to be earned, as is more common in Protestant religions (Weber, 1958). The good is already in the present, in how one lives life. What one does today is one's life and who one is—the quality, not necessarily the quantity or objective success (Giorgi, personnal communication, 1993). It is an unrepeatable gift, as Professor Z said.

Clearly, as the number of believers and practicing Catholics decreases (Cantoni, 1992), the meanings around life, death, illness, and suffering break from their traditional moorings. The effects of the traditions linger on as embodied ways of being. Though we found a large number of professionals believe in "something after death" (Appendix, Q9.3), those who specifically believe in another spiritual life after this one maybe significantly fewer (Cantoni, 1992). Proposed is a decline in the power of the meanings of life as a divine gift and suffering as a means to a better afterlife (Mori, 1992), so that all investment is placed in living this life to the maximum.

When one lives in a particularly embodied rather than a disengaged way, the prospect of a future separation may be experienced more immediately in the here and now. The present is a major stage for the past, present, and future. It is the scene where the good is conveyed and lived. When the future is lived less as an abstract entity but more as an immediate present, words can have particular power to create in the present that to which they refer. It is perhaps in this way that speaking about cancer and death evokes the anticipated separation and brings it into the present, and how not speaking about them keeps them out. Living the continuity of the family, sustaining life as normally as possible, actualizes the hope of life, of continuity, and connection with one's social group (Paci, 1993). This very hope is enacted.

The Problem of Suffering. Suffering is essentially useless in this traditional world (Appendix, Q6.2) and in this social way of being presents some problems. It of course tears a smooth social fabric and, worse, creates suffering in others. Because seeing others suffer causes suffering in oneself, each person has the responsibility to spare others suffering, often through silence and through responding to others who are suffering by drawing them out of it, by being for them in that moment a person who is not suffering. One does not join the sufferer and be "with" him or her, embrace or absorb his or her pain by "expressing it" or by problem solving; rather, one helps the sufferer leave it.

Nor is this suffering solely possessed by the individual. It is a shared, group responsibility, and others must help prevent and remove it.

Publicly expressed suffering is viewed as an embarrassment, a failure of the group to protect or remove another's suffering, or as selfishness on the part of the individual, who makes others suffer by expressing his or her own suffering. With the decrease in the power of Roman Catholicism, suffering, like death, has become untethered from meaning and has become an awkward problem (Mori, 1992). No longer meaningful in terms of a future world, it remains as an embarrassment, a failure, or useless. In contrast to the view of illness and suffering as the failure of the individual (see chapter 12 of this book), suffering here is viewed more as the failure of the group to protect or remove the suffering, or as selfishness and lack of control on the part of the individual. That there is suffering and always will be suffering appears to be taken for granted.

Hope. Hope around death, within a background of accepted death, irresolvable problems, and relative uncertainity about the future, appears to be absent from the background and must be in the foreground; it becomes essential for coping and continuing when life is lived so fully in the present. Hope is more for continuity of the family and normal everyday life, for a particular quality of life free of concern about finitude and suffering, than for longevity or control of life. Starkly absent are the meanings of being in charge, of choosing and controlling and perhaps managing illness, death, or suffering.

In this relational context, hope lies in staying connected and avoiding potential individuation that could result from either the announcement of death or a separation. This is less hope in progress or technology, hope for the control of nature, hope in the challenge of "beating the odds." Hope is not thrust onto the future; it is very much in the present and in a social world. Much more is at stake in taking away hope than in giving "false hope."

Language and Communication Styles. In considering some of the characteristics of communication that relies on ambiguity, the unstated, the indirect, the masked, and the implicit, we may note that such communication generally:

- relies more on face-to-face interaction and is more in the present and embodied because it relies more on comportment
- is possible most among communities of relatively long standing, situations of "high" versus "low context" (Hall, 1977) because they take much for granted
- allows for and requires more interpretation

- creates and fosters unequal, differentiated relationships, wherein some people know more or less than others
- highlights a distinction between social space and personal space, between inner and outer

Ambiguous, indirect communication takes its meaning more from the context; statements are considered not independent in and of themselves but as indexical, open to interpretation, without sharp unambiguous confines. Here, words are lived less as neutral things in themselves, whose existence is based on a correspondence theory of word and "objective reality," as in naturalism. Words can and are used for social means, and "truth" is defined more in these terms than in the correspondence between word and "objective" reality. For example, the common understanding that telling a cancer patient a different diagnosis in order to protect him is not a lie (Appendix, Q2.3) reveals a social definition of truth.

Clear, explicit communication puts something into social space, creates social facts and public space (Taylor, 1985) and allows for more equality. It can be more disembodied communication, relying more exclusively on words for understanding, and it tends to fix and define things rather than leave them open. Precise language and complete knowing can be experienced as having distinct borders, requiring minimal interpretation, and as standing independent on their own—that is, as being relatively autonomous of relationship and context. The word *cancer* in Italy is an example of not only a powerful negative word but, still for some people, a word with very clear meanings of death and suffering.

The Enlightenment view of language as representational, in which words are understood to correspond to a particular objective reality and communication consists of the transmission of information about that reality, leaving as few traces on the message as possible and presenting clear facts, is of course illusory. In this world, language and reality are understood to be blatantly socially constructed.

Conclusion:
World, Possibility, Culture,
and the Human Condition

Different positions regarding disclosure offer different possibilities and preclude others. The availability of possibilities depends much on world, on what can enter and be lived as existential possibilities, as "live options."

Culture provides limits and possibilities, but so does being human. And so we find that within the clarity and illumination of the Enlightenment tradition, people who want to know precisely and be self-determining sometimes feel that they are told too much and would like more uncertainty and more hope (M.J.D. Good, 1993; R. MacIntyre, 1993) and that for some, the protective vagueness and silence in the Italian situation means that one is not recognized "as a person," a good as fundamental as hope. "Recognition as a person," hope, identity, truth, certainty and uncertainty—these are all necessary for people but may be provided in a wide variety of ways, as we have discussed: one may have not the truth about one's diagnosis but the truth of social commitment; one may have not the certainty of knowing what illness one has but have the certainty of knowing who one is.

Whether a tradition tries to deny social and cultural constitution, as in the Enlightenment tradition, and promotes "self-determining acts" such as those currently blossoming in the United States, or whether it recognizes and cherishes social and cultural roots at the expense of emphasizing individual creativity and choice, in the end, people are tied to their pasts and also free to move from them. Whether reality is understood explicitly to be socially constructed in a particular moment, or objective, it is both. Whether emotions are considered to be the private inner possession of the individual or socially constructed and very contagious, they are both. And whether life is considered basically controllable and predictable or basically uncontrollable and unpredictable, it is both. Clearly, emphasis on one side of the equation tips the balance even more in favor of making life show up in the assumed way. But some part of life always escapes and continues to exist unofficially, mystified, called by another name, unnamed.

This brings us back to those "in-between spaces" where for many in this context hope is allowed to exist. Perhaps it is no accident that an Italian anthropologist, Pandolfi (1990, 1991) charts so beautifully and fluidly a geography of the in-between spaces in women's lives, the folds and interstices that defy our dichotomies and that harbor life excluded from more open and sunny terrain. In psychiatry, Weisman (1972) spoke of this zone as "middle knowledge." Recently such terrain has been further delineated by Comaroff and Comaroff (1989, 1991) as they speak of the space between consciousness and unconsciousness where human perception is neither articulate nor absent, but is in shadow, in nuance, in metaphor, in what is unsaid yet clearly felt.

These in-between spaces take on particular life in very social, hierarchical contexts, not only unofficially but officially, as in this context. They constitute a zone well recognized in this local world for its everyday possibilities, where the light of the Enlightenment is not blinding, where encroachment and colonization of the life world by science is incomplete (Comaroff &

Comaroff, 1989). This in-between space may allow room for freedom and fantasy and survival, particularly in its unofficial use. Its official use, however, may foster loneliness, privatizing of experience, confusion, and lack of recognition for the individual. It may be lived as the silencing of the individual, the weak, and the unwanted for the sake of the group and the powerful.

Though in-between spaces always exist, though ambiguity is inherent in human relationships and communication, though vagueness can be understood precisely, though people are constitutively part of each other, the prevailing myth of autonomy and control, scientific clarity and precision, and technological control creates an image of accuracy and precision that may be equally uncertain (Barnes et al., 1993; M.J.D. Good, 1993). It may work to some extent, until it reaches its limits within a particular human ontology and history and begins to be experienced as "inhuman." The prevailing myth that you are always a part of a larger whole, that others should decide, take care of you, protect you, and keep silence over the situation can also work only within given limits of a particular human ontology unitl history enters; and it too can come to be felt by some as too extreme, eclipsing some too-fundamental humanity.

Cross-cultural study of shared human conditions, such as those dealing with severe illness, suffering, and death, helps reveal the elasticity of human beings, our limits, and our commonalities (Kleinman & Kleinman, 1991). It shows us the mutually constituting relationships between a good life, world, and human ontology. It shows us how a practice such as "informed consent" is not monolithic but is set in a whole field of practices, whole ways of being. Disclosure or nondisclosure must be "a caring practice" in MacIntyre's (1981) and Benner's (1990) terms, with inner standards of excellence, skills, and habits. It must reflect not just the "right thing to do" but the "good way to be." "Right" practice that does not address "the good life" becomes, in the end, empty technique. This, of course, is the challenge in situations of change, such as those in present-day Italy.

Notes

1. In a national study in 1988, for example, Moscone et al. (1991) found that only 47% of 1,171 women in a clinical trial for stage I, potentially curable breast cancer were told their real diagnosis.

2. Specifically these studies include semistructured interviews with over 100 "healthy" woman about cancer and prevention (Gordon et al., 1991); an in-depth, open-ended interview study of the experiences of over 20 women with breast cancer (Gordon, 1989, 1990; Paci & Venturini, 1989); a study of family members around the death of loved ones with cancer

(Cardosa et al., 1989); an ethnographic study of 20 women with breast cancer (Gordon, 1991, in press); an ongoing ethnographic study of the cultural basis of noncommunication around cancer based on 50 physician interviews and 20 interviews with other professionals (Gordon, 1991); work with and observations of over 20 nurses and paraprofessionals around their difficulties in working with cancer patients (Gordon, 1990, 1991; Cordoso et al., 1989); and, finally, the questionnaire survey regarding disclosure described in this chapter (Gordon & Paci, 1993; Gordon, in press).

3. It is the distinct impression of clinicians working with women who have had a conservative breast operation, for example, that women express their concern for the cancer and the resulting physical alteration through sensations in their arm—that their arm is bigger and more distorted than it is, that they are more handicapped than they are, and so forth (G. Guasparri, personal communication, 1993; M. Muraca, personal communication, 1993). Headaches, body aches, and excessive pain around the wound have also been noted as possibly emotionally related. Finally, though the numbers are small, 5 of the 20 women I followed took some kind of psychotropic medication and or sleeping pills.

4. This may be an important common denominator among communities that continue with nondisclosure. See, for example, Beyene, 1992; Feldman, 1985, 1992; Holland et al., 1987; Long and Long, 1982; Muller and Desmond, 1992; Ohnuki-Tierney, 1984; and Orona, Koenig, and Davis, in press.

5. This section particularly benefited from interpretive suggestions from Patricia Benner.

References

Barnes, D. M., Koenig, B., Mirande, A., & Davis, A. (1993, March). *Telling the truth about cancer. The ambiguity of prognosis for culturally diverse patients.* Paper presented at the Society for Applied Anthropology, San Antonio, TX.

Benner, P. (1990). The moral dimensions of caring. In J. S. Stevenson & T. Tripp-Reimer (Eds.), *Knowledge about care and caring* (pp. 5-17). Washington, DC: American Academy of Nursing.

Benner, P., & Wrubel, J. (1989). *The primacy of caring: Stress and coping in health and illness.* Reading, MA: Addison-Wesley.

Beyene, Y. (1992). Medical disclosure and refugees—Telling bad news to Ethiopian patients. *Western Journal of Medicine, 157,* 328-332.

Cantoni, L. (1992). Ricerca qualitativa. In G. Di Mola (Ed.), *Qualità della vita e morte individuale: Una nuova cultura del morire?* (pp. 25-49). Milan: POLITEIA.

Cardoso, P., et al. (1989). Per un progetto sperineutale di assisteura continuativa ed integrata al malato oncologico. Fireure: Lega Italiana per la Lotta Coutro i Turnori.

Carroll, R. (1987). *Cultural misunderstandings: The French-American experience.* Chicago: University of Chicago Press.

Cattorini, P. (1993, April). Il consenso informato dalla teoria alla prassi. *Toscana Medica,* pp. 14-16.

Caudill, W. (1976). The cultural and interpersonal context of everday health and illness in Japan and America. In C. Leslie (Ed.), *Asian medical systems* (pp. 159-183). Berkeley: University of California Press.

Comaroff, J., & Comaroff, J. (1989, November). *Anthropology and the nature of consciousness.* Paper presented at the Annual Meeting of the American Anthropology Association, Washington, DC.

Comaroff, J., & Comaroff, J. (1991). *Of revelation and revolution: Christianity, colonialism and consciousness in South Africa* (Vol. 1). Chicago: University of Chicago Press.

Comitato Nazionale per la Bioetica. (1992). *Informazione e Consenso All'atto Medico.* Rome: Author.

Crapanzano, V. (1990). Introduction. Traversing boundaries. *Culture, Medicine and Psychiatry, 14*(2), 145-152.

Desjarlais, R. R. (1992). *Body and emotion: The aesthetics of illness and healing in the Nepal Himalayas.* Philadelphia: University of Pennsylvania Press.

Dreyfus, H. L. (1991). *Being-in-the-world: A commentary on Heidegger's "Being and time, Division I."* Cambridge: MIT Press.

Dreyfus, H. L., & Wakefield, J. (1988). From depth psychology to breadth psychology: A phenomenological approach to psychopathology. In S. B. Messer, L. A. Sass, & R. L. Woolfolk (Eds.), *Hermeneutics and psychological theory* (pp. 272-288). New Brunswick, NJ: Rutgers University Press.

Dumont, L. (1970). *Homo hierarchichus.* London: Granada.

Feldman, E. (1985). Medical ethics the Japanese way. *Hastings Center Report, 15,* 21-24.

Feldman, J. (1992, December). *An American anthropologist in a Paris clinic: Ethical issues in the French doctor-patient relationship.* Presented at the Annual Meeting of the American Anthropology Association, San Francisco.

Gaines, A. D. (1985). The once and the twice-born: Self and practice among psychiatrists and Christian psychiatrists. In R. Hahn & A. D. Gaines (Eds.), *Physicians of Western medicine.* Dordrecht, Netherlands: D. Reidel.

Gaines, A. D., & Farmer, P. E. (1986). Visible saints: Social cynosures and dysphoria in the Mediterranean tradition. *Culture, Medicine and Psychiatry, 10,* 295-330.

Giorgi, S. Personal Communication, 1993.

GIVIO (Interdisciplinary Group for Cancer Care Evaluation, Italy). (1986). What doctors tell patients with breast cancer about diagnosis and treatment: Findings from a study in general hospitals. *British Journal of Cancer, 54,* 319-326.

Good, B. (1993). *Medicine, rationality and experience: An anthropological perspective.* Cambridge, UK: Cambridge University Press.

Good, M.J.D. (1990). *Oncology and narrative time.* Paper presented at the Annual Meeting of the American Anthropology Association, New Orleans.

Good, M.J.D. (1993, November). *The political economy of hope.* Paper presented at the Annual Meeting of the American Anthropology Association, Washington, DC.

Good, M.J.D., Good, B. J., Schaffer, C., & Lind, S. E. (1990). American oncology and the discourse on hope. *Culture, Medicine and Psychiatry, 14,* 59-78.

Good, M.J.D., Hunt, L., Munakata, T., & Kobayashi, Y. (1993). A comparative analysis of the culture of biomedicine. In P. Conrad & E. Gallagher (Eds.), *Sociological perspectives on international health.* Philadelphia: Temple University Press.

Gordon, D. R. (1989). "Vivendo questa nostra storia:" La voce delle donne. In E. Paci & A. Venturini (Eds.), *Dall'esperienza di malattia una nuova cultura* (pp. 17-57). Firenze: Lega italiana per la lotta contro i tumori.

Gordon, D. R. (1990). Embodying illness, embodying cancer. *Culture, Medicine and Psychiatry, 14,* 273-295.

Gordon, D. R. (1991). Culture, cancer, and communication in Italy. In B. Phleiderer & G. Bibeau (Eds.), *Curare, 7,* 137-156.

Gordon, D. R. (in press). La modalità della comunicazione della malattia cancro e lo sfondo culturale. Aspetti psicologici, culturali, e etici nella comunicazione della diagnosis. In G. Invernizzi (Ed.), *Aspetti psicologici, sociali, ed etici della comunicazione della diagnosi di cancro.* Milan: Guiliani.

Gordon, D. R., Belloni, L., & Allamani, A. (1990). *La comunicazione con pazienti con neoplasia.* Firenze: Regione Toscana.

Gordon, D. R., & Paci, E. (1993). Aspetti culturali nella modalità della comunicazione della diagnosi e prognosi di tumore. In G. Invernizzi (Ed.), *Psico-oncologia negli anni '90.* Milan: Guiliani.

Gordon, D. R., Venturini, A., Rosselli Del Turco, M., Palli, D., & Paci, E. (1991). What healthy women think, feel and do about the prevention of breast cancer. *European Journal of Cancer, 27,* 913-917.

Hall, E. T. (1977). *Beyond culture.* Garden City, NY: Doubleday.

Heidegger, M. (1962). *Being and time* (J. Macquarrie & E. Robinson, Trans.). New York: Harper & Row. (Original work published 1927)

Holland, J., Geary, M., Marchini, A., & Tross, S. (1987). An international survey of physician attitude and practice in regard to revealing the diagnosis of cancer. *Cancer Investigation, 5,* 151-154.

Kleinman, A., & Kleinman, J. (1991). Suffering and its professional transformation: Toward an ethnography of experiences. *Culture, Medicine and Psychiatry, 6,* 4-23.

Lombardi-Satriani, L. (1979). *Il silenzio, la memoria, lo sguardo.* Palermo: Sellerio.

Long, S. O., & Long, B. D. (1982). Curable cancers and fatal ulcers: Attitudes toward cancer in Japan. *Social Science and Medicine, 16,* 2101-2107.

MacIntyre, A. (1981). *Beyond virtue.* Notre Dame, France: University of Notre Dame Press.

MacIntyre, R. (1993). *Sex, drugs, and T-cells.* Unpublished doctoral dissertation, University of California, San Francisco.

Merleau-Ponty, M. (1962). *The phenomenology of perception* (C. Smith, Trans.). New York: Routledge & Kegan Paul.

Miller, S. (1987). *Painted in blood: Understanding Europeans.* New York: Atheneum.

Mori, M. (1992). Idee per una nuova cultura della morte e del morire. In G. Di Mola (Ed.), *Qualità della vita e morte individuale: una nuova cultura del morire?* (pp. 50-64). Milan: POLITEIA.

Moscone, P., Meyerowitz, B. E., Liberati, M. C., & Liberati, A. (1991). Disclosure of breast cancer diagnosis: Patient and physician reports. *Annals of Oncology, 2,* 273-280.

Muller, J., & Desmond, B. (1992). Ethical dilemmas in a cross-cultural context: A Chinese example. *Western Journal of Medicine, 157,* 323-327.

Ohnuki-Tierney, E. (1984). *Illness and culture in contemporary Japan.* Cambridge, UK: Cambridge University Press.

Orona, C. J., Koenig, B., & Davis, A. (in press). Cultural diversity and informed consent. *Cambridge Quarterly of Health Care Ethics.*

Paci, E. (1993, November). *The disclosure of the cancer diagnosis and the discourse on competence in Italian medicine.* Paper presented at the Annual Meeting of the American Anthropology Association, Washington, DC.

Paci, E., & Venturini, A. (Eds.). (1989). *Dall'esperienza della malattia una nuova cultura.* Firenze: Comune di Firenze.

Pandolfi, M. (1990). Boundaries inside the body: Women's suffering in southern peasant Italy. *Culture, Medicine and Psychiatry, 14,* 255-274.

Pandolfi, M. (1991). *Itinerari delle emozioni: Corpo e identità femminile nel sannio campano.* Milan: Franco Angeli.

Rubin, J. (1988, January). *Ethics and the concept of the person.* Lecture series at the University of California, San Francisco.

Ruddick, S. (1989). *Maternal thinking.* Boston: Beacon.

Sandel, M. J. (1982). *Liberalism and the limits of justice.* Cambridge, UK: Cambridge University Press.

Singer, M. K. (1988). *Bamboo and oak: Differences in adaptation to cancer between Japanese-American and Anglo-American patients.* Unpublished doctoral dissertation, University of California, Los Angeles.

Spinsanti, S. (1992). Obtaining consent from the family: A horizon for clinical ethics. *Journal of Clinical Ethics, 3*(3), 188-192.

Surbone, A. (1992). Truth telling to the patient. *Journal of American Medical Association, 268,* 1661-1662.

Tamburini, M., Gamba, A., Morasso, G., Selmi, S., & Ventafridda, V. (1988a). Comunicazione della diagnosi di cancro e terapia dei malati in fase terminale. *Federazione Medica, 41,* 487-492.

Tamburini, M., Filiberti, A., Gamba, A., Perry, L., & Ventafridda, V. (1988b). *La comunicazione della diagnosi di cancro.* Milano: Lega Italiana per la lotta contro i tumori.

Taylor, C. (1985). *Philosophical papers* (Vol. 1). Cambridge, UK: Cambridge University Press.

Taylor, C. (1989). *Sources of the self.* Cambridge, MA: Harvard University Press.

Taylor, C. (1991). *The malaise of modernity.* Concord, Ontario: Anansi.

Taylor, K. (1988). Physicians and the disclosure of undesirable information. In M. Lock & D. R. Gordon (Eds.), *Biomedicine examined* (pp. 441-464). Dordrecht, Netherlands: Kluwer.

Thomsen, O. O., Wulff, H. R., Martin, A., & Singer, P. A. (1993). What do gastroenterologists in Europe tell cancer patients.? *Lancet, 341* (Feb. 20), 473-476.

Weber, M. (1958). *The Protestant ethic and the spirit of capitalism.* New York: C. Scribners.

Weisman, A. (1972). *On dying and denying.* New York: Behavioral Publications.

Appendix

RESULTS FROM BIOETHICS QUESTIONNAIRE
Percent in Agreement

Case Example:

	"Traditional"[a]	"Nontraditional"[b]
Physicians ($n = 81$)	51%	49%
Nurses et al.[c] ($n = 158$)	29%	71%

a. "Traditional" = agrees with behavior and reasoning of Dr. J, that is, not informing patient with lung cancer and metastasis about diagnosis or prognosis

b. "Nontraditional" = not in agreement

c. "Nurses et al." = 71% nurses, 8% psychologists, 8% social workers, and others

---

1.4 If a patient does not follow the treatment decision of the physician, it is because the physician was ineffective in convincing him.

	Trad.	Nontrad.	Total
physicians	75%	53%	63%
nurses et al.	55%	48%	50%

1.5 I try to instill in my patients, more than anything:

	tranquillity and serenity			a combative spirit		
	Trad.	Nontrad.	Total	Trad.	Nontrad.	Total
physicians	88%	76%	81%	12%	24%	17%
nurses et al.	69%	61%	63%	31%	39%	37%

2.1 Especially when the patient has a potentially fatal illness, I tend to give the family information that I don't give to the patient.

	Trad.	Nontrad.	Total
physicians	78%	46%	63%
nurses et al.	62%	31%	41%

2.2 Even when a patient with a serious illness wants to know the seriousness of his condition, it is more important that he is serene, even if that means keeping the truth from him.

	Trad.	Nontrad.	Total
physicians	71%	11%	42%
nurses et al.	52%	8%	21%

2.3 If I feel it is better to protect a patient from painful information, I do not consider telling a different diagnosis or prognosis as lying.

	Trad.	Nontrad.	Total
physicians	88%	50%	70%
nurses et al.	84%	39%	52%

2.5 When facing a serious illness, it is the relationships one has with one's family and health care professionals that count more than the "truth" that one is told.

	Trad.	Nontrad.	Total
physicians	67%	64%	66%
nurses et al.	72%	53%	59%

3.1 To tell the truth about a diagnosis of malignant tumor to a patient effectively amounts to "giving him a sentence."

	Trad.	Nontrad.	Total
physicians	44%	23%	34%
nurses et al.	49%	28%	35%

4.1 It takes much courage on the part of the patient with a potentially fatal disease to want the truth of his or her diagnosis.

	Trad.	Nontrad.	Total
physicians	94%	84%	90%
nurses et al.	80%	83%	83%

6.2 Suffering serves little. I try to help my patients avoid emotional suffering as much as possible.

	Trad.	Nontrad.	Total
physicians	98%	78%	88%
nurses et al.	81%	83%	82%

6.3 You should never refuse the request for reassurance by patients regarding the seriousness of their illness, even if that means not telling the truth.

	Trad.	Nontrad.	Total
physicians	82%	48%	67%
nurses et al.	81%	43%	54%

8.2 You can never give much weight to what people say. It is the nonverbal communication that makes you understand what a person wants to say.

	Trad.	Nontrad.	Total
physicians	76%	64%	70%
nurses et al.	72%	70%	70%

9.2 I don't think anyone can really accept the idea of his or her own death.

	Trad.	Nontrad.	Total
physicians	55%	42%	49%
nurses et al.	74%	58%	62%

9.3 I believe in something after death.

	Trad.	Nontrad.	Total
physicians	60%	50%	56%
nurses et al.	53%	65%	62%

9.4 The ideal death is to live as normally as possible until the end, then dying without being aware of it.

	Trad.	Nontrad.	Total
physicians	73%	56%	65%
nurses et al.	63%	50%	54%

10.5 When I see someone "down," I usually try to distract him, to "pick him up," even by changing the topic.

	Trad.	Nontrad.	Total
physicians	85%	66%	76%
nurses et al.	86%	61%	68%

10.6 If someone is crying, sad and depressed, someone who cries with him can only worsen the situation.

	Trad.	Nontrad.	Total
physicians	68%	68%	68%
nurses et al.	73%	68%	70%

10.7 Speaking about painful topics only makes one feel the pain more.

	Trad.	Nontrad.	Total
physicians	58%	34%	47%
nurses et al.	60%	22%	33%

10.8 Emotions are basically "contagious."

	Trad.	Nontrad.	Total
physicians	95%	62%	79%
nurses et al.	82%	69%	73%

11.6 I feel very close to my family of origin.

	Trad.	Nontrad.	Total
physicians	78%	89%	84%
nurses et al.	89%	92%	94%

11.9 When I have a problem, I tend to hide it from the persons closest to me in order not to weigh them down.

	Trad.	Nontrad.	Total
physicians	67%	47%	52%
nurses et al.	47%	38%	40%

12.2 It is we who create reality for each other. For example, if a patient with a serious illness sees you tranquil, he thinks, if he is so calm that means that the situation is not so serious."

	Trad.	Nontrad.	Total
physicians	89%	73%	82%
nurses et al.	86%	75%	78%

13.1 Call it what you will, I believe in some kind of destiny.

	Trad.	Nontrad.	Total
physicians	60%	46%	54%
nurses et al.	57%	59%	65%

13.2 In essence, life is a flow of unpredictable events, that at best we can face spontaneously as they arise.

	Trad.	Nontrad.	Total
physicians	76%	65%	71%
nurses et al.	79%	76%	77%

14.3 I prefer not to worry about my health; if I get sick, then I'll think about it.

	Trad.	Nontrad.	Total
physicians	54%	48%	51%
nurses et al.	37%	25%	29%

15.2 My identity is strongly defined by the people with whom I am emotionally involved.

	Trad.	Nontrad.	Total
physicians	61%	61%	60%
nurses et al.	59%	42%	47%

15.4 In the final analysis, people are quite fragile.

	Trad.	Nontrad.	Total
physicians	56%	56%	56%
nurses et al.	61%	40%	46%

16.3 I was always taught to avoid causing a person to suffer.

	Trad.	Nontrad.	Total
physicians	96%	70%	85%
nurses et al.	77%	67%	70%

16.6 I feel very grateful and obliged to my parents.

	Trad.	Nontrad.	Total
physicians	83%	84%	84%
nurses et al.	84%	75%	78%

16.7 In my family (of origin), there was a tendency to keep one's deep emotions to oneself.

	Trad.	Nontrad.	Total
physicians	69%	64%	67%
nurses et al.	44%	44%	44%

20.3 On a gut level, notwithstanding all the progress in the field, when I hear the word *cancer,* I feel it's an incurable disease.

	Trad.	Nontrad.	Total
physicians	54%	54%	54%
nurses et al.	75%	53%	60%

15

❖

Narrative Methodology in Disaster Studies

Rescuers of Cypress

CYNTHIA M. STUHLMILLER

Researchers agree that natural and human-created disasters have a strong psychological impact on individuals, communities, and those who become involved in helping in disaster recovery. They disagree, however, about the nature, extent, and consequences of these events. Traditionally, two competing positions have guided inquiry and conclusions in this area. Most researchers believe that disasters create adverse psychological reactions both immediately after the impact and for a long period—perhaps for the individual's entire life span. The less popular position holds that although some individuals experience adverse reactions, research has greatly overstated the extent of those negative consequences and has overlooked some positive outcomes: the enhanced coping abilities with which many victims and helpers emerge from their experience.

Disaster studies in the past decade have largely followed the rational-empirical school of thought and typically have attempted to answer causal questions in order to explain negative consequences in terms of the canons of positivistic science. These decontextualized and objective views have limited our ability to grasp the range of common and idiosyncratic interpretations of disaster in the flow of human experience.

If a goal of nursing science is to uncover not only factors that compromise well-being but also those that facilitate it, then discovering the personal and cultural meanings and strategies that enable individuals to cope with crisis in constructive, self-enhancing ways is essential.

On October 27, 1989, an earthquake measuring 7.1 on the Richter Scale struck the San Francisco Bay Area, causing the collapse of .76 miles of a double-decked roadway known as the Cypress Street viaduct and resulting in the tragic death of 42 people. This event provided an opportunity to examine the experience and effects of rescue work as it was lived and given meaning. These rescue workers are a rich source of practical knowledge that can be used to reconcile an overly individualistic pathological view and an overly social view that excludes personal meanings and experience.

An interpretive study was conducted among rescue workers who were directly exposed to the life-threatening conditions created by the disaster. The data included participant observation, document analysis, and interpretive analysis of semistructured interviews with 42 rescue workers, including coroner-investigators, transportation workers, military pararescuers, and firefighters. The study explored the rescuers' motivations, actions, coping strategies, interactions, and understanding of their responses to the event, as well as the practical wisdom each acquired.

This chapter uses the narrative data to describe the specific work meanings and practices of two occupational groups, illustrating how those meanings shaped forms of involvement, issues of stress, and sources of coping and influenced the experience of rescue work in this disaster. The careful study of individual narratives permits the discovery of what a particular event meant to its participants.

To understand the experience of these rescue workers, an in-depth exploration of them as individuals was the first step. Each person described their life history embedded in a network of meaningful relationships provided by membership in a culture, community, job, and family. Their narratives revealed individual and shared concerns based on occupational roles, demands, and prior experience. The first section describes work responsibilities, socialization into work practice, and work sustenance, or that which keeps people involved in their projects. The following section that illustrates how specific work meanings and practices guided involvement and issues of stress at Cypress. The final section summarizes the importance and relevance of uncovering occupationally based meanings and practices and the significance of narratives to this project.

Pararescuers: "We Do This So That Others May Live."

Pararescuers, or PJs, are an elite group of highly trained men attached to various military outfits. They were formerly known as Parajumpers (thus the abbreviation PJ) because their function was to serve as special forces medics, responding to rescue and recovery of wounded soldiers behind enemy lines. Today there are approximately 500 PJs in the country. In peacetime they train extensively for the rescue and recovery of civilians. If assigned to the National Guard, they are under the jurisdiction of the state. Those attached to the Air Force are governed and regulated by the federal government. One informant gave further explanation:

> We have a combat mission, our mission is to rescue downed air crew members behind enemy lines, so if war breaks out, a guy goes out and gets shot down, it's our job to get in there any way we can and bring him back. And that means get in with scuba diving, with mountain climbing, with parachuting, high altitude drops, whatever it takes to get there is what we have to do to recover them. Then we treat them medically. So that's our job. The offshoot of that is the fact that when war is not happening, we do a lot of civilian rescues. When we're not doing civilian rescues, we're training. We go to climbing schools in British Columbia and Scotland and Wales, go glacier training in Iceland and Greenland, go all over the world for all sorts of emergency medical training courses, winter survival, summer survival.

Though the personal backgrounds of these men vary widely, it is striking to hear how each one comes to share in a common concern to save life. Their motto, "We do this so that others may live," is proudly worn in the form of a pin on the beret of each PJ, symbolizing their hard-earned special status. Each member, through rigorous training, indoctrination, and socialization, comes to know, understand, and embody this motto. The narratives of these men provide illumination as to how their personal and occupational backgrounds and concerns set up what is salient or stressful about a situation. Using the words of three informants, the following excerpts offer a representative glimpse into the background histories of PJs, including why or how each became involved in the work.

Becoming a PJ

Tom entered the military during the Vietnam conflict because of the patriotic influence of his small hometown community. He found the paramedic aspect of basic training very exciting and decided, "It would be more appealing to be on the rescue end than to be on the other end of the rifle." In describing the missions he was part of in southeast Asia, he spoke fervently of the high degree of commitment, professionalism, and intelligence of his peer group: "The camaraderie, the adventure, excitement . . . something to belong to, with the goal of helping others." These things have become important to Tom and he continues to seek them in his work and life.

Upon return to the States, he returned to school, explaining that school for him was a wonderful way to reintegrate into civilian life after returning from the hostilities and insanity of war. After working in the Sheriff's Department, Fire Department, and an ambulance service, because he was bored and newly divorced, he rejoined the Air Force.

He talked about his years of involvement in important rescue missions all over the world with pride and enthusiasm. In fact when asked what motivated him, he slammed his beret on the table and pointed with tears in his eyes to the emblem that says, "We do this so that others may live."

Ralph, the youngest PJ, reported his reasons for being in pararescue:

> I've always liked to help people out, basically anyone who is feeling ill or in trouble, and a friend told me about pararescue. I also read about it in some magazines. So when I came into the Air Force, I kind of had the idea I wanted to be a pararescuer. I got involved in a training program, which was quite a hard program. It took me a year and it was mentally demanding, and I liked that—that and helping people.

When asked where that comes from, he answered, "Probably from my mother and father. They are very giving people, always wanting to help someone out. . . . That's probably where I got it." Although he speaks of his parents with admiration, it is evident that he is somewhat emotionally distant from them. Later on he offered:

> I pretty much grew up on my own. I mean I was pretty much a loner when I was younger. I never really related to people that much. I was pretty much on my own, doing my own thing. . . . My best friend died on me when I was 16. We were really close and he had got in a motorcycle accident and drowned. That's one of the reasons why I wanted to get into helping people.

In talking about getting into pararescue work, he said, "Well, it was a challenge to me as well. I really enjoy challenges. If a person is not challenged, he has no self-development—that's what I feel. So I always tried to find challenges. It just kind of fit the framework."

Ralph also described the grueling indoctrination for PJs that includes what are known as crossovers, where the indoctrinee swims back and forth under water with the instructors pulling off his face mask, disconnecting the oxygen tanks, and attempting to drown him. He explained, "It's just mind games is what they play with you. Considering the job and how stressful it is, you have to be mentally stable."

Ted, a PJ of 15 years, also revealed a background history suggestive of the challenge that typically lures PJs into the field. Even early on, Ted was confronted by some tough moral issues.

Father was very ambitious and motivated by material things; Mother was strictly motivated by her children—the love she got from her children kind of sustained her. I ended up seeing, on one hand, that material possessions were nice, but, on the other, a gut feeling that what was important was not the material things. As a result, I think I learned the two sides of the situation. It gave me an insight that I think I might not have had otherwise.

Ted ran away from home at 17 because of the conflicts and abuse his father began to show his sister after their mother died of cancer. "When I was 14 . . . things kind of went to crap at home. I was like a zombie at the time, everything happened in slow motion, I was almost not feeling at all." Ted pursued a music career at a prestigious music school, partying extensively until he flunked. Having lost his study grant, he decided to join the Air Force to take advantage of the GI Bill. "All of a sudden I realized the jobs were boring, [and I] asked the recruiter, 'Do you have anything like special forces?' and he said, 'Yeah, we have these guys called PJs but they're superhuman. You're never going to be able to do that.'" Having been an athlete in high school, Ted decided that he could meet any physical demands, so he said, "Put me in that, that's what I want to do." He didn't have a love relationship with pararescue at the time; for him the decision was strictly one of economics and travel: "I wanted to travel and see the world. So I ended up passing the program, and after a year and a quarter of training, I made pararescue and put on the beret. After about a year I started to realize this was just a fantastic career field."

Analysis

Analysis of the narratives of PJs shows that several striking similarities stood out in their backgrounds. All of them had experienced a significant loss by death or separation as children or young adults. For example, Tom talked about his fallen comrades in Vietnam, Ralph's best friend died in a drowning, and Ted's mother died of cancer. Every other PJ of the sample as well described family backgrounds of premature loss of parents to cancer, divorce, and alcoholism. In addition, each discovered in their work adventure, challenge, and/or the call to help others.

There are two levels of possible explanation in operation here—psychological and cultural. Psychologically, the desire to help others could result from the individual's need to compensate for the sense of vulnerability, helplessness, and powerlessness experienced in those earlier losses. On the cultural level, gaining mastery is part of the individual's quest to overcome chaos and adversity. The PJs' training and rites of passage reflect this shared value, which is essential to success in their work.

For PJs, the crossover indoctrination typifies the psychological test that separates the strong from the weak. Each individual, having withstood the rigors of training, shares in a common bond of competency and excellence. Though teamwork is essential for success in missions, the emphasis seems to be on the fortitude of the individual. Ultimately the team is only as strong as its individual members.

Sustenance of a PJ

Besides the fun, challenge, and excitement of pararescue work, at least two deeper reasons seem to keep people in the field. Membership in an elite group is one. Two excerpts illustrate this notion of exclusivity.

> I think in pararescue you're trained to such a point where you're going to be doing that job no matter what. You're sacrificing your life to save somebody else's, and I think that's how pararescuers are different from any other person in the Air Force, from any other person in the Department of Defense, the SEALs, Army Special Forces, Army Rangers, Reckon in the Marines. . . . Pararescue is a different breed than most Joe Blows.

The following statement also speaks to this level of specialized commitment.

> We train to go in where other people can't. That's basically our job . . . and we've got the individuals who can go in, we identify with our motto, "So that others may live." And speaking for myself and any of the PJs here, we will sacrifice ourselves no matter who it's for. We're ready to represent pararescue.

Perhaps the most crucial sustaining element of pararescue work lies in the rewards of the practice itself. PJs typically recalled their first live rescue experience as an epiphany that solidified their commitment to the work.

> It was the best one, you know. You save someone's life. . . . First one was a guy that fell down 6 feet deep in a steel hole and was all busted all up. We had to do everything. . . . I think the most satisfying thing was . . . after we started working on him he started responding, "Hey, yeah, how's it going, oh, trippy, man." So, I always had a very satisfied—good work, guys, look, you saved me! I think everyone feels satisfaction in doing things like that.

A 15-year veteran PJ reflected:

> I think what got me addicted was the first couple of saves I experienced. The adrenalin-releasing act of the mission itself. When the mission breaks and you find out you have an injured person at sea, then you have to put all your gear together, you jump on in, you're out there for days treating this individual on the open ocean, you get across the ocean any way you can to save the guy's life. Then the feeling that you get as a result of having done that, when he says, "God bless you," or "Thank you, if you hadn't done that I would be dead by now." It's almost like an addiction. I think this is what truly made me decide that this is what I wanted to do.

Individuals who find their work meaningful are inclined to continue that work. To save a life makes any and all efforts worthwhile. The seasoned PJ continued:

> I think that life is very, very important, and I have that feeling that what I do matters. I know that when I go out there and I'm going to rescue an individual, that I'm going to bring him back to children that love him and a wife that needs him. The essential fact is that it's just the right thing to do, and that gives me a purpose in my life that I think is very important.

If the concern to save life even at risk to self defines and sustains the pararescuer, it stands to reason that retrieval of dead bodies would define what becomes stressful. Death is final, leaving the pararescuer no opportunity to intervene, alter the course of outcomes, or "make a difference." Because these options have been eliminated, a feeling of helplessness and depression can result unless a purpose and meaning for the work can be generated. The following excerpts from a 23-year PJ illustrate this struggle to find meaning when it is not readily apparent.

> Rescue, the thing of living, gives you the esprit. And in recovery, they died and now you are going to live with that. The body, you just pick it up, it is never going to live and you're always going to believe in that. . . . We have a little thing that those that fought for life have a feeling that they are protected from everything [are invulnerable]. So when you are out there and you've got Joe Shmo somewhere, you are going to go in and get that guy. But when you are going in after dead bodies, it's rough because you know they are not going to live. . . . People have to have a reason, I think, for being there. Now when you are there for rescue, you have a clear mission a hand and good rescue guys will do anything for someone alive even if they put their own life in jeopardy—this is continuous throughout their life.

Having a purpose for the work is also essential. As in the case of retrieving dead bodies, a reframing of the mission is often required. The following conversation with a PJ involved in rescuing five people from a drowning accident illustrates the shifting of focus onto those who remain.

> That had a decent effect on my life in terms of—four adults went in to save three children. . . . I think the innocence of the children will get to you . . . right in the prime of their life going down. . . . Yeah, that kind of gets to you. You know they are dead, there is nothing you can do. All you are trying to do is save a family more grief. The family is on the side of the lake. You're acting as professional as you can, because you know they're listening to everything that goes on. . . . It's just the job that was expected of us and we got out of there. That's where I think we somewhat excel, because pararescue guys . . . can actually separate emotions from the scientific or whatever you want to call it approach, that's where I think we might differ from the average.

Saving the family more grief became the purpose in this mission. Reframing the purpose, along with keeping emotions separate, allowed this pararescuer to do his work. PJs also discuss the strong foundation of character and habits from which they derive motivation to save life at all costs.

> What are you going to do when all of a sudden the weather goes to shit and the guy's life is in danger. It seems to me that for some reason the very qualities that made this guy on a daily basis give a crap about completing his schedule, performing, being punctual, also are what carries him through in a stress situation. In contrast, if they are motivated by the fact that visibility and heroics and the self-fulfillment of maybe doing something that they think is important, and then that falls by the wayside. It's varying degrees where it just seems to not work for them. All of a sudden, the ones that it works for are the ones that you kind of knew all along it would. Consistency, performance, reliability, dependability, the very things that on a daily work basis these people exemplify, in a stress situation seems to be the very things that you knew you could depend on them for.

Analysis

Are the characteristics of these individuals inherent or developed through the rigors of training or experience? These narratives suggest both. Each person reveals something that explains their reasons for becoming involved in the work, as well as the sustaining features of that "live find" that keeps them involved. For the PJs, there is no doubt as to the purpose or goal of pararescue. "To save life" is a society-sanctioned function of utmost importance. To do so at risk to self suggests a heroic quality and thereby must attract individuals with special needs and capabilities. To stand out as someone courageous in facing death with a special mission might be acknowledgment enough to keep anyone involved, but when the status or mission is threatened, the individual must create a new purpose and goal. It is then that the individual is challenged to draw on his or her personal beliefs, commitments, habits, and convictions to endure the unpleasant demands of the work.

Firefighters:
"We Help People, We Make a Difference."

The firefighters in this study come from the City of Oakland Fire Department. This department is considered to have some of the toughest runs of any department in California and perhaps the entire United States. The firefighters serve a community with a very high crime rate threatening the value of a human life. Actual firefighting constitutes a small percentage of their calls. They primarily respond to medical emergency calls, initiate first aid, and control traffic and crowds until police and paramedics arrive. Despite the constant exposure to the down side of life, their stories express a love for their work and for each other.

Besides 10 weeks at a training academy and a written examination, the tradition of firefighting is handed down from the "old-timers." For example, there is the old-timers' model of how to handle emotions in difficult situations. One young firefighter reported: "The old-timers' thing of not letting your emotions show and all that, and it's kind of like don't let it affect you emotionally because if it affects you emotionally, you are going to be affected—your whole performance is going to be affected." The fire department policies also foster a particular acculturation that influences how business is conducted. The Oakland Fire Department, like other departments, schedules work in shifts of 24 hours every third day. Though there has been some discussion of changing the schedule to the more conventional 8-hour, 5-day-a-week routine, this idea has been met with opposition by the firefighters themselves. There are several reasons for this sentiment. The most frequently mentioned reason for keeping things as they are is, "The hours are great. . . . I love my time off. . . . The scheduling is one of the job's attractions."

The 24-hour shift may also serve a vital support and team-building role because of the nature of the work and the tight interdependent relationships that develop as a result of living and working together over the extended period of time. Besides each firefighter's particular work role, he or she must additionally contribute to the day-to-day tasks involved in living together.

Household chores such as meals, shopping, cleaning, repairs, and general environmental maintenance provide the firefighters an opportunity to really get to know and care about one another. Caring about and for oneself in this type of setting becomes synonymous with caring about and for each other. Trust and bonding between firefighters are essential ingredients in the success of their work. Firefighters state that the dangers they face are eased by knowing they are a member of a team they know and have confidence in. The intensity of the work is shared and absorbed by this interdependent family system in a way that would not develop without the 24-hour shift.

Because the job is physically demanding, firefighters must keep healthy and fit. When not out on calls, they engage in exercise such as weight lifting, running, basketball, and other sports in order to keep in good shape. These activities foster camaraderie through fun and team building and allow individuals to feel good about themselves and their bodies. Indoctrination and socialization of firefighters therefore seem to be on the job rather than in training and testing processes.

Becoming a Firefighter

Very few of the firefighters interviewed set out with firefighting as a career goal. Their background histories indicate, however, that after becoming a firefighter, each developed a commitment to the work. Using a few examples, the stories below provide the varied motivations that attracted them to the work.

Pete feels he is a natural for the job.

> Reacting in a stressful situation was something I realized early in life that I could do. I used to tell my mother when I was a kid that I wanted to be an efficiency expert when I grew up because I liked the idea of putting a number of things on and have them come to fruition at a certain given point in time. That was my title when I was 10 or 12 years old, I'd get up and cook the whole family breakfast, and I actually got a charge out of making the eggs come out at the same time when the toast popped up and when the bacon was done. I like the plan that comes together.

Pete described his experience serving as a medic in the Vietnam conflict.

> I worked in surgery, which was a good experience. . . . I liked the team spirit. If you know anything about the military it's obvious there is a chain of command—do what you're told when you're told—but I was working with a group of doctors . . . and I liked it. . . . I further liked the feeling of making a difference . . . accomplishing something very visible.

Pete also described the constant uneasiness of Vietnam, which he coped with by staying centered. "When something happened I'd find a center point in whatever the situation was . . . just to make it out alive. So it worked, I made it back."

He joined the Oakland Fire Department in 1986 after working a number of years in the "sterile environment of computers." He explained how fortunate he feels:

> I made it just in time—so I think I got in just under the wire, I found my niche. . . . It's wonderful. . . . I'm with good people, I do a good job. . . . I don't know how to describe how I got to this, other than [there were] certain things I wanted to accomplish. One of those things would be extending my feelings of self-worth. . . . I feel good about myself, and when you feel good about yourself, you want to pass it around. . . . Mine's a free spirit tempered with some discipline. I think it sounds probably a little hokey or folksy to say, I guess I'm just tying to make a better world.

Growing up in a close family provided him with a strong foundation of being able to work with people.

> I just remember having a good time growing up, good memories and a close family, close friends, other families who were close friends, which I think helped a lot. It reinforced what was already a solid foundation of being close to other families, so maybe that's why I like what I'm doing so much. It's the same principle, in a way, as networking with each other in the station for some common goals. I guess I've always liked working with people, I like making a difference, that's another thing, and I also like the immediate gratification, I like to see what I've done or haven't done fairly quickly. I guess I've been very fortunate in my life to work in areas that interest me.

Rick, born and reared in Oakland, also described a very close family background. His father was a firefighter for 28 years who died on the job in 1975. "At the time I wasn't in the department and I had not really had a childhood desire to be a firefighter. It was just the right time to examine this area." Rick has a law degree but chooses to continue firefighting. "I enjoy the job. It's been very rewarding for me and I really get a lot out of it. I'm happy with it."

Charles went to Catholic school, which he claimed had an effect on him—"that stands out, leaves an impression." From there he went into the Navy, and was in from 1967 to 1971. He was in Vietnam, stationed in D'nang doing aircraft maintenance. Before getting out of the Navy, he took the firefighter's test, "then 2 months after I got out I came on at the fire department, so it was a real nice transition. It was nice, from a Catholic school to the service to, at least when I came in, an all boys' atmosphere."

> I could have been a GS worker and gone right back to developing test programs for electronics and stuff, but I was kind of burned out on that and this service thing and I wanted some personal feelings back, all that kind of stuff. . . . So it wasn't that I wanted to be a fireman, or wanting to help people and all that kind of stuff, it was pretty much just a thing that I kind of fell into by taking the test.

Seth was in the Coast Guard for a while. "The military was kind of my cup of tea. And so I kind of liked the field and I kind of pursued it, so I was taking tests before I got out of the military." He worked for the county coroners and then an ambulance service before getting his job with the fire department.

Seth enjoys his work, equating it to playing on a football team.

> I find a lot of satisfaction in supporting the team and stuff like that because we're a team. It's not to be overlooked, it's just like they say, you know you hear in all the papers about the quarterback of the team. And he always says, "There's a lot of guys that were behind me."

Vince is third oldest of a family of 12. Because his parents didn't speak English and because he was the most outspoken and aggressive, he served as their interpreter.

Vince grew up in a part of town where it wasn't unusual to walk over a dead body or see someone get shot or stabbed.

> The fire department was pretty noticeable because of all the work that they had to do, and I was always amazed. That's what I wanted to be. I wanted to be a fireman when I was about 14 or 15. I asked some firemen that used to work out at the YMCA what it took to be a fireman, and one guy looked me dead in the face and said, "Son, you'll never be a fireman." Now I don't know why he said that. I don't know if it was racially motivated or if he just felt that I wasn't going to grow or whatever, I really don't, and I just said, "okay."

He described how he feels about his work:

> I've always had a level head in an emergency, even as a child, so when I was assigned to this station I was very fortunate because at the time this was the most experienced crew in the whole city. You feel good when people acknowledge that you've done something good, but whether people acknowledge me or not, I feel good about myself and about what I'm doing. That's the bottom line.

Analysis

These firefighters have differing backgrounds and motivations for being involved in their work. From Vince's lifelong desire to be a fireman to Charles's "just falling into it," each has come to enjoy the challenges and teamwork.

There are similarities and differences between what attracts and sustains firefighters and PJs in their jobs. The "all boys" atmosphere and military or quasimilitary atmosphere stand out as one overlap. A majority of the firefighters are military veterans. Another similarity seems to be wanting to help serve or work with people. Both career fields provide challenge and excitement.

There are several differences between the two professions. Firefighters make substantially higher wages than PJs. The 24 hours every third day shift work of firefighters is also a major attraction of the job. Some of the PJs described actively seeking out their jobs and have an ingrained purpose to save life. Much of this clarity seems to come from their intense training and indoctrination, but it is additionally reinforced by the nature of the situations they respond to. In contrast, most firefighters developed the love for their work on the job, despite some of the meaningless situations they become involved in. This distinction will become clearer in the next section, which discusses what sustains firefighters.

Sustenance of Firefighters

As with PJs, firefighters especially feel the rewards of their work when they are able to save a life. One firefighter explained:

He didn't have a pulse and we'd revive him. It's the kind of thing I felt warm about. It hasn't happened as much lately, but it's the type of thing that reaffirms, rekindles. In a way we all look for the times when we can make a difference. I think that's a real underlying and unifying thread through most of the guys' attitudes about the job.

This passage illustrates the major reward of the job: making a difference. The possibility of saving life does not often present itself to these firefighters. More often, they are faced with the challenge of improving a bad situation or trying to make a difference. As one firefighter said, "You're there to actually try and make something of the emergency situation already there. There's nothing you can do about that, what you have to do is make the best of what's there."

Firefighters are in the business of helping people and protecting property. The call to do so provides purpose for their work. However, when the situations prove to be bogus or are acts of violence, the narrowed possibilities for successful intervention are met with mixed emotions.

> I think you get agitated when you go out there. I think it's a level of caring, caring about what level of service you give, not taking seriously the things that you encounter. . . . You start looking at 75%, 85% of them are just useless things that you go out on. For example, somebody's got a kid that's got a cold. Well, how long's the kid had the cold? Well, for two weeks. Well, have you taken him to the doctor? No, we haven't. Why not? Well, we just haven't gotten around to it. Well, take your kid to the doctor, do what normal people who raise kids would do. I mean, the kid's not going to die, so unless they're going to die, there's no reason for calling us. We're not here to take care of your headaches and constipation and colds and those kinds of things, and I think that if you went throughout the department you would find that most people kind of feel that way. You sit in a firehouse and watch the people who work in a firehouse and see how they react when a call for a fire comes in, and watch how they react for a call for an EMS, and it's totally different. I mean the effort given to speedily get to the rig and leave the firehouse, there's a great difference.

Another firefighter described:

> For 16 years I've worked in one of the busiest firehouses the city's got going. Oh, I had four triple murders, and probably 10 or so double murders and so many singles that I can't even count them. . . . It's part of life. You know, it's east Oakland. It's living in east Oakland. Death is a real meaningless item down here. Life is not a high-priority item. This city is in the top 10 in the nation per capita in murders.

This firefighter summarized what the others have expressed about dealing with acts of violence:

> I think what you have to do is realize what goes on is part of life. You can't control the things that happened, all you can do is try to help people, and if you aren't there to help them, you don't feel guilty about things. You don't feel like anything was your fault . . . and I think you feel good if you can help them a little bit, so the fact that you can go in there and help people quite often helps you deal with that type of situation. We do see a lot of pain and misery, but at least we can do something to help that.

The following statements express the predominant outlooks of firefighters that serve to sustain them:

> I think it takes a certain kind of character to be an effective fireman. It takes a certain kind of personality to be—you know, if you get one of these individuals that's so intellectual he's going to rationalize and weigh things out and all this, he's going to be useless. I mean, when they swore me in, it was to save lives and to protect property. That's what this is all about. To save lives. That doesn't mean that I'm going to go in and sacrifice my life to try to save someone else's. That'd be stupid. But, at an instant, I can make a judgment call on whether or not I'm able to do this successfully. My captain, my chief, anybody can tell me, hey, go do that, but if I don't think I can do it successfully, fuck you, you do it, because I'm not going to sacrifice myself for anybody.

Analysis

What sustains firefighters in their work is similar to what sustains pararescuers. However, because firefighters face more bogus calls and have less opportunity to save life, they tend to be more experienced in shifting meaning and goals. "To make a difference" tends to be their call to duty: "To improve a situation but not at cost to self." The last phrase underscores the caution with which firefighters approach their jobs. Unlike pararescuers, firefighters don't engage themselves unless the odds are in their favor. The notion of teamwork is also more important to firefighters than to pararescuers.

The physical and mental challenge, the adrenalin rushes, the close-knit working conditions, the time off, the good salary, and the help they are able to render the community keep these firefighters engaged. Threats to these conditions define appraisals of stress.

The firefighters' stories depict an esprit de corps indicative of the nature of their work. Their indoctrination and socialization are based on the concept of teamwork. Because many of their calls are medical and often bogus, they find meaning in assisting the community by making a difference.

Their stories also reveal patterns that link these separate individuals to each other in ways based on occupational roles, demands, and experiences. The PJs entered their jobs to "save life" and described the strong personal and professional commitment required to withstand the rigorous demands of the work. They are socialized and indoctrinated to be self-reliant and determined because they often work separately. As PJs tell a story of a successful mission, the rewards and sustaining aspects of the work become extremely clear.

These oral accounts reveal the common and unique perspectives, backgrounds, and experiences from which these individuals came to participate in the significant event of Cypress. The following section continues tracing the distinct patterns of meaning, involvement, and concern related to occupational affiliation that accounts for variation in experience.

Pararescuers' Involvement:
Obligation to Heroism

The roles and functions of the PJs define a pattern focusing on the obligation to heroism. Their motto, "We do this so that others may live," embodies their existence. They come to know that the team is only as strong as the individual and that success in their work depends on their dependability, consistency, determination, courage, and selfless dedication—qualities that emphasize the importance of saving life at risk to self. Early in training, the PJs learn to overcome their fear so that they can come through in the tight situations they will face and may often face alone.

The self is central in their projects. Ultimately, their commitment to saving others is self-defined, self-motivated, and self-sustained. The determination to "press on" keeps individuals focused on their goal and reminds them that they dictate their own choices. The very presence of PJs at Cypress was the result of a PJ's following his own convictions. The prime example was Ted, who disobeyed orders, put his job on the line, and did what he thought was right, taking a team uninvited to the Cypress site.

Ted: "We Are Probably the Most Qualified, Highly Trained Individuals Available."

We ended up responding, but only in an air capacity [originally dispatched by helicopter to survey areas of damage]. They used our equipment, and we ferried VIPS around while people on the ground were dying and needed help. The mentality of the people that had command of our unit was that we were an air resource and were doing our job. The mentality of the pararescue unit was what the hell are we doing here, man? We are probably the most qualified, highly trained individuals available. We were extremely irritated that all we were doing was fulfilling a nonessential function. . . . So at the end of a particularly frustrating first day, . . . I said, screw this bullshit. I formulated in my mind that I was going to get off the plane when I was released, I was going to get the truck, and I was going to head out to the areas of devastation.

Upon arrival at Cypress, Ted witnessed techniques that bothered him because he knew a better way to do it.

I jumped down and said, "Whoa, man, back off, what are you doing?" A guy goes,"What do you mean, what am I doing?" And I said, "Hey, you recover bodies like this, you got to take it easy, buddy. This guy is crushed. You're going to start dismembering his body real quick." So all of a sudden the coroner comes over. The coroner remarked, "Do you know that we have only recovered five people all day?" Inside of about 4 hours, pararescue recovered 17 people because we got up inside these structures and rigged up a system to get them down. We did this all through the segments of the bridge.

The situation at the Cypress, it was just important to me that I participated in some way, and if that meant only getting bagged bodies to the relatives, then that was important enough. That's all we did, we didn't save lives—there was nobody alive, but always in the back of our mind was the fact that there *might* be somebody alive. There was a chance that could have happened.

Ted defined, accepted, and carried out the obligation he felt, using self-initiative and determination. A quality of elitism is evident in Ted's statement, "We can do it better than any one else." The superior value of the pararescuers is also highlighted through performance contrasts, such as accomplishing more rescues in a shorter period of time.

Sam: "I Am Really a Firm Believer That If They Had Let Us Go in Right Then and There to Do Our Jobs, There Would Have Been More Lives Saved."

Sam's story also highlights the elite, egoistic nature of the PJs' outlook. He expressed feelings of resentment that a dog was sent to do the work of the most highly trained individuals.

We started pulling bodies out, and I am really a firm believer that if they had let us go in right then and there, to do our jobs, there would have been more lives saved. . . . We were putting bodies in bags and lowering them down just one, two, three, one right after another. I think within an hour and a half we extracted about five or six bodies. Boom, boom, boom, right down the line. To me that was really important, to get those bodies off that bridge and to go in there to check to see if there's anybody alive.

I think the whole procedure took way, way too long. Once things started settling down a little bit, I was really, really angry and upset and empty. Here I'm qualified to do something, I'm willing to give everything I got and put everything on the line, and I wasn't able to do something I have trained for years to do. It's what we're ready for. I still have some feelings of anger. I don't know if the right word is anger or frustration. I hope the next time will realize they can use us. They were pretty much in awe of the assists which we set up, because we were in there and out of there.

Sam's narrative is remarkably similar to Ted's. He believes that he is trained and qualified better than anyone to do the job. Those that know what

PJs do, such as the coroner, realize this too. In his statement, it is fact, not speculation. Frustration and anger are focused and personalized. He is blocked from doing what he lives to do and knows no one else can do it as well. "I'm able to put everything on the line and I wasn't able to do something I have trained for years to do." All was not for naught, though, because Sam proved to himself as well as others that he could do it. "They were pretty much in awe of the assists, I hope next time they will realize they can use us."

The following case further substantiates the prevalent heroic, self-encompassing attitude the PJs share. Good and bad feelings are defined by what they were allowed to do and what they were prevented from doing. Because success and accomplishment in their work are major sources of self-esteem, the assaults are directly to their egos and become assimilated in highly personalized ways.

Ralph: "I Felt Good Because We Were the People That Cleared the Whole Bridge."

I just basically wanted to get in there and save people because that is what I've been trained to do, so I was really eager to get going and do things. It seemed that we were really hampered by a lot of people because they really didn't know who we were and what our abilities were. . . . I feel personally if we had gotten in there earlier we would have been able to save a couple of people. Which is kind of a bummer.

They really didn't draw a conclusion about our worth until a couple of days later. We did a majority of the work at the end. Plus, they started realizing what an asset they had. The first couple of nights, though, there was a lot of sitting around. I found myself very frustrated. It was a big time, and I wasn't doing what I wanted to be doing. I wanted to be there searching for people and treating people.

These excerpts have an egocentric quality. Most of the appraisals organize information around the self-system. Stress is that which discounts personal capabilities. Given the requirements of motivation and perseverance necessary for success in pararescue, it makes sense that individuals interpret information in ways that enhance self-esteem; otherwise that information might stymie involvement.

Because the situations the PJs find themselves in are often life threatening, the PJs' reliance on aggrandizing self-centered beliefs of personal control and optimism increases the likelihood that they will realize their goals. In other words, the goal of saving others is best accomplished through successful mastery of the challenges to which a PJ has pledged himself.

His obligation allows him to serve the values of his society. His individualistic heroic creed and practices tell him that he cannot need others, submit to their wishes, or depend on their judgment. His behavior is based not in selfishness but rather in a heroic selflessness, and he accepts the crusade of justice and excellence as the creed he lives by and is willing to die for.

These individuals are reminiscent of the mythic American individualist hero known as the cowboy. Like the cowboy, the PJ is a self-made person taking on self-appointed tasks. PJs are the most highly qualified and trained individuals who, standing outside in a unique position and uninvited, take on Cypress. An excerpt from Tom's narrative reveals this interpretive parallel to the cowboy. The stage is set as they were wrapping up their work, completing the final search.

> We walked up from the end all the way back to where the main area was, and the place was completely deserted. There wasn't one piece of power machinery running, and there was light shining through the thing in an eerie way. We kind of spread ourselves across the road and walked our way on up, and I said, "If they ever made a movie it would be really something." . . . "How would it be?" someone asked. . . . I said, "This is it, we've got the PJs here, we've got Nancy nurse, and the psychologist. . . . This is great."

The scene resembles the classic movie image in which the cowboy blows the smoke off his gun after a hard day's shooting and rides out of town into the sunset. The PJs' unique pattern of operation at Cypress was defined by their role as well as by what the situation held for them. Their narratives depict their overriding obligation to heroism, an obligation that drove their involvement, set the style of their responses and behaviors, and defined the issues of stress in an overwhelming situation.

Firefighters' Involvement: Obligation to Each Other

Firefighters provide a contrast to the PJs in involvement and conduct, yet like the PJs their patterns were determined by their identity as a group and their experiences at Cypress. Firefighters generally operated as a closely knit team, a pattern highly consistent with their day-to-day functioning. For them, the team is stronger and more valuable than the individual. Membership, participation, and concern for coworkers and friends are most important, as reflected in the shared sentiment, "Don't sacrifice the crew for a save."

The following excerpts portray the obligation that firefighters feel to each other.

Larry: "There Were Two of Us, and It Made It Real Comforting."

As Larry describes the life-threatening conditions he is in while rescuing trapped motorists, he mentions:

> What I didn't like is, we were so spread thin, the uniformed personnel. I didn't like the fact that none of our guys really knew where I was at. They might have known, but they weren't really sure. That I didn't like. . . . There were two of us, which made it real comforting, I mean having somebody I know and work with makes a difference. But it's also comforting to know that my guys know where I'm at because if anything would have happened, I feel real confident that they would have focused on me to get me out. And it's a little reassurance. Not to put anybody else down or whatever, but it's like if one of my guys were, if Chester got trapped on the other side of Dorothy [rescuee], I would have had to go right to Chester. I mean, nothing against Dorothy, but I would have made sure I got Chester out first, and that's just the way it is.

Larry's statement provides an example of how his concerns were mitigated by the support of his peers. Anxiety shifted to comfort when he realized that although his team was spread thin and wouldn't know where he was if something were to happen to him, his partner Chester knew where he was and would save him. His friendship with Chester and the support of his team strengthened him despite a sense of vulnerability and provided a sense of connection and continuity.

Brief excerpts from Roy, Charles, and Greg also illustrate the strength of friendships and the central importance of peer relationships—themes that are pervasive throughout all the firefighters' narrative accounts.

Roy: "I Became More Concerned About the People We Had in There and Their Lives."

Roy, who became the officer in charge of a particularly dangerous and lengthy rescue, was responsible for the fate of his crew and made decisions accordingly. At about 3 hours into it, Roy called for a doctor because if they couldn't get the rescuee out they were going to cut her foot off. He was not concerned about her foot.

> I became more concerned about the people we had in there and their lives, because it doesn't do any good for us to sit in there and this thing comes down

around our ears, for all of us, and yet if we could cut her foot off, cut our losses at that, everybody else gets out of it, then we've accomplished something. She's alive. We've all won.

There was no question for him that risking his whole crew wasn't worth the loss of a foot, but in listening to him defend his decision, I felt that he was concerned about how other people would view his decision. Although he claimed otherwise, he was in a difficult, if not unpopular, position. At stake was his crew as well as his sense of competency as an officer. In the aftermath, coping for him meant reviewing and providing sufficient evidence and justification to support his primary obligation to his crew. His assessments, involvement, and decisions were closely tied to the needs of his fellow firefighters.

Greg: "I'm Proud of the Guys I Work With, I'm Proud of Myself, I'm Proud to Be Part of the Crew."

Roy and Charles and I went up and in [the structure], and at the time we went in, I remember thinking, I don't want to go in here, but I don't want Charles to go in either. I mean, he's my son's godfather and he's got a small daughter my daughter's age, and we're not going to go anywhere without Roy, and Roy is, you know, the pedal to the metal, he's not going to back down for anything. So we went in and I remember thinking, climbing over the rail where the upper section had come down, this is the worst thing I've ever been in. I thought about my wife and my kids. But once you got in there and started working, you're concentrating on what you're doing. I worked with these guys for so long (over years), you're just used to working. You don't really think about it.

After finishing up in that area, they went back to where Roy was working.

I really didn't want to go, but Roy was still in there, and there were a number of guys still in there, and it was the thing to do . . . just did it. I think I felt like if I didn't go back in there I'd feel bad about it the next day. . . . I might have hesitated if I wasn't working with my right-wing crew, but I've known Roy since high school, and Charles and I are real good friends. It was just something, you had to do it, had to do it.

I think I'm pretty upbeat about it. I'm proud of the guys I work with, I'm proud of myself, I'm proud to be part of the crew. I think we do a good job. We've always done a good job. There's nothing to hold back. The things that we do are necessary, and I think what we did that night was, what's the word, exemplary—because we were able to go to work and we knew what needed to be done.

Notice the frequent use of the word "we" in contrast to the consistently dominant use of the pronoun "I" in the PJ accounts. Coping for the firefighter is done as a team, sharing in a stressful encounter and realizing the crew may die together, but that that is the way it should be. Greg was able to overcome his reluctance to enter the structure only when he considered who he was with and could forecast how he would feel later if he didn't join them. The bonds of friendship and camaraderie made no other choice possible for him. Even though Cypress was the worst situation he had ever been in, the comfort of being with his "right-wing" crew allowed him to do the job. He is still proud of himself and his crew and realizes that the success of the effort was the result of teamwork.

Charles: "He Wanted Us to Die Together as a Crew.
I Could Understand—I Would Do the Same."

As Charles remembered it, when the structure moved, he immediately thought about his peers and even prioritized their value.

All this stuff started crumbling over my shoulder and everything and I could feel it moving. So they were screaming, "Get out, get out." And that's where I just thought, shit, I lost Greg. I mean I haven't liked Jeff all that much, but Greg—I know his kid and his wife and his new kid, and they just flashed in front of me and just—so anyway we got out of there.

The guys there are having a tough time getting the hoses hooked up, so Greg says screw it, he hops on the ladder and goes up, so then I follow him up, and then right at that point Roy had sent somebody to go get us because, he told us, he figured if he was going to die in that thing he wanted us up there, he wanted us to die together as a crew. I could understand—I would do the same.

Then I get back and then I start working on her again [the Dorothy Otto rescue]. . . . Roy kept saying, "Well fuck the vitals, you know, I don't want to die up here and she's gonna die up here if we don't get her out of here real soon." . . . Then I kind of said, "Well, let me try this." She had a flat-heeled shoe on, and it stuck—I couldn't even get the shoe off her, the toe was caught that much. So I stuck my thumb in and grabbed around the heel part of her heel and grabbed the top of her foot and put my foot on the thing and actually tried to pull her toes off . . . but at that point I really didn't care about her. I just wanted to relieve this situation of me and these other guys having to be in there. I didn't really care about her. In fact, I told Gary, "I'm going to go get an axe and cut her goddamn foot off. I don't give a shit about her foot, I wanna get out of here."

The three firefighters shared an internal debate between not wanting to enter the structure and not wanting to stay behind and have to live to explain their comrades' fate. After a close encounter with the crumbling structure, the two friends acknowledged their confrontation with mortality but felt they had to go back in because "we're a team." Fear and threat motivated action, including attempts to pull the rescuee's foot off—which, incidentally, was spared. The value of the crew outweighed the value of saving the victim's foot. The bonds of friendship were so tight that it was better to die together as a crew than to have to bear the burden and guilt of survival.

Ben: "Did I Let Them Down or Did I Do Good?"

Ben worked in a support capacity during one of the live rescues. His story demonstrates how questions of uncertainty about fulfilling his obligation to his crew created stress.

> It was a difficult position to be in because I wanted to be in there and help them, but I also didn't want them to need something and not have somebody there they could rely on. . . . I almost felt like I wasn't doing anything, I was like a sissy and I wasn't doing anything, and I almost had to constantly remind myself that what I'm doing is really the best thing for the crew and don't worry about it. I had a lot of problems dealing with that later, I think, and that was one of the things that I really needed to resolve was that I did do the best thing in the long run.
>
> I know they need me, and I got to get in there and find out what they need. And you do it for the crew as much as anything. I remember one of my other friends was talking about how the guy that he was working with went in, and he thought, now if I don't go in there with him and this thing falls down on top of him, then I'm going to have to go tell his wife that he's dead, and I'd just as soon die with him than have to face his wife. So, you know, there's a real sense of not letting the crew down and going in and supporting them. That's the way I felt. . . . It was difficult for me to talk about my role and my feelings of not being able to contribute. That was the thing that was the hardest for me to get out.
>
> I think for me, the most difficult thing to resolve in the whole thing was, did I let them down or did I do good. Just dealing with amputating the kid's leg and cutting the woman in half and things like that, I think that those are the things, for firemen, are the easiest thing to deal with.

Ben was most distressed about his role as a crew member during the operation. He later described having spent a lot of his time reviewing his participation and subsequently experiencing personal growth as a result of confronting issues of fear, control, and his need to contribute. He even talked with members of the crew about his bad feelings. They reassured him that he had played an integral role in the success of the work through his support.

Ben's story highlights the firefighters' strong sense of obligation to the team and illustrates how a perceived violation of that code both created stress and sustained him in the situation.

Just as PJs are indoctrinated to function with self-reliance, firefighters are socialized to perform interdependently as a team. It is not surprising that the theme of social support surfaces in these accounts. By watching out for others, for the crew, each was watching out for himself. The ingrained concept of group affiliation characterized the perspective from which firefighters defined their work priorities at Cypress—first to each other, then to any others.

As with all rescuers, social support also played a major role in coping. Social support, defined as stress-related interpersonal aid, clearly motivated firefighters to get involved and complete work they were hesitant to do and might not have done otherwise. The statement "I really didn't want to go, but Roy was still in there, and there were a number of guys still in there, and it was the thing to do" suggests that the power of personal relationships transcended acknowledged threats and enabled participation.

The comfort they derived from being with their right-wing crew was also the result of an increased sense of predictability, stability, and control, proven in previous work interactions. Therefore the sense of support was not only a result of friendships developed over time but also the product of a history of stress-related helping transactions developed through the practice of firefighting. This inherent obligation to each other fostered confidence and bolstered the firefighters' ability to cope with the imposed demands, even reducing appraisals of threat and helping to redefine the risks of the situation. As Rick succinctly stated:

> Well, it was being surrounded by a tremendous support network of talented people; there is no way one person could have performed the rescue. Without a doubt, it exceeded any skills that any one person could have. It was being part of a good team and I'm thankful for that. . . . Just the slip of a tool would have taken off a person's leg.

Seth: "If I Could Have Only Done More."

Seth's story seems to provide a contrast to the "obligation to each other" paradigm that drove the involvement of the firefighters at Cypress. It is presented here to illustrate how contrast cases in narrative methodology make particular patterns stand out more clearly.

> I'm crawling around back in there, I can't see nothing. There doesn't seem to be anybody just beyond the smoke, and back in there I can hear something

like rubble moving. There's a point that I told myself, get out of here. Just get out of here. It's full of smoke and you could be trapped. That's kind of frightening in itself. The other thing is if I got trapped they were going to have to be coming after me. One of the things is the feeling of being trapped and no one knowing about it.

You should kind of buddy up. So what I feel in retrospect is, I was kind of cowboying it up a little bit there, but then I came to my senses and I said, let's get out of here. I kind of beat myself up about that a little bit later.

I got stuck on the rappel [rope transport system] because the line down below wrapped on something. It wasn't that far, so I was just going to release everything and hang out a bit and drop, which wouldn't hurt me or anything. Someone helped me, and so with that action right there, one of the officers saw it and they wrote me up for a silver medal of valor. What I felt is that, I got in there, I kind of wasted some time, didn't rescue anybody, and I could have lost some resources. I'm usually still somewhat hard on myself in situations like this, and now they're giving me a medal, like I'm almost embarrassed to get this. I had to face it. I guess it is somewhat heroic to do that and just go on in where I did. I looked around and I did prove that pretty much there was nobody in there that would be salvageable.

In the back of my mind, if I had just gone a little bit farther I would have found a person—I could have stayed up there a little bit longer. While I was there, I might as well have just gone and crawled way back in there.

My overall feeling . . . is, you just feel like, God, if I only could have done more. You couldn't do enough. It was like things were getting done, but not any one single person was doing it. It's kind of a team effort. You kind of felt powerlessness over the whole thing. You just felt kind of weird, like maybe I should have done more.

Seth's story sounds much like one of the PJs'. He participated from a solo heroic stance, charging in to save life as if he could undo the tragedy. He knew he should buddy up, but he "cowboyed it" and even received a medal that embarrassed him because he knew he had violated firefighting practices. "If I could have only done more" echoes the PJs' "I could have done more." Seth doesn't experience strength in being a team member; instead, he feels powerless.

Interestingly, however, Seth is a former paramedic and relatively new to firefighting. The fact that paramedics operate independently may account for the way he perceived and related in this emergency, drawing on prior experience. He attempted to deal with his sense of powerlessness through action, but unlike the actions of his peer group, his actions were self-absorbed, with little consideration of the ramifications for his team. Thus an example that seemed to contradict the firefighters' creed may represent only a case of incomplete indoctrination.

Summary

This chapter traced the occupational backgrounds and experiences of two groups of rescue workers. Narrative excerpts demonstrated that individuals have strong ties to their work, ties formed and strengthened by indoctrination, other milder forms of socialization, and practices specific to their occupations. The rescue-related events they defined as stressful involved threats and challenges to the expectations, mores, and goals of each occupational practice in relation to the disaster work. The value and meaning of the work and personal understanding of role obligations also helped to determine the form of involvement at Cypress and the definition of stress.

The PJs stood out as members whose personal identity was closely related to their occupations. They are devoted to their call to save lives. When not on a mission, they keep physically fit and practice rescue operations. Self-reliance is essential for success and is encouraged and valued in the practice. The PJs consider stressful any events that threaten the success of a mission and all insults to their abilities. The majority of the PJs reported that at Cypress, stress was having to prove themselves as valuable members of the rescue effort. Coping involved doing what needed to be done in the situation using the familiar strategy of "press on"—a determined intent to use their training and skills in the operation.

Firefighters have a strong team affiliation with built-in socialization practices that encourage and support that team identity. "Making a difference" is the role of firefighters, who respond to the public in situations that are often devoid of apparent meaning (e.g., senseless shootings). Stress was identified by firefighters as whatever threatens the team and its members or undermines their ability to intervene. Stress at Cypress, especially during the early hours, related to safety of the team. Coping involved weighing the risks and making decisions accordingly—always watching out for one another.

As the individuals of this study reconstructed events through narratives of experience, they made sense out of what happened to them in relation to their past and present life stories. Although participation at Cypress was only a brief moment in each individual's lifetime, it has the potential to exert tremendous lasting influence. The collection of rescuers' stories not only allowed the extraction and comparison of various influences but had therapeutic value as well. The simple acknowledgment that their story was important, that they had something worthwhile to offer others, allowed individuals to come forth and share their experiences. Allowing informants to describe their feelings and responses also gave credence to the value and meaning they described in their encounters—in contrast to other research techniques that strictly guide what information is elicited and therefore what information has value.

There are several other reasons for preserving these rescuers' narratives. They serve as a means of transmitting cultural experience, providing historical continuity. The informants' narratives reflect courage and human possibility as well as fear and a sense of vulnerability. Their accounts provide visions of the value and integrity of life. The most striking thread throughout the Cypress story is the reservoir of shared cultural meanings related to personal commitment, dedication to saving human lives, avoiding suffering, facing death, and comforting families from which these people drew to help their fellow beings. In a pluralistic society that struggles in its search for common meanings and mores, these stories capture a sense of community and solidarity that prevailed in one particular moment in history.

Appendix

DOCTORAL DISSERTATIONS USING INTERPRETIVE PHENOMENOLOGY

Brykczynski, K. (1985). *Exploring the clinical practice of nurse practitioners.* Unpublished doctoral dissertation, University of California, San Francisco.

Chesla, C. (1988). *Parents' caring practices and coping with schizophrenic offspring, an interpretive study.* Unpublished doctoral dissertation, University of California, San Francisco.

Darbyshire, P. (1992). *Parenting in public: A study of the experiences of parents who live-in with their hospitalized child, and of their relationship with paediatric nurses.* Unpublished doctoral dissertation, University of Edinburgh, Edinburgh, Scotland.

Doolittle, N. D. (1992). *Life after stroke: Survivors' bodily and practical knowledge of coping during recovery.* Unpublished doctoral dissertation, University of California, San Francisco.

Dunlop, M. (1990). *A phenomenological investigation of clinical knowledge evident in university curricula in Australia.* Unpublished doctoral dissertation, University of California, San Francisco.

Haberman-Little, B. (1993). *The experience of Parkinson's disease in middle life: An interpretive account.* Unpublished doctoral dissertation, University of California, San Francisco.

Hartfield, M. (1986). *Coping with anger in normotensive and hypertensive samples.* Unpublished doctoral dissertation, University of California, San Francisco.

Kesselring, A. (1990). *The experienced body, when taken-for-grantedness falters: A phenomenological study of living with breast cancer.* Unpublished doctoral dissertation, University of California, San Francisco.

Leonard, V. (1993). *Stress and coping in the transition to parenthood of first-time mothers with career commitments: An interpretive study.* Unpublished doctoral dissertation, University of California, San Francisco.

MacIntyre, R. (1993). *Sex, power, death and symbolic meanings of T-cell counts in HIV+ gay men.* Unpublished doctoral dissertation, University of California, San Francisco.

MacLeod, M. L. P. (1990). *Experience in everyday nursing practice: A study of "experienced" ward sisters.* Unpublished doctoral dissertation, University of Edinburgh, Scotland.

Madjar, I. (1991). *Pain as embodied experience: A phenomenological study of clinically inflicted pain in adult patients.* Unpublished doctoral dissertation, Massey University, Palmerston North, New Zealand.

McKeever, L. (1988). *Menopause: An uncertain passage.* Unpublished doctoral dissertation, University of California, San Francisco.

Popell, C. L. (1983). *An interpretive study of stress and coping among parents of school-age developmentally disabled children.* Unpublished doctoral dissertation, Wright Institute Graduate School of Psychology, Berkeley, California.

Schilder, E. J. (1986). *The use of physical restraints in an acute care medical ward.* Unpublished doctoral dissertation, University of California, San Francisco.

SmithBattle, L. (1992). *Caring for teenage mothers and their children: Narratives of self and ethics of intergenerational caregiving.* Unpublished doctoral dissertation, University of California, San Francisco.

Stainton, C. (1985). *Culture and cue sensitivity: A phenomenological study of mothering.* Unpublished doctoral dissertation, University of California, San Francisco.

Stuhlmiller, C. M. (1991). *An interpretive study of appraisal and coping of rescue workers in an earthquake disaster: The Cypress collapse.* Unpublished doctoral dissertation, University of California, San Francisco.

Warnian, L. (1987). *A hermeneutical study of group psychotherapy.* Unpublished doctoral dissertation, University of California, San Francisco.

Wnos, P. L. (1993). *Behind the curtain: Nursing care of dying patients in critical care.* Oregon: Oregon Health Science University.

Wrubel, J. W. (1985). *Personal meanings and coping processes: A hermeneutical study of personal background meanings and interpersonal concerns and their relation to stress appraisals and coping.* Unpublished doctoral dissertation, University of California, San Francisco.

Name Index

Subject Index

About the Contributors

Gay Becker, Ph.D., a medical anthropologist, is Professor in Residence, Social and Behavioral Sciences and Medical Anthropology, University of California, San Francisco. The primary theme in her research is the process by which individuals acquire and live with health conditions that create unforeseen paths in the course of life. Her particular emphasis is on the experience of illness. In addition to her work on asthma with Janson-Bjerklie, Benner, and Ferketich, she has conducted research on aging and the life span; chronic and disabling conditions, including life after a stroke; reproductive health problems, including the experience of infertility; and chronic health problems as they are experienced by ethnic minorities. She is the author of three books and numerous papers in social science journals.

Patricia Benner is a Professor in the Department of Physiological Nursing, University of California, School of Nursing, San Francisco, California. Her current research examines expert ethical comportment of nurses and focuses on engaged clinical and moral reasoning. She has conducted research in stress and coping in persons with a chronic illness. She is the author of *From Novice to Expert: Excellence and Power in Clinical Nursing Practice* (1989) and, with Judith Wrubel, *The Primacy of Caring: Stress and Coping in Health and Illness* (1984).

Catherine A. Chesla, R.N., D.N.Sc., is Assistant Professor at the Department of Family Health Care Nursing, University of California, San Francisco. She teaches family theory and family intervention to graduate family nurse practitioner students. In her research she examines family responses over time to the chronic illness of a member, using a hermeneutic approach. To date she has examined family patterns of response to schizophrenia and Alzheimer's disease. She additionally worked with Drs. Benner and Tanner in a hermeneutic investigation of clinical judgment and skill development in nursing practice. A study of Pilipino-American family responses to the care of a member with schizophrenia is in progress. Next, she plans to conduct, with a multidisciplinary research team, a combined hermeneutic and model-testing investigation of family processes and coping with the diagnosis of diabetes in a primary care population. She has recently published in such journals as *Family Relations, Journal of Community Health Nursing,* and *Image.*

Philip Darbyshire is Lecturer in Health and Nursing Studies at Glasgow Caledonian University. His clinical background is in learning disability and pediatric nursing. He holds a master's in nursing from the University of Glasgow and a doctorate from the University of Edinburgh. He is a frequent contributor to a range of nursing books and journals, and has most recently published in *Nurse Education Today* and *Journal of Advanced Nursing,* where he serves on their editorial boards. He also writes a regular review column called "Media Watch" for *Nursing Times* and is the Consulting Editor for their regular "Telling Stories" series of nurses' narratives. As an educator he is committed to promoting interpretive and narrative approaches within undergraduate and postgraduate education. His current research interests involve an interpretive appraisal of a new course called "Understanding Caring Through Arts and Humanities," which he cocreated and teaches, and an interpretive study that looks at the process of becoming a nurse teacher. He is a frequent presenter at nursing conferences and forums in the United Kingdom and abroad and has recently presented his work in Canada, the United States, Australia, and New Zealand. In 1994 he will be returning to the University of Wisconsin-Madison for a second term as a Visiting Scientist.

Nancy L. Diekelmann, R.N., Ph.D., F.A.A.N., is a Helen Denne Schulte Professor at the University of Wisconsin-Madison School of Nursing, a Fellow in the American Academy of Nursing, and a past president of the Society for Research in Nursing Education. A noted authority for her work in nursing education and primary health care, she received two Book of the Year awards from the *American Journal of Nursing* for her textbook *Primary Health Care of the Well Adult.* In addition, and as the coeditor of *Transforming RN Education: Dialogue and Debate.* Her current research uses Heideggerian hermeneutics to explicate the narratives of teachers, students, and clinicians. Dr. Diekelmann has described an alternative approach for nursing education in her educational program *Narrative Pedagogy: Caring, Dialogue and Practice.*

Nancy D. Doolittle, R.N., M.S., Ph.D., received her master's degree and doctorate in nursing from the University of California, San Francisco. Her primary research interest is qualitative study of living with neurologic illness. The focus of her doctoral dissertation was the bodily experience of recovery following stroke. Her contribution to this book is based on the dissertation findings. Publications related to this work can be found in the *Journal of Neuroscience Nursing* (1991) and *Rehabilitation Nursing* (1992). She is currently a research nurse in the Department of Physiological Nursing, University of California, San Francisco. She serves on the editorial boards of *Journal of Stroke and Cerebrovascular Diseases* and *Rehabilitation Nursing Research.* She has presented her research findings on recovery after stroke to national and international audiences.

Margaret J. Dunlop is Foundation Professor and Head of Australia's newest school of nursing at Griffith University in Queensland. She is preparing a monograph that critically evaluates the relationship between nursing and hermeneutics and is also involved in a major funded research study on nursing specialty education in universities in Australia. Her research interests are in structuring of nursing knowledge, women and health care, midwifery, nursing history, and nursing education. She has recently published *Shaping Nursing Knowledge: An Interpretive Analysis of Curriculum Documents from NSW Australia* (1992) and has contributed a chapter to D. Gaunt's *A Global Agenda for Caring* (1993).

Sandra Ferketich, Ph.D., R.N., F.A.A.N., earned a B.S.N. and a B.A. in Fine Arts from the University of New Mexico, a master's degree from Indiana University, and a Ph.D. in Nursing with a minor in Statistics from the University of Arizona. She is Professor and Project Director for the Institutional NRSA program in instrumentation (funded by National Institute of Nursing Research) at the College of Nursing, University of Arizona. She has numerous publications, which focus on measurement issues in nursing research. She edits the column "Focus on Psychometrics" in

Research in Nursing and Health. In addition, she publishes and speaks extensively on model respecification, with a particular emphasis on the use of graphic residual analysis. Dr. Ferketich has a sustained publication record on the effect of antepartum stress on families. Her current research funding centers on the evaluation of community-based nursing intervention studies. She is funded by the Agency for Health Care Policy and Research to study the effectiveness of a comprehensive multi-level practice model for rural Hispanics and by the National Institute of Nursing Research to examine the effectiveness of an aggressive nursing contact intervention for homeless on prophylactic medication for Mycobacterium Tuberculosis.

Ragnar Fjelland is Professor of Philosophy of Science at the Center for the Study of the Sciences and the Humanities, University of Bergen, as well as Director of the Center. In 1990, he was a Visiting Scholar at the University of California, Berkeley. His current topics of interest include the relation between science and technology, the possibility of an "alternative science," philosophical implications of chaos theory and fractal geometry, and philosophical problems of quantum mechanics. He is a member of the National Research Ethics Committee for Natural Science and Technology and has written several books on philosophy of science, technology, and human values in Norwegian.

Eva Gjengedal is Assistant Professor at the Center for Continuing Education, the University of Bergen. She received her master's degree in nursing from the University of Oslo in 1987 and has just finished the work on her doctoral dissertation. Included among her recent publications is an article in the *Scandinavian Journal of Caring Science.* Her main interests are methodological and theoretical problems in nursing science, in particular phenomenology as a justification for the uses of qualitative methods in empirical research.

Deborah R. Gordon is Research Consultant in Medical Anthropology at the Center for the Study and Prevention of Cancer in Florence, Italy, and International Affiliate with the Center for the Study of Medicine and Culture, Harvard Medical School, Boston. She holds a Ph.D. in Medical Anthropology from the University of California, San Francisco/Berkeley. Her recent ethnographic research in Tuscany, Italy, has focused on communication around cancer and the local cultures of cancer prevention, death and dying, home care, and bioethics, as well as on Italian women's experience with breast cancer. Her research interests include cultural—

particularly cultural phenomenological—studies of biomedicine, bioethics, technology, illness, and distress, with special attention to spiritual/religious dimensions of Western medicines and cultures.

Susan Janson-Bjerklie, D.N.Sc., A.N.P., F.A.A.N., received the B.S.N. and M.S. degrees in nursing from the University of Michigan and her doctoral degree from the University of California, San Francisco. She is a Professor in the Department of Physiological Nursing and an Adjunct Professor in the Department of Medicine at the University of California, San Francisco. She is the Director of the Pulmonary Graduate Nursing Program. Dr. Janson-Bjerklie is a pulmonary clinical nurse specialist and certified nurse practitioner and a nationally known expert in care of people with asthma. She was a member of the Expert Panel on Diagnosis and Management of Asthma, National Asthma Education Program, NIH-National Heart, Lung, and Blood Institute. Her current research is focused on the biobehavioral markers of airway inflammation in asthma and the impact of patient education. She maintains a faculty practice in the Division of Pulmonary Medicine, specializing in care of adult patients with asthma.

Sui-Lun Lam is an Information Processing Consultant for the Alice Simonds Center for Instruction and Research in Nursing, School of Nursing, University of Wisconsin-Madison. He specializes in computer networks and in the development of software for research applications. He has degrees in mathematics and in engineering with a focus on robotics and computer applications.

Victoria W. Leonard recently completed her doctoral work at the University of California, San Francisco. Her doctoral work focused on stress and coping of first-time mothers with career commitments in the transition to parenthood.

Karen A. Plager is a master's-prepared family nurse practitioner and doctoral candidate in nursing science currently completing her dissertation research at the University of California, School of Nursing, San Francisco. She specializes in family primary care nursing and family health promotion.

Robert Schuster is the Director of the Alice Simonds Center for Instruction and Research in Nursing, School of Nursing, University of Wisconsin-Madison. He has developed several hundred instructional programs, has authored numerous corporate films, and has coauthored *Natural Landscaping: De-*

signing With Native Plant Communities. His graduate work was in American literature, with a focus on the American transcendentalists.

Lee SmithBattle, R.N., D.N.Sc., is Assistant Professor at Saint Louis University School of Nursing, in St. Louis, Missouri, where she teaches community health nursing. Her research interest in teenage mothering as shaped by family and community contexts and ethics of care has drawn upon extensive community health nursing experience. Her current study examines the life course and caregiving practices of former teenage mothers and their family members.

Cynthia M. Stuhlmiller, R.N., M.S., D.N.Sc., is affiliated with the University of San Francisco, Department of Veterans Affairs, Palo Alto, California, and the American Red Cross, Palo Alto, disaster action team. She is a private consultant and lecturer and has worked as a clinical nurse specialist with Vietnam Veterans with PTSD at the National Center for Post Traumatic Stress Disorder Clinical Laboratory and Education Division (formerly the Vietnam Veterans Inpatient Treatment Program). Her experiences in those 10 years have generated her concern for the pathologizing of psychological responses to trauma. In her participant observation and ongoing research on rescue and emergency workers, she seeks to uncover the salutary aspects of extreme experiences and incorporate them into treatment.

David C. Thomasma, Ph.D., is the Michael I. English Professor of Medical Ethics and Director of the Medical Humanities Program at Loyola University, Chicago Medical Center, and also Chief of the Ethics Consult Service and a member of the Hospital Ethics Committee. He has served on the Technical Advisory Panel for Biomedical Ethics of the American Hospital Association, and the Theology and Ethics Advisory Committee for the Catholic Health Association. He is Editor-in-Chief of *Theoretical Medicine*, Coeditor of *Cambridge Quarterly for Healthcare Ethics*, and Section Editor of *The Journal of the American Geriatrics Society*, has written an Ethics Column for *Healthcare Executive*, and is on the editorial boards of four other journals. He has published more than 200 articles and 15 books. His most recent books are *Human Life in the Balance* (1990); with Edmund Pellegrino, *The Virtues in Medical Practice* (1993) and *For the Patient's Good* (1988); with Glenn Graber, *Theory and Practice in Medical Ethics* (1989) and *Euthanasia: Toward an Ethical Social Policy* (1990); and with John Monagle, *Medical Ethics: Policies, Protocols, Guidelines, and Programs* (1992). In 1992 he was named Director of the International Bioethics Institute.

Peggy L. Wros is Assistant Professor of Nursing at Linfield College, School of Nursing, in Portland, Oregon. She obtained her B.S.N. from the University of Wisconsin-Madison, and her M.S.N. from Marquette University, Milwaukee, Wisconsin. She recently completed her Ph.D. in nursing at Oregon Health Sciences University. Her dissertation work focused on nursing care of dying patients in critical care, and continuing research interests include bedside nursing ethics and phenomenological methods. She is also interested in the implementation and evaluation of new paradigm curriculum change and teaching strategies in nursing education. She is currently involved in the ongoing phenomenological analysis of an existing data set concerning the development of clinical judgment in critical care nurses (Drs. Patricia Benner and Christine Tanner, Co-Investigators). The present analysis is focused on learning from clinical practice and on the relevance for nursing education.